EVALUATION
OF BEHAVIORAL
PROGRAMS

in Community,
Residential
and School
Settings

The Fifth Banff International Conference on Behavior Modification

edited by
Park O. Davidson
University of British Columbia
Frank W. Clark
Leo A. Hamerlynck
University of Calgary

Research Press
2612 North Mattis Avenue
Champaign, Illinois 61820

CONTENTS

RA790
.5
.B28
1974

Preface   xi

Introduction   xv

Contributors   xix

1 Design and Analysis Problems in Program Evaluation   1
Richard R. Jones

Evaluation Designs   3
   N=one vs. Group Designs   5
   N=one *and* Group Designs   9
Effectiveness Analysis   11
   Treatment Effectiveness
      and Causation Between Two Constructs   12
   Generalization of Program Treatment Effects   20

2 Who Benefits from the Program? Criteria Selection   33
Siegfried Hiebert

Introduction   33
The Patient's Point of View   34
Clients Other Than the Patient   39
Society's Point of View   41
The Therapist's Point of View   45
Conclusion   51

3 Process Control: A Guide to Planning   55
Bryan C. Smith

Introduction   55

131683

A System   55
System Approach   56
System Analysis   57
Network Based Systems   59
Conclusion   62

4   Considerations in the
    Implementation of Program Evaluation   65
    Aldred H. Neufeldt

Problem Sources   66
    Example 1   66
    Example 2   67
Dimensions of Implementing Program Evaluations   68
Implications for Implementing Program Evaluations   69
    Instrumental Elements   69
    Expressive Elements   73
Summary and Concluding Remarks   79

5   Evaluating Community-Based Psychiatric Services   83
    Peter D. McLean

Contemporary Evaluation
    of Private-Practice Psychiatry in the Community   84
The Shift from the Private-Practice
    to Community Mental Health Model   85
Evaluation of Community
    Mental Health Programs and Organizations   87
Evaluation Strategies   88
    Evaluation of Program Structure   89
    Evaluation of Program Process   89
    Evaluation by Outcome   90
    Cost-Effectiveness Analysis   94
    Systems Analysis   96
The Choice of Evaluation Procedure   97

6   Behavioral Measurement
    in a Community Mental Health Center   103
    Robert Paul Liberman, William J. DeRisi, Larry W. King,
    Thad A. Eckman, David Wood

    Mental Health Setting   105
    Staff Training   105
    Patients   107
    Behavioral Measurement   107
    Behavioral Progress Record   108
    Experimental Designs for Individual Patients   109
    Behavior Observation Instrument (BOI)   114
        Procedures   118
        Observer Reliability   118
        BOI Settings   119
        BOI Categories   119
        Results of Group Observation   119
        Observations of Staff Behavior   126
        Observation Procedures   127
        Results   127
    Discussion   129
    Summary   135

7   Methodological Issues and Problems
    in Evaluating Treatment Outcomes in the Family
    and School Consultation Project, 1970-1973   141
    Srinika Jayaratne, Richard B. Stuart, Tony Tripodi

    Study Design I (1970-71)   142
        Design Implementation and Reality Problems   144
        Selection of Outcome
            Variables and Measurement Problems   148
        Analysis and Conclusions   154
    Study Design II (1971-72)   158
        Therapist Variation   159
        Final Outcome Measures   160
        Analysis and Conclusions   162
    Study Design III (1972-73)   163
        Design Modifications   164
        Measurement Refinements   166
    Recommendations   167

8 Benefit-Cost Analysis and the
  Evaluation of Mental Retardation Programs   175
  William B. Neenan

  Introduction   175
  Benefit-Cost Analysis   175
    Basic Concept   176
    Price Signals   177
    Program Benefits   178
    Program Costs   179
    Discount Rate   180
    Criteria for Choice   181
    Constraints and Suboptimization   182
    Distributional Pattern   182
  Human Investment and Program Evaluation   184
    A Specific Program Evaluation   185
    Conley's Analysis   186
  Concluding Critique of Benefit-Cost Analysis   189

9 Evaluation of Living Environments:
  The MANIFEST Description of Ward Activities   201
  Michael F. Cataldo, Todd R. Risley

  The Need for an Assessment
    of Living Environment Quality   202
  Prior Research of Living Environments   204
  The Resident Activity MANIFEST   205
    Stimulation Measure   206
    Interaction Measure   212
    Activity Measure   216
  Summary   218

10 Evaluation of Mental
   Health Programs for the Aged   223
   Robert L. Kahn, Steven H. Zarit

   Types of Studies   224
     Intra-institutional Studies   224
     Effect of Changes in Institutionalization: Relocation   230
     Admission to Institutions: Alternative Treatment   230

Alternatives to Institutionalization   232
Alternatives to
    Institutionalization: Community Programs   234
Evaluation Criteria: Further Issues   236
    Community Mental Health Programs   236
    Value Judgments:
        The Contented vs. the Angry Patient   237
    Deterioration   237
        Covert Deterioration: Limited and Basic Goals   239
Conclusions   243

11 Evaluation Process and Outcome
    in Juvenile Corrections: Musings on a Grim Tale   253
    Rosemary C. Sarri, Elaine Selo

Issues and Dilemmas in Evaluation   254
    Recidivism: A Criterion for All Seasons   256
    Experimental Design Dilemmas   258
    Humaneness and Justice vs. Effectiveness   259
Program Goals—Can They Be Measured?   261
A Critique of Five Studies in Juvenile Corrections   262
A Summary Critique   281
A Plan for Comparative Assessment   285
    Program Outcomes   287
    Detention Programs   288
    Processing Programs   289
    Change and Control Programs   289
    Exit Management and Reintegration Programs   290
    Organizational Processes and Efforts   291
    Inter-organizational Processes and Efforts   293
Conclusion   293

12 Cost Efficiency and Effectiveness
    in the Early Detection and
    Improvement of Learning Abilities   303
    H. S. Pennypacker, Carl H. Koenig, W. H. Seaver

The Program   311
The Evaluation   313

**13 Evaluating Individualized
    Education in Elementary School   323**
    William W. Cooley, Gaea Leinhardt

How Real Is the Need?   324
What Priority Does the Need Have Relative to Others?   327
Do the Proposed Means Achieve the Desired End?   328
How Competitive Are the Proposed Means?   336

**14 System-Wide Analysis of Social
    Interaction and Affective Problems in Schools   339**
    James R. Barclay

Part I   339
Multiple Needs Assessment in Elementary Schools   339
    Instrumentation   340
    Method   343
    Results   350
Part II   379
A Model for Policy-Making   379
    1. Preventive Intervention   380
    2. Policy-Making   384
Summary   386

**15 Evaluating Program
    Evaluation: A Suggested Approach   395**
    Charles Windle, Peter Bates

Introduction   395
The Framework of Values
    of Program Evaluation Research   395
    A Value Identification Approach   395
    The Schematic Representation of
        Values Surrounding Program Evaluation   396
Experiences with Program Evaluation Research   403
    Factors in the Success of Applied Research Grants   405
    Literature on Research Utilization   405
    Factors in Success of Evaluation Contracts   406
    Disjunction Between Program
        Decisions and Formal Evaluation Efforts   410

Feedback from Evaluation Research Feedback   415
Support for Automated Psychiatric Record Systems   420
Criteria for Program Evaluation Research   420
   Ultimate Criteria   422
   Process Criteria   423

Author Index   437

Subject Index   445

PREFACE

This is the fifth volume in a continuing series of publications sponsored by the Banff International Conferences on Behavior Modification. The conferences are held each spring in Banff, Alberta, Canada, and serve the purpose of bringing together outstanding behavioral scientists to discuss and present data related to emergent issues and topics in the field of what is now termed Behavior Modification. Thus the International Conferences as a continuing event have served as an expressive "early indicator" of the developing nature and composition of behavioristic science and scientific application.

Distances, schedules, and the restricted audiences preclude wide attendance at the conferences. Consequently, this series of publications has equal status with the conference proper. Past conference topics and faculty were:

1969: I.   Ideal Mental Health Services*

Nathan Azrin	Todd Risley
Ogden Lindsley	Richard B. Stuart
Gerald Patterson	

1970: II.   Services and Programs for Exceptional Children and Youth*

Loren and Margaret Acker

Wesley C. Becker	Ogden Lindsley
Nancy Buckley	Patrick McGinley
Donald Cameron	Nancy J. Reynolds
L. Richard Crozier	James A. Sherman
David R. Evans	Richard B. Stuart
Leo A. Hamerlynck	Walter Zwirner

1971: III. **Implementing Behavioral Programs for Schools and Clinics***

Joe A. Cobb	Jack L. Michael
Rodney Copeland	Gerald R. Patterson
R. Vance Hall	Ernest G. Poser
Ogden Lindsley	Roberta S. Ray
Hugh McKenzie	Richard B. Stuart
Garry L. Martin	Carl E. Thoresen

1972: IV. **Behavior Change: Methodology, Concepts, and Practice**

Eric J. Mash	J. B. Reid and
S. M. Johnson and	A. F. C. J. Hendriks
O. D. Bolstad	R. B. Stuart
K. D. O'Leary and R. Kent	Lee C. Handy
K. Skindrud	H. M. Walker and H. Hops
R. R. Jones	J. LoPiccolo and W. C. Lobitz
L. A. Hamerlynck	D. L. Fixsen, M. M. Wolfe and
G. C. Davison	E. L. Phillips
G. R. Patterson	R. L. Weiss, H. Hops, and
H. Hops and J. A. Cobb	G. R. Patterson

To continue the annual role of the Banff International Conference on Behavior Modification as a medium for behavioral scientists and applied professionals, many people have donated their energies and talents. Foremost certainly, must be the guest faculty who develop, present and discuss the topics found in this volume.

Secondly, it should be gratefully noted that the material support and technical guidance of The University of Calgary's Division of Continuing Education has again for the past conference been of a typically high order. Dr. S. Chapman and Donna Fraser have been the persons responsible for making this extraordinary service an everyday occurrence. Continuing a tradition from last year, Dr. David Leighton and the staff of the Banff Centre insured that the physical environment for the conference was enjoyable and facilitative. A special contribution by the Province of Alberta is also gratefully acknowledged.

Other members of the editorial board and conference planning committee deserve to be singled out for their substantial help and guidance. They are Dr. Lee Handy, Educational Psychology and Counselling Service and Dr. Eric Mash, Psychology. Our special thanks to Miss Ruth Craig for secretarial assistance.

Finally, it is impossible to conclude our acknowledgements without thanking our colleagues and conference participants who guide our efforts by their feedback, and our families, who have continually refreshed our efforts.

P. O. D.
F. W. C.
L. A. H.

*The publications from 1969 and 1970 are currently out of print. With the 1971 proceedings, Research Press became the publisher, and *Implementing Behavioral Programs for Schools and Clinics* is the first of the series contracted.

INTRODUCTION

The central topic of this book is program evaluation in social and health settings. It is primarily intended to be used as a contemporary text on the subject in colleges and universities, and as a reference source for program managers in establishing evaluation units or procedures in applied settings.

Program evaluation is an activity which is qualitatively different from assessment or behavioral measurement as typically understood by behavioral scientists. It is also distinct from the familiar evaluation of research designs used in rather circumscribed and controlled laboratory settings. In spite of these important differences, administrators frequently expect the behavioral scientist (because of his perceived expertise in behavioral measurement and research design) to accept primary responsibility for designing and executing program evaluation. The rapidly accelerating demand for this new type of output from behavioral scientists has stimulated the growth of a new technology to meet this demand.

Early attempts at program evaluation tended to be primarily descriptive. One major focus involved attempts to operationalize the goals of programs by developing behavioral descriptions of the program objectives. A second major focus was on the analysis of the relationship of the program's intent and the program resource allocation. This analysis typically occurred at the conclusion of the program or, occasionally, at choice points determined by program renewal budget reviews made by funding bodies. At the present time, as represented by the chapters contained in this volume, behavior scientists are bringing to the task of program evaluation their spirit of scientific enquiry and the conceptual and operational tools which have proven to be of value in the experimental investigation of complex human behavior. A large part of the challenge of program evaluation is to use and modify these tools to build bridges between the behavioral sciences and those allied disciplines (such as economics and business administration) which also have contributions to make in developing technologies for program evaluation.

Program evaluation is not a technology which "belongs" to any one discipline. There is not yet a sufficient body of knowledge in this area for it to be considered interdisciplinary but, to the extent that it requires knowledge and skills from several disciplines, it is clearly a multidisciplinary endeavour. For the neophyte or student, a multidisciplinary area is hazardous since it requires a flexibility of viewpoint and it lacks a common or unifying vocabulary.

Because contributors to this volume come from diverse backgrounds in economics, psychology, social welfare, psychiatry and education, no attempt was made by the editors to impose a single viewpoint or system of terminology on the contributors. In spite of this, the reader will note a consistency of theme and communality of viewpoint in many of the chapters. Where the terminology is distinctive, the authors have generally attempted to clarify it by supplying explanations or examples. While the editors acknowledged the somewhat wistful hopes of some readers (and occasionally of the editors themselves) that this book might represent a "how-to-do-it manual" which would lead an evaluator step-by-step through the procedures and problems of evaluating his own program, we rapidly decided that such hopes were at best premature and probably impossible (because of the unique problems involved in every individual program evaluation). What we have attempted instead is to provide the reader with a variety of program evaluation strategies demonstrated across a wide range of behavioral programs. The reader can therefore extrapolate across procedures and problem areas to develop the most suitable tools for the particular evaluation problem at hand. Thus while Neenan, for instance, discusses a cost-benefit analysis within the context of evaluating mental retardation programs, the cost-benefit procedures could certainly be used in evaluating juvenile correction programs or education programs. On the other hand, individuals concerned with evaluating a particular mental retardation program might prefer to use the multi-trait, multimethod principles discussed by Barclay, although these are introduced within the context of assessing elementary school educational programs. All of the selections in this volume are original contributions by individuals who have had experience in practical aspects of program evaluation. They have, in addition to outlining various strategies, pointed out difficulties and pitfalls that they have encountered which may be avoided or circumvented by others.

Contained in the chapters to follow are a number of noteworthy and original ideas related to program evaluation. For example: the need to intermix individual and group treatment designs; a method for inferring caused factors from correlational analysis; an assertion of the necessity for the evaluation of implementation variables related to the costs and benefits of moving research and demonstration projects into the field; the generalization of program effects through direct intervention; a growing awareness of how the structure of service delivery systems either facilitates or impedes program evaluation; an identification of macro-social or societal factors influencing service delivery; attention to the "expressive" or human factor aspects of program evaluation as well as to the "instrumental" or design and analysis issues; and, in addition to procedural guidelines for the conduct of program evaluation, some guidelines for the evaluation of evaluation designs.

While each contributor deals to a large extent with many facets of program evaluation, the contexts are generally arranged to allow the reader to move through the following sequence: first, design and analysis issues, and then examples of program evaluations including discrete local programs, regional approaches, and national perspectives.

We believe that students and professionals alike will find in this book stimulation and assistance for developing evaluation programs in operational settings and for improving existing evaluation programs. Finally, and most importantly, it is the belief and hope of the authors that improved feedback to social, educational, and health organizations can result in more effective and personally satisfying services to persons in our society.

Park O. Davidson

CONTRIBUTORS

James R. Barclay
University of Kentucky, Lexington

Peter Bates
University of Denver, Denver

Michael F. Cataldo
University of Kansas, Lawrence

William W. Cooley
University of Pittsburgh, Pittsburgh

William J. DeRisi
Oxnard Community Mental Health Center, California

Thad A. Eckman
Oxnard Community Mental Health Center, California

Robert P. Hawkins
Western Michigan University, Kalamazoo

Siegfried S. Hiebert
The University of Calgary, Calgary

Srinika Jayaratne
The University of Michigan, Ann Arbor

Richard R. Jones
Oregon Research Institute, Eugene

Robert L. Kahn
The University of Chicago, Chicago

Larry W. King
Oxnard Community Mental Health Center, California

Carl H. Koenig
Behavior Research Company, Florida

Gaea Leinhardt
University of Pittsburgh, Pittsburgh

Robert Paul Liberman
Oxnard Community Mental Health Center, California

Peter D. McLean
University of British Columbia, Vancouver

William B. Neenan
The University of Michigan, Ann Arbor

Aldred H. Neufeldt
Department of Public Health, Saskatoon

H. S. Pennypacker
University of Florida, Gainesville

Todd R. Risley
University of Kansas, Lawrence

Rosemary C. Sarri
The University of Michigan, Ann Arbor

W. H. Seaver
New London, North Carolina

Elaine Selo
The University of Michigan, Ann Arbor

Bryan C. Smith
University of Florida, Gainesville

Richard B. Stuart
The University of Michigan, Ann Arbor

Tony Tripodi
The University of Michigan, Ann Arbor

Charles Windle
National Institute of Mental Health, Maryland

David Wood
Oxnard Community Mental Health Center, California

Steven H. Zarit
The University of Chicago, Chicago

Design and Analysis Problems in Program Evaluation[1] 1

Richard R. Jones

Program evaluation, the theme of this book, can mean different things to different people. For this writer, that part of social science research which has come to be known as evaluation has as its central concern the study of behavioral change: behavioral change that is public and hence observable, and behavioral change that is either directly or indirectly due to some form of programmatic manipulation. Assessment of behavioral change is taken as the main focus of evaluation research because virtually all social programs seek to change the order of things in people's lives, whether it is to increase the school readiness of disadvantaged children, improve the economic power of minority groups, reduce rates of delinquency, or ameliorate the mental health problems of the public at large. Demonstrating that behavior has changed as a result of programmatic interventions serves as the major mandate for virtually all program evaluators, and producing that behavioral change is the major mandate for all program planners and directors.

But here there are two very thorny matters to be faced by all behavioral researchers, and particularly by evaluation specialists. If our concern is with behavioral change due to programmed intervention, then first we are confronted with problems in the *measurement of behavioral change,* and second by the problems in identifying the *causes of behavioral change.* Even if all the methodological difficulties in the measurement of behavioral change were solved, which of course they are not (e.g., Cronbach and Furby, 1970; Harris, 1963), there is the added necessity of clearly showing that whatever change does occur, occurs as a result of the particular social or behavioral innovation being evaluated. Both the measurement and causation issues abound with methodological pitfalls, pitfalls which are all too quickly noted by critics of social programs, and which can so feed the fires of political, bureaucratic, and operational debate as to obscure often real gains to society accruing from even weak social innovations (e.g., Williams and Evans, 1972).

Social researchers and program directors must solve as many of the methodological shortcomings of program evaluations as possible, and thereby obviate some of the adverse criticism which in the end can abort even the most well conceptualized project. The experimental design and statistical analysis tools readily available to social program evaluators have definite shortcomings when it comes to the measurement of change and the demonstration of causation (Harris, 1963; Holtzman, 1963; Kahneman, 1965; Meehl, 1970). Hence, just as social scientists, politicians and bureaucrats can and must be innovative in designing social and behavioral programs, researchers, evaluators, and statisticians must become innovative in providing the techniques needed to answer the many questions surrounding the measurement of change and the demonstration of causation associated with social programs.

Parenthetically, we would discount for this discussion the skeptic's charge that social programs are solely political gambits with little, if any, real intention of producing important social and behavioral change. Notwithstanding the immense difficulties encountered in trying to demonstrate the effects of program manipulations, it is taken here that all programs do in fact have the primary goal of achieving change in the social or behavioral order of things. It is, of course, the very immense difficulties encountered by evaluation researchers in proving that programs do work which have served as a partial impetus for the series of papers comprising this volume.

The function of research design in proving that programmatic innovations have their intended impact is much the same as the role that experimental design plays in testing scientific hypotheses. In fact, much of the rationale underlying, and even specific approaches toward, evaluation design derive directly from experimental design as used in the psychological laboratory and communicated to students in graduate school texts. Hence, design means the same thing in evaluation research as in experimental or laboratory research. It is a formal plan for systematically studying the effects of some intrusion into a psychological phenomenon. Analysis, on the other hand, refers to the particular statistical, mathematical, logical, or inferential procedures used to determine whether or not the formal plan or design had its intended impact on the psychological phenomenon under study. While it is possible to discuss on a conceptual level the design of evaluation research separately from the analysis of the data, these two topics are actually so interwoven in their application that decisions regarding design clearly influence data analysis procedures, and to some extent the reverse as well.

Unfortunately, many problems with analysis of program data often do not appear until after design decisions have been made, and even worse, after information has been collected. Virtually every statistics or design textbook in use today warns that data analysis procedures should be well thought through *before* programs are started and data are collected. Of course, the exigencies of field research often require changes in planned projects, but this does not preclude the responsibility of the program director and evaluation researcher to insure as much as possible the desired compatibility between design, data collection, and statistical analysis. The likelihood of problems with analysis after the data are collected is increased in little traveled research areas (e.g., social interventions) where in truth the evaluator sometimes does not know what to expect. But even here some attention to the most likely forms of data and peculiar needs for their analysis can prevent many after-the-fact methodological headaches. The point is that evaluation design and data analysis decisions should be considered together from the outset; hence, any discussion of methodological problems necessarily combines the design and analysis components.

For purposes of exposition, however, this chapter is arranged in two sections: Evaluation Designs and Effectiveness Analysis. The specific topics the reader will encounter under each of these broad headings reflect the writer's experience in designing and conducting evaluation studies (Jones, 1968a, b; Jones, 1969a, b; Jones and Burns, 1970; Jones and Popper, 1972) and in playing the role of in-house evaluator for an extensive project at Oregon Research Institute under the direction of Dr. Gerald R. Patterson (Gallon and Jones, 1972; Jones, 1972; Patterson, 1972; Patterson, Cobb, and Ray, 1972; Patterson and Reid, 1972). No claims are made for the broad scope generalizability of these ideas and procedures. If, however, it is correct that the needed methodological and theoretical developments in program evaluation research and practice will evolve gradually, as have other developments in social science, then these modest contributions may find a place in that evolution.

Evaluation Designs

Research design issues permeate social and behavioral programs ranging in scope from the largest national demonstration projects to the smallest experimental laboratory studies. Projects conducted under relatively naturalistic conditions, in contrast to strict laboratory environments, seem to be particularly susceptible to design problems, and since this presentation is intended to cover such problems, most of the discussion will emphasize social or behavioral projects conducted under essentially field conditions. This is not to imply that laboratory investigations are devoid of design or analysis problems, since they clearly are not. However, it does seem that projects conducted under natural conditions need more methodological innovations (Meehl, 1970). Also, this chapter will focus on evaluation of behavior therapy projects as opposed to broad aim programs of national or regional scope. And, in so focusing, we shall be concerned mostly with change in individuals rather than institutions, recognizing with Rossi (1972) that programs designed to change individuals typically are more difficult to evaluate than programs designed to change institutions.

The primary goal of most clinical or academic intervention projects using behavior modification techniques is to change specified behavior(s) in the subject(s). The design of evaluation research for such projects should be aimed toward demonstrating and proving that the intervention in fact had the desired effect on the subject's behavior. The nuclear consideration in the choice of design has to do with the matter of control, control of possible outside influences which might have caused an observed change, but not be detected as the cause, such as the possible influences discussed as threats to internal and external validity of quasi-experiments (Campbell and Stanley, 1963). The importance of control of extraneous influences in social experiments is highlighted by the fact that this aspect of design is one frequently open to criticism. In some ways it is unfortunate that the ideal designs, i.e., those least objectionable from the standpoint of control, are those that originated in the laboratory setting. These designs are often unfeasible for the field experiments characteristic of many social or behavioral intervention projects (Weiss and Rein, 1969).

Solutions to this dilemma arising from the needs of naturalistic experimentation and the restrictions of traditional experimental design have taken various forms. One solution, borrowed from the animal laboratory, has been to largely avoid statistics and comparison groups (Bijou *et al.,* 1969; Sidman, 1960). This approach has given rise to a class of procedures known as "*n*=one" or reversal designs, in which the effects of environmental manipulations on behavior are studied for one subject over a series of time periods. The alternative to reversal designs is the use of variously formed comparison groups of multiple cases, some treated and some not, an approach which approximates the traditional experimental designs from the laboratory but often falls short due to mismatches between the restrictions of the statistical models and the nature of the data collected under field conditions. Selected characteristics and problems of *n*=one and group designs are discussed in the following sections.

N=one vs. Group Designs

One need not read very far into the literature of behavior modification, or clinical psychology in general for that matter, without encountering these two quite distinct approaches to the design of therapeutic intervention studies (e.g., Garfield, 1972; Zubin, 1972). Group designs are those taught to most of us in graduate schools. They require multiple subjects arranged into different treatment groups. The standard statistical procedures used to analyze the data generated in group studies is the analysis of variance and its variants, such as the analysis of covariance.

The second kind of study design is not as frequently taught in graduate schools, although at least passing mention is made of this strategy in most curricula. It is the so-called "n=one" design, and in expanded form is known as the reversal design. Readers of the *Journal of Applied Behavior Analysis* will recognize this design as the preferred method of analysis of behavioral data for that publication. There are no standard statistical procedures known to this writer for the analysis of data generated in the n=one reversal design, although ANOVA has been suggested, possibly inappropriately (Gentile *et al.,* 1972; Jones, Vaught, and Reid, 1973; Shine and Bower, 1971), as well as various kinds of descriptive statistics (Bijou *et al.,* 1969). In lieu of statistical analyses of n=one data, effects typically are evaluated visually by references to changes in the dependent variable which occur at appropriate points during the course of treatment. Usually, a baseline phase is used to establish "typical" rates of the target behavior and/or to establish the environmental control needed to obtain stable behavioral scores. Then an intervention phase occurs, followed by a return to baseline conditions (removal of the treatment conditions). The changes in the behavioral score for the subject are inspected for evidence of treatment effectiveness. Only one subject is analyzed at a time, and if several cases are treated in a similar manner, the analysis is handled separately for each. Sidman's (1960) classic book, *Tactics of Scientific Research*, provides the essential arguments favoringtthis method, and an article by Bijou *et al.* (1969) expands this strategy to the study of observational data collected on young children in natural settings.

The design and analysis problems attendant on the group and n=one designs differ substantially. Where the user of group data should be sensitive to the restrictions and assumptions underlying the statistical inference models used to analyze multiple subject data, the user of the n=one, reversal designs can ignore such considerations since inferential statistics typically are not employed in the analysis of single subject data. On the other hand, the visual inspector of n=one time series data can only be sure of his treatment effects when the changes in the dependent variable are so obvious that no critic would contest the researchers' conclusions that treatment had had its desired effects. One wonders how many n=one studies have gone unreported because the changes in the subject's behavioral scores were not extreme enough to allay the possibility of critical review. The same can be said, of course, about group studies which often yield non-significant or negative findings and also go unreported. There is some small advantage accruing to the latter, however, since some information about the magnitude of effect needed for significance is obtained from the unsuccessful group analysis (Cohen, 1969), while the power of the n=one visual analysis is always the same, meaning that the next study can only try to do the same things again, but more so, to obtain the desired effects (Bijou *et al.*, 1969).

Control over variables other than those under experimental manipulation differs in these two kinds of designs. The n=one or reversal design uses each subject as his own control, in the sense that changes in behavior brought about by the intervention are compared with what the behavior looked like prior to intervention (the baseline phase) and again following the intervention (return-to-baseline phase). The experimenter gains control over the behavior by providing appropriate envionmental contingencies and demonstrates this control by manipulating the behavior of the subject away from baseline or "typical" performance. Since the only (programmed) change in the subject's environment is the intervention, it is concluded that whatever behavior changes do occur are due to the manipulation.

The efficacy of the n=one design for proving the effectiveness of program intervention resides in the capability of the experimenter to control the various and perhaps unknown environmental contingencies that can influence the target behavior. In contrived, laboratory-like settings this control is easier to achieve than in more naturalistic settings. In principle, if not in practice, attributing changes in behavior to the programmatic intervention becomes more problematical as the direct experimental control over the environmental influences lessens. As a method, then, of general application in evaluating the effectiveness of social intervention programs in open field settings, reversal designs can be seen as somewhat limited. Of course, these designs were not originally intended for such use, but as the functional analysis of behavior proceeds out of the laboratory into the real world, it is likely that the experimental design and analysis methods used in the laboratory will follow. Whether these approaches will be as successful in

6

evaluating the impact of social programs as they have been in the functional analysis of behavior cannot be determined in advance.

But there are other reasons why the *n*=one design may prove less valuable in social program evaluation than the more traditional group designs. For example, as now used, reversal designs are applied to one subject at a time. But socially or behaviorally innovative programs in the field will have to deal with large samples, even whole populations of subjects, if any impact of such interventions is to be felt on the main fabric of society. For obvious reasons, the one-subject-at-a-time approach characteristic of reversal designs will have to be changed to accommodate usage on a large social scale. Modifications of the *n*=one design for use with multiple subjects, including the development or adaptation of statistical procedures would be a substantial accomplishment, with important payoffs both for research methodology in general, and evaluation procedures in particular.

Another difficulty with *n*=one designs in field experiments involves the experimenter's ability to return the subject to actual baseline conditions during the reversal phase(s) of the design. In the laboratory there is much more control over environmental influences on the target behavior than in the field, and unless these influences are controlled the return-to-baseline phase may not constitute a true reversal of the behavior, and/or the environmental conditions, to the pre-intervention baseline state. The most important component that might not return to original baseline conditions is the conditions related to the intervention, if, for example, the subject's behavior continues under the control of the manipulation, even though it has been removed (e.g., Bijou *et al.,* 1969). This may happen even under relatively controlled laboratory conditions, but seems particularly likely in the field where the experimenter does not have total control over the reinforcing contingencies in the environment, including perhaps those contingencies which are integral parts of the manipulation. Phenomenally, it can be argued that the subject is never actually returned to baseline conditions, if only because time has changed. And, to the extent that time is a factor in the behavior of the subject, reversals will be incomplete. But the more important problem seems to be the likelihood that there will be carry-over of some kind from the last trials of the intervention phase into the first trials, or perhaps the complete set of trials, of the reversal-to-baseline phase. The influence of such carry-over on the subject's behavior probably is largely indeterminant, and clearly presents an interpretational problem for the reversal design, since it cannot be stated whether incomplete returns-to-baseline are due to carry-over of treatment effects *per se*, or to the simple inability of the experimenter to reproduce true baseline conditions.

Whichever kind of design is considered, n=one or group, they both are based on the simple rationale that to evaluate change in some phenomenon, e.g., the behavior of people, comparisons of various kinds must be made. The most essential kind of comparison is between assessments of status prior to an intervention and assessments following the application of the intervention. But simple pre- vs. post-intervention comparisons for either single individuals or groups of individuals are not sufficient scientific evidence to support claims for significant change. The reason, of course, is that any observed change might have occurred anyway, and that there really occurred only a simply coincidence between the planned intervention and some other unknown cause of the observed change. The solution to this impasse in evaluating "real" change is the use of some kind of comparison group, i.e., individuals who are observed in the same way as the target cases, but who are not treated in the same way. The most scientifically rigorous kind of such a comparison group is the randomly created control group, where each member of the control group is drawn at random from the same population of individuals comprising the also randomly selected treatment group. Individuals selected into treatment and control groups in this random fashion have an equal chance of assignment to either group, hence there are only chance differences in the composition of the groups and the characteristics of the individuals within the groups. Thus, when assessments of pre- and post-intervention status are compared, the effectiveness of the intervention should appear in the treatment group and not the control group, and this should be the only reason for any difference between the groups, since they were randomly equivalent before the intervention.

This treatment vs. control group design represents the best of all worlds from the standpoint of evaluation methodology. When such a design is possible, all of the traditional statistical and data analysis techniques taught to us in graduate school apply. But, evaluators are frequently called on to analyze the effectiveness of interventions when this random assignment of individuals to treatment and control groups is not possible, for practical, moral, ethical, or economic reasons. The most frequent situation encountered is when it is necessary to employ previously constituted groups of individuals as comparison samples in evaluation designs. Examples come readily to mind, e.g., separate classrooms of pupils, schools, hospital wards, etc. Such preformed groups usually differ from one another in many ways, some of which may be critical to the evaluation of the effectiveness of treatment applied to one and not the other of such pre-existing groups.

One particularly crucial way that preformed groups can differ from each other is in status on the pre-intervention measures. Truly randomly selected groups will vary only according to chance on pre-test status, but naturally formed groups can, and often do, vary importantly on pre-test status. This will interfere with comparisons between pre- and post-test scores (Elashoff, 1969; Lord, 1958; Werts and Linn, 1971) and comparisons among groups on post- or gains scores because often it is the case that the amount of change is associated with the subject's status on the pre-intervention measure. For example, subjects already scoring high on some dependent variable can change less in terms of measured score units than some subject with initially low score status. So, if the mean pre-intervention scores for one preformed group is importantly lower than the mean for another preformed group, and one group is treated while the other is untreated, and then comparisons are made between post-treatment score means, the observed difference could be due simply to the differences that existed on the pre- measures and have nothing to do with the effectiveness of treatment. The simple correlation between pre-test and gains (post- minus pre-test scores) scores will usually tell whether or not this particular problem exists in any actual evaluation problem.

N=one and Group Designs

There is a very definite "either-or" quality to discussions of n=one vs. group designs, and the schism between the two strategies of research is noted even in the editorial policies of professional journals. One seldom finds group studies reported in *JABA*, or n=one studies in the *Journal of Abnormal Psychology*. There would seem to be considerable merit in the joint usage of these two methods, at least in some contexts, and the argument for this approach might take the following form.

In virtually any group study, there will be subjects for whom the intended treatment effects are greater than for other subjects. Perhaps it is even the case that some subjects are not affected by the treatment at all, or minimally at best (e.g., Eyberg, 1972). When such is the case in the analysis of data in group designs, the small-change subjects attenuate the magnitude of the average effect for the group. If the separate subjects were treated as n replicates of the treatment design, some of the cases would show large changes due to treatment while others would show small or nil effects of treatment. In a replicated n=one analysis such as this, note that the results for the "large-effect" subjects only would be likely to appear in journals according to current editorial practice, and therefore, the subjects who did not change much, or changed only a little, would be viewed as unsuccessful. In a group analysis of the same data, the unsuccessful subjects could reduce the overall impact of the treatment for the group, while in the n=one strategy they would probably be ignored.

But something should be learned from the failure of the procedures to work with some cases, while working successfully with others. Rather than either ignoring such instances, or resigning oneself to a reduced treatment effect due to the inclusion of unsuccessful cases in a group analysis, investigators could try to understand why some cases were unsuccessful. What is suggested here is an analysis of the failures in an intervention study, something which may well be done on a *post hoc* basis by some investigators, but which typically is not reported. A search for characteristics of the cases, of the treatment, or of the case by treatment interaction which would distinguish among the successes and the failures in program intervention work should repay the efforts handsomely. For example, one possibility is that some interaction has occurred between individual characteristics or their socio-psychological situations and the treatment conditions. Understanding the nature of this interaction(s) would provide suggestions for the design of subsequent programs, indicate the appropriate client populations for the treatment that was used, or at least permit a "moderated" conclusion from seemingly negative evaluation findings.

A possible methodological approach to studying this set of questions could be to develop a multiple regression model for "predicting" (really post-dicting) the outcome of treatment. The dependent variable would be the success or failure with each case. The independent variables would include many classes of variables, e.g., therapist characteristics, patient characteristics, family characteristics, intake test scores for the child and parents, demographic and environmental variables, etc. In effect, virtually all of the measurable variables noted in reviews of the literature on psychotherapy effectiveness (e.g., Fiske *et al.,* 1970; Kiesler, 1966) could find a place in this multiple regression model for predicting the effectiveness of any kind of psychological intervention. Presumably those variables that were not related to the outcome of the treatment (as measured by the successes vs. the failures) would drop out of the regression equation since they would not carry any predictive weight. Those that remained could provide some indication of what particular characteristics of the entire therapeutic situation were important from the standpoint of effectiveness.

Conceptually this suggestion makes sense as a procedure for understanding in some detail what components of intervention programs are more important than others for the success of those programs. But as a practical matter, the technique probably would be useful only with comparatively large projects involving many cases. In order for the regression model to "work," large samples of subjects would be necessary. But consider, for example, large-scale programs like Head Start, Sesame Street (Ball and Bogatz, 1972), and Project Follow-Through (e.g., Porter, 1972). Here, given solutions to various measurement problems, it would be possible to run this regression model to ascertain what, if any, characteristics of these programs discriminated between successes and failures. This kind of *post hoc* analysis could usefully replace the often extended polemics surrounding ambiguous results from studies in which the effects of treatment varied considerably among subjects.

Effectiveness Analysis

The following two sections deal with approaches for demonstrating *(a)* the causal relationship between variables, when one of the variables has been the object of a programmatic manipulation; and *(b)* the generalization of treatment effects across settings. The latter topic represents the issue of ultimate concern to program designers and evaluators, viz., to what extent is the impact of treatment observed in settings other than those in which the intervention occurred. Criminologists are concerned with this issue when they study recidivism rates in "rehabilitated" penal institution releasees. Behavior modifiers should be concerned with this issue when they treat children in a school setting and assume that their therapeutic efforts will extend into the home.

The first topic, concerned with the causal relationships among variables studied in treatment programs, provides the framework for suggestions about analyzing data to "prove" that interventions have produced the hypothesized effect, or even more basically that the theoretical underpinnings of certain kinds of manipulations are sound. The essential question here concerns an appropriate demonstration that changing behavior in desired ways has the expected effect on some other behavior, either in the same person, or in some other person.

Treatment Effectiveness and Causation Between Two Constructs

In some behavioral programs, the intention of the treatment is to change the behavior of one person in order to alter the behavior of another person. An example is training parents in child management techniques, the focus of the family intervention work ongoing at Oregon Research Institute (ORI) under the direction of Dr. Gerald R. Patterson. The part of this treatment model of concern for this presentation involves teaching parents how to consequate the behavior of their deviant children such that rates of deviant behavior in the child will be reduced. There is an obvious causative relationship implied by this model. *If* the parents learn the appropriate consequation skills, *then* the effects of this change in their behavior will be observed in lowered rates of deviant behavior in the child. Demonstration of this multiple effect is not as straightforward as might seem to be the case, nor is its evaluation.

To begin, analysis of variance (ANOVA) models might be used to show that the parent training had a significant effect on the rates of consequating behaviors for the mother and father. And, a separate ANOVA might also show a significant decrease in the children's rates of deviant behavior. But, neither of these results, taken separately or together, proves that a causative connection was established between the parent's consequating behavior and the child's deviant behavior. Consider the following arguments and possible solution to the analysis dilemma.

When parents bring their children to the ORI Social Learning Project for clinical help, it can be reasonably assumed that an extensive history of unproductive parent-child behavioral interactions has occurred. Although the primary hypothesis suggests that the behavior of the parent influences the behavior of the child, it is quite possible that the behavioral history of parent-child interactions has been such that the child's behavior is a stimulus for the parent's behavior as well as the reverse. For example, deviant acts by the child, instigated for any of a variety of reasons, could "tip off" the parent's inappropriate consequating behavior, which in turn serves as a stimulus for more deviancy from the child, etc. This historically evolved interaction among parents and children can be construed as a looping or closed circle kind of behavioral phenomenon. What the parent does starts the child off, and what the child does starts the parent off, and the circle of interaction continues. Given such a situation, it would be very difficult to clearly identify which agent was the primary causative agent of the other's behavior, the parent or the child.

Now, if successful, the treatment (being to train the parents in appropriate consequating skills such that the child deviant behavior is brought under control) should produce the hypothesized causal connection between what the parent does and what the child does. In fact, the demonstration that what the parent does directly influences what the child does is a necessary demonstration of the effectiveness of treatment, at least of a kind that is proposed in the present treatment model. Simply showing that the child's deviant behavior drops from pre- to post-treatment is not evidence that the causal connection between the parents' behavior and the child's behavior has been established. Nor does showing that the parents' training was effective in increasing the parental skills in consequating behaviors. Either could have occurred, but not in concert with the other. But, by the following application of cross-lag panel correlation technique (Campbell, 1963; Campbell and Stanley, 1963), in conjunction with the traditional ANOVAs to show changes in means due to treatment, the issue of causation can be directly and logically attacked.

Before detailing the approach, an overview should help the reader anticipate some of the arguments, and hopefully reduce the burden of details that will be necessary to explain the technique. First, if the behavioral history has, in fact, generated a reciprocal or looping connection between parent and child behavior, then the crossed and lagged correlations in the diagram (Figure 1, p. 14) should not be different from each other, and should be positive. That is, according to the logic of the CLPC technique, neither parent nor child behavior can be seen as a temporally preceding causative influence on the other's behavior. So, if assessments of the two agents' behaviors are obtained at two points in time, say during baseline and later, just prior to the institution of treatment, then it should not necessarily be possible to ascertain which causes which using the CLPC technique.

Now, following the collection of these data, treatment is started, treatment designed directly to change the parents' consequating skills, since the therapeutic model assumes that such changes will directly cause changes in the deviant behavior of the child. And, in this treatment situation the child is given relatively little direct treatment designed to change his behavior *per se*. It should now be the case that if the treatment of the parents is effective, there will be a decrease from pre-treatment to follow-up in the parents' average rate of inappropriate consequations. There also should be a decrease in the children's deviant behavior rates. Can we say that the parents' changes in behavior have been such that there is now a causal connection between what the parent does and what the child does?

Figure 1 Cross-lagged panel correlation paradigm for assessing causal relationships between two variables.

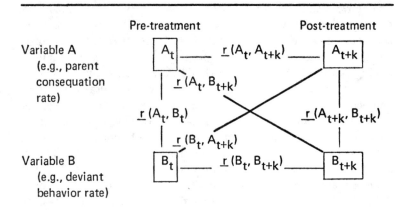

If the two crossed and lagged correlations now stand in a certain relation to each other, the matter of causation can be argued. Briefly, the parents would have been trained to manage their children's behavior by appropriately consequating deviant and pro-social acts. Also, they would have been trained *not* to respond to their children's behavior as they had been doing prior to treatment. Those responses were, as already argued, serving as often as not to inappropriately reinforce the child. Hence, there would have been no difference between the two crossed and lagged correlations between parent and child behavior scores from baseline to pre-treatment. Now, however, if the causal connection between parent and child behavior has been established by treatment, the same two correlations computed from pre-treatment to post-treatment should show that the parents are causers of the child's behavior and the children are *not* causers of the parents' behavior. Specifically, the correlation between parent at pre-treatment and child at post-treatment should be significantly greater than the correlation between the child at pre-treatment and the parent at post-treatment. If this inequality holds, *and* there are significant changes in mean levels of both parent and child behaviors, it seems quite appropriate to conclude that not only was treatment effective in reducing deviancy, but that also it was effective in establishing the causal connection between what the parent does and what the child does.

The foregoing approach to the analysis of causation in behavioral studies was recently used by the writer (Jones and Cobb, 1973) to evaluate the following proposition:

It has been suggested (Cobb, 1969, 1971; Cobb and Hops, 1972; Hops and Cobb, 1972) that particular classroom behaviors, called survival skills, may be causally related to academic achievement as measured by standardized tests. Survival skill behaviors include *Attention*, *Volunteering*, and not *Looking Around*. Correlations between behavioral survival skill scores and scores on standardized achievement tests have been significant and positive, while experimental treatments have produced increases in survival skill behaviors, with accompanying increases in academic achievement. Hence, both correlational and experimental studies suggest that if pupils' overt survival skill behaviors increase over time, due either to spontaneous development, maturation, or experimental manipulation, there will also occur an increase in the pupils' academic achievement test performance. (Jones and Cobb, 1973. P. 1)

As reviewed by Cobb and Hops (1972), correlations between each of the individual behaviors classified as survival skills and first grade reading achievement are in the approximate range from .40 to .60. These correlations provide the descriptive underpinnings for the hypothesis that survival skills may be causally connected with academic achievement. Other studies have shown positive effects of various classroom interventions on survival skill behaviors. Putting these two sets of results together suggest the possibility that increasing the level of survival skill behaviors via direct classroom intervention may produce a change in academic achievement. Two studies (Cobb and Hops, 1972; Hops and Cobb, 1972) report the results of just such a manipulation, and the reanalyses reported in the present paper are based on the data from these investigations. (Jones and Cobb, 1973. P. 2)

The data from Hops and Cobb (1972) were reanalyzed according to the paradigm and arguments presented above. Each pupil had pre- and post-treatment scores on both the survival skills (SS) and reading achievement (RA) measures. Hence, the four scores for each subject can be displayed and analyzed according to the cross-lagged panel correlation technique shown in Figure 1. Results will be presented separately for the 20 control subjects and the 42 combined experimental samples, providing two replications of the findings.

Figures 2 and 3 show the correlations among the four scores displayed according to the cross-lagged panel correlation paradigm, for the control subjects and experimental subjects, respectively. Consider the results for the control group first. Looking only at the concurrent correlations between SS and RA for baseline ($r = -.20$, ns) and post-intervention ($r = .72$, $p<.01$), only the latter coefficient supports previous studies showing a significantly positive relationship between survival skills and achievement. No immediate explanation is available to account for the nonsignificant, and negative (!) correlation obtained between survival skills and reading achievement during baseline.

Figure 2   Cross-lagged panel correlations for control group (N = 20).

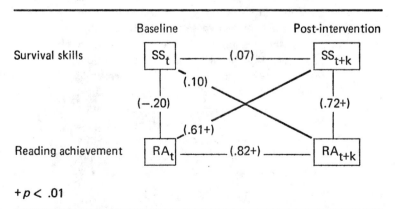

+$p < .01$

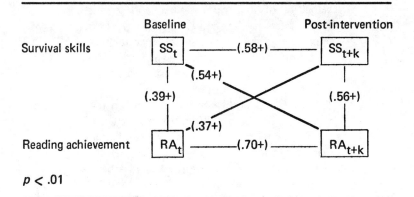

Figure 3   Cross-lagged panel correlations for experimental group (N = 42).

Baseline   Post-intervention

Survival skills SS_t ———(.58+)——— SS_{t+k}

(.54+)

(.39+)   (.56+)

(.37+)

Reading achievement RA_t ———(.70+)——— RA_{t+k}

$p < .01$

Next, consider the baseline vs. post-intervention correlations for each variable, which can be viewed as stability or test-retest reliability coefficients. Survival skills scores were virtually unrelated over time in this control sample ($r = .07$, *ns*), but the achievement scores were substantially reliable ($r = .82$, $p < .01$). Again, the unexpected low stability for SS in unexplainable.

Now, turning to the two cross-lagged correlations in Figure 2, the expected inequality between them did not appear; in fact, the reverse was obtained. Instead of r (SS_t, RA_{t+k}) being larger than $r(RA_t, SS_{t+k})$, indicating support for the primary hypothesis that SS caused RA, the present results suggest just the opposite! The crossed, lagged correlation between RA_t and SS_{t+k} was .61 ($p < .05$), while the correlation between SS_t and RA_{t+k} was only .10 (*ns*). Hence, it would appear that in this control group, RA was causally related to SS, and *not the reverse.*

The findings for the subjects in the experimental group were rather different. As shown in Figure 3, both concurrent correlations

(rs = .39 and .56, $p<.01$) support the previous work showing significantly positive relationships between SS and RA. Also, the temporal stabilities of the two measures appear satisfactory (rs = .58 and .70, $p<.01$). Most importantly, the two cross-lagged correlations were both positive and significant, and as predicted by the primary hypothesis, the correlation between SS_t and RA_{t+k} was larger (r = .54, $p<.01$) than the correlation between RA_t and SS_{t+k} (r = .37, $p<.01$). However, a test of the difference between these two correlations was not significant, suggesting the plausible rival hypothesis that a reciprocal or reverberating relationship exists such that SS and RA have mutually facilitating effects. The other rival hypothesis that RA causes SS, as suggested by the results in the control group, is not supported by the findings in the experimental group. (Jones and Cobb, 1973. Pp. 11-12)

The foregoing discussion illustrates the use of cross-lagged panel correlation technique to evaluate the causal connection between two behaviors within subjects (the Cobb and Hops reanalysis) and between the behavior of two different subjects (the example involving the consequating parent and the deviant child). However, CLPC techniques, like other data analysis procedures, should not be employed uncritically. An important restriction in the interpretation of CLPC results has been raised by Pelz and Andrews (1964), which also has implications for assessing the effects of any program manipulation. These authors note the important distinction between *intervals of causation* and *intervals of remeasurement.*

Consideration of these two intervals seems crucial in any evaluation study involving repeated assessments of program effectiveness. The interval of remeasurement means simply the period of time intervening between the repeated assessments, typically and most simply, the interval between pre- and post-treatment testings. The interval of causation is less clearly defined, referring to the period of time between pre- and post-testings which is optimal for the effects of the intervention to be reflected in the behavior of the subjects.

In terms of the previous examples, concern for the appropriate interval of causation would be reflected in the following questions.

Given that changes in reading achievement can be produced by manipulating survival skill behaviors, what is the optimal period of time following the intervention needed to observe this effect? And, given that changing parental child management skills will produce changes in the deviant behavior rates of children, what is the optimal period of time following intervention needed to observe this effect?

If the intervals of remeasurement and causation are not suitably matched, the CLPC technique probably will yield ambiguous findings. Of course, if the desired results are obtained in any particular study, it seems safe to assume that the optimal interval of causation was in fact selected and the repeated measurements were suitably timed to that interval. But in addition to serving as a critical proviso in the use of CLPC technique in program evaluation, the issue of appropriate intervals of causation and remeasurement has important implications generally for program design and evaluation.

Designers and evaluators of social programs should try to develop either theoretical, intuitive, or empirical ways of estimating the optimal period of time required for a particular manipulation to have its impact on the clientele served. Whether one is evaluating relatively small scale behavior modification projects dealing with single cases or large scale social engineering programs, an inappropriate interval of causation used for retesting could produce negative results when an appropriately chosen interval would show positive effects of the programmatic manipulations. Of course, intervals of causation will vary substantially from project to project, depending on the particular behavioral or social problem under study, and the type of manipulation employed. And specification of appropriate intervals of causation is certainly a complicated matter. Consider the following remarks regarding this issue as applied to the example involving survival skills training and reading achievement gains.

It seems obvious

> ...first that the acquisition of survival skills via programmed intervention requires some (unspecified) period of time. Second, once acquired, the beneficial effects of survival skills must somehow accumulate to the point where they are reflected in achievement test performance. Most probably this step involves the learning of scholastic material which would have been less well learned in the absence of the acquisition of appropriate survival skills.

Certainly these rather complex learning, memory, assimilation, and recall processes must take more than a trivial period of time. What, then, is the optimal length of time following the acquisition of survival skills before effects of these behavioral changes will be clearly seen in improved achievement test performance? It can be argued that our knowledge of the complexities of human cognitive learning is not sufficient to answer this question with any real precision. (Jones and Cobb, 1973. P. 16)

When remeasurement intervals cannot be precisely specified, it probably makes sense to employ as many spaced repeated assessments of outcome variables as feasible, since then one has the opportunity to determine empirically the interval(s) which demonstrate the greatest effect of treatment. The practicality of this suggestion will vary from study to study, but the general point remains: Evaluation of program effectiveness would be substantially enhanced if (a) intervals of causation can be specified on *a priori* bases before data collection is started, or (b) multiple-occasion measurements of critical outcome variables can be obtained during the life of the project.

Generalization of Program Treatment Effects[2]

Our final concern with the analysis of program effectiveness is perhaps the most important from the standpoint of overall impact on client populations. While it is often shown that interventions of various sorts do, in fact, have their planned effect on clients within the therapeutic setting, and at the particular time of their application, it is another matter entirely to show that these effects will show up in, that is generalize to, different settings and times.

Reviews, studies, and discussions concerned with treatment generalization abound in the professional literature (e.g., Baer, Wolf, and Risley, 1968; Bandura, 1970; Birnbrauer, 1968; Bucher and King, 1971; Gruber, 1971; Kuypers, Becker and O'Leary, 1969; O'Leary and Drabman, 1971; Patterson, 1971; Redd, 1970; Skindrud, 1972; Wahler, 1969; Walker and Buckley, 1972; Walker, Johnson, and Hops, 1972). A widely accepted conclusion, based on both theory and data, is that to insure generalization of behavior change, stimulus and response generalization decrements should be minimized (Gruber, 1971). And, following the advice of Baer, Wolf, and Risley (1968), the most promising way to minimize stimulus and response generalization decrements is to program generalization across settings, just as treatment effects are programmed within the therapeutic setting. Conceptually, this advice is most reasonable—programming across settings should improve the likelihood of generalization of behavior change. But it is quite another matter to manipulate the relevant environmental contingencies in (often) diverse extra-therapeutic settings. This practical matter seems to represent the Achilles' heel of the generalization issue in behavioral treatment programs. We seem to know what should be done (at least theoretically), but actually doing it often presents formidable difficulties, some of the reasons for which follow.

Stated in perhaps oversimplified fashion, behaviorally oriented treatment programs are designed to change characteristics of the stimuli, responses, or reinforcement schedules peculiar to a certain behavioral problem or class of problems. The desired changes are brought about by direct manipulation of observable events in the environments of the clients. As examples, stimuli which may set the occasion for a deviant response are altered vis-a-vis their potency or relevance for that response; or, the subject is taught a competing response to substitute for a deviant act; or, a reinforcement schedule which has historically supported a deviant response is altered such that extinction takes place. Each of these kinds of manipulation takes place within some specified environmental setting—perhaps a clinician's office or a special classroom, a client's home, or an institution. And the environmental characteristics in each of these settings may be quite different from those in other settings. Most would agree that lack of generalization of behavioral change across different settings, given effective treatment within the therapeutic setting, probably is due to dissimilarities in the environmental characteristics of extra-therapeutic settings. This, of course, is a behavior theory explanation of why rehabilitation of criminals in prisons often shows little carry-over or generalization to previous neighborhoods. Appropriate behaviors learned in one setting may not be performed in another setting when the stimulus, response, and reinforcement schedule parameters of those settings vary; and these parameters typically do vary across the numerous natural environments within which most people behave.

It is this across-setting variability of relevant behavior-controlling parameters which presents often formidable practical problems for the theoretically sound strategy of programming generalization in extra-therapeutic settings. Suppose, for example, that treatment consists largely of altering a reinforcement schedule which historically has maintained a particular deviant behavior. Such manipulation has been shown to be relatively easy to accomplish and effective in changing behavior within a therapeutic setting. For this behavior change to generalize, the therapist must obtain control over reinforcement schedules in extra-therapeutic settings, such as the school classroom, the home environment, or the neighborhood playground. If control of the reinforcement schedules in different settings is incumbent upon the therapist, and not on the client, then as a practical matter such across-setting programming of generalization seems unfeasible. Similar conclusions could be easily drawn from examples of behavioral therapy which focus not necessarily on reinforcement schedules, but on manipulations of responses (such as training competing behaviors) or on alterations of stimuli which set the occasion for deviant behaviors. For whatever strategy of treatment, focusing either on stimuli, responses, or reinforcement schedules, if the therapeutic manipulation is primarily in the control of the therapist or some other significant agent in the client's environment, and that agent is unable to produce the therapeutic manipulations across a variety of environmental settings in which the subject may behave, the likelihood of generalization of behavior change seems low.

If it is agreed that the likelihood of generalization of behavioral change is low unless control over environmental contingencies is obtained in most settings encountered by the subject, the question, then, is how to obtain such control. From the foregoing, it seems both unreasonable and impractical to expect that the therapist or some other social agent can be effective across the numerous settings in which clients will find themselves.

A more reasonable alternative is to provide clients with the ways and means of exercising their own contingency control across diverse settings. This notion would seem to underlie recent suggestions in behavior modification and social learning theory which have focused on self-management of behavior (e.g., Bandura, 1970; Kanfer, 1970; Mahoney, 1972). The apparent goal of this internalization strategy for insuring generalization of treatment effects is to provide clients with various techniques for manipulating environmental contingencies which control their behavior in various settings. For instance, clients might be taught the behavioral principles required to control reinforcement schedules; or, to control the stimuli which set the occasion for undesired responses; and also be taught how to apply this knowledge across a variety of environmental settings. Such cognitive control of behavior represents an awareness by the client of the functional relationships between stimuli, responses, and reinforcement. This awareness is quite different psychologically from situation-specific and simple stimulus-response-reinforcement connections established within a confined therapeutic setting. For this self-management strategy to be effective, therapy must produce changes in the cognitive apparatus of the client and such changes must be enduring across time and settings, thereby providing the client with the necessary skills for manipulating environmental contingencies without the assistance of outside therapeutic agents.

A crucial question, however, is concerned with what treatment we should be attempting to teach the client. More generally, it would appear that the client must change or improve his skills in perceiving the relevant stimulus, response, and reinforcement parameters of novel environments vis-a-vis his particular behavioral problem. This clearly implies an awareness of the functional relationships between the client's behavior and the numerous events which control that behavior in diverse environments.

Curiously, however, the identification and measurement of important characteristics of environmental stimuli has not been much emphasized in behavioral research concerned with generalization. Therapists, researchers, and clients must somehow learn more than is now known about the environmental contingencies which directly influence behavioral outcomes in both treatment and extra-treatment settings. Clients obviously cannot be trained in the recognition of controlling environmental events unless the salient characteristics of stimuli can be identified and measured. In the past, moderate success has been achieved in identifying and measuring response characteristics and parameters of reinforcement schedules. The same kind of effort now must be focused on the characteristics of controlling stimuli which occur in both therapeutic and natural environments.

The first and most critical problem to be addressed in this quest for information about controlling stimuli concerns the identification of potent or relevant stimuli for a particular client's behavioral problems. That is, which of the numerous environmental events influencing a subject are the crucial ones for controlling the client's target behavior. Once these relevant or potent stimuli have been identified for a particular case, then the kinds of procedures used previously to measure responses and reinforcement schedules could be applied. For example, stimulus density, duration, and intensity characteristics could be used to describe and classify the stimuli relevant for a particular behavioral problem. Assuming for the moment that such identification and measurement procedures can be worked out, two major problems will have to be solved both theoretically and methodologically in order for work on stimulus generalization to fulfill its promise of insuring generalization of treatment effects.

The first problem that will be encountered will delight those holding an idiographic view of behavior and be a constant enigma to those with a nomothetic approach to psychological theory and data. It seems likely that there will be little comparability across clients with regard to the salient stimuli and characteristics of those stimuli, even for very similar clinical problems. That is, the environmental stimuli which seem to set the occasion for one child's social aggression probably will be quite different from those environmental stimuli which set the occasion for another child's social aggression. If this prediction proves true, then much of the nomothetic tradition in psychology, with its theoretical and methodological notions and techniques, will not directly apply to the stimulus generalization issue in treatment evaluation. However, it may be possible to generate classes of stimuli which seem to be related to classes of behaviors across subjects, but it may well turn out that for such across-subjects generality to be obtained, the classes of behavior and stimuli will have to be so broad as to be relatively meaningless from a clinical or practical point of view.

And, as if incomparability of stimulus characteristics across subjects was not enough of a problem, a second difficulty may provide methodological headaches for the single subject researcher and practitioner. There is little reason to expect the salient characteristics of potent stimuli, or even their potency *per se,* to be invariant across settings. Stimuli which set the occasion for a target response either may differ themselves across settings, or their peculiarly relevant characteristics may differ across settings. This possible problem rings of the situational specificity of behavior noted by others (e.g., Mischel, 1968, 1973), and will be a stumbling block in the way of assessing stimulus generality across settings.

It would be constructive to provide some suggestions which might obviate some of the problems highlighted above. Unfortunately, I am not able to do that. I can only suggest some general strategies, particularly for research activities, over the next decade. The primary recommendation is to free our research thinking, strategies, and procedures from the relatively standard techniques that we have learned as students in psychology. For example, strict adherence to the prevalent nomothetic tradition in psychology probably will prevent researchers from coming to grips with the identification and measurement problems attendant on a concern with stimulus generalization. If the predicted lack of comparability of both relevant stimuli and their properties across subjects proves true, this would largely preclude the application of many statistical models and other traditional ways of thinking about behavioral data. But there will be problems with a purely idiographic or functional analysis style of research, also. If stimuli and their properties vary within the subject across settings, there would be little hope that time series analyses, whether based on visual or statistical inspection of data, would provide a viable test of behavioral generalization for the single subject. Overall, it would appear that very different ways of thinking about behavior and its controlling environmental contingencies may be necessary to overcome the very real problems encountered by present day analyses of behavior change which rely on traditional or quasi-traditional methods and procedures.

This discussion has painted a rather black picture, but it is still possible to close on an encouraging note. The behavioral and social problems with which behavior modifiers and designers of social action programs deal are very real; some would argue that if these problems are not treated effectively, the ultimate outcome for society will be disastrous. So, clearly the challenge is there, and to meet this challenge new ways of thinking about and new methods for dealing with society's problems, both in practical and research contexts, should evolve. While many present methods and techniques do not adequately serve the needs for evaluation of social programs designed to produce behavioral change, the inadequacy of present techniques will become more strongly felt in the future. Hence, now is the time to begin encouraging methodologists and theoreticians alike toward the development and implementation of novel approaches to the treatment of behavioral problems and evaluation of behavioral change programs.

Footnotes

1.   This study was supported by Grant No. MH 15985 and MH 12972 from the National Institute of Mental Health, U. S. Public Health Service.

2.   These remarks have benefitted substantially from discussions with Dr. John B. Reid and Mr. Robert Sanson-Fisher.

References

Baer, D. M., Wolf, M. M., and Risley, T. R. Some current dimensions of applied behavior analysis. *Journal of Applied Behavior Analysis,* 1968, *1,* 91-97.

Ball, S. and Bogatz, G. A. Research on Sesame Street: Some implications for compensatory education. Paper presented at the Second Annual Hyman Blumberg Symposium on Research in Early Childhood Education. Johns Hopkins Press, 1972.

Bandura, A. *Principles of behavior modification.* London: Holt, Rinehart and Winston, 1970.

Bijou, S. W., Peterson, R. F., Harris, F. R., Allen, K. E., and Johnston, M. S. Methodology for experimental studies of young children in natural settings. *The Psychological Record,* 1969, *19,* 177-210.

Birnbrauer, J. S. Generalization of punishment effects—A case study. *Journal of Applied Behavior Analysis,* 1968, *1,* 201-211.

Bucher, B. and King, L. W. Generalization of punishment effects in the deviant behavior of a psychotic child. *Behavior Therapy,* 1971, *2,* 68-77.

Campbell, D. T. From description to experimentation: Interpreting trends as quasi-experiments. In C. W. Harris (Ed.), *Problems in measuring change.* Madison: University of Wisconsin Press, 1963.

Campbell, D. T. and Stanley, J. C. Experimental and quasi-experimental designs for research on teaching. In N. L. Gage (Ed.), *Handbook of research on teaching.* Chicago: Rand McNally, 1963.

Cobb, J. A. The relationship of observable classroom behaviors to achievement of fourth grade pupils. Unpublished Doctoral Dissertation. University of Oregon, Eugene, 1969.

Cobb, J. A. The relationship of discrete classroom behaviors to fourth-grade academic achievement. *Journal of Educational Psychology,* 1972, *63,* 74-80.

Cobb, J. A. and Hops, H. Effects of academic survival skill training on low achieving first graders. *The Journal of Educational Research,* 1973, *67,* 108-113.

Cohen, J. *Statistical power analysis for the behavioral sciences.* New York: Academic Press, 1969.

Cronbach, L. J. and Furby, L. How should we measure "change"—or should we? *Psychological Bulletin,* 1970, *74,* 68-80.

Elashoff, J. D. Analysis of covariance: A delicate instrument. *American Educational Research Journal,* 1969, *6,* 383-401.

Eyberg, S. An outcome study of child-family intervention: Effects of contingency contracting and order of treated problems. Unpublished Doctoral Dissertation. University of Oregon, Eugene, 1972.

Fiske, D. W., Hunt, H. F., Luborsky, L., Orne, M. T., Parloff, M. B., Reiser, M. F., and Tuma, A. H. Planning of research on effectiveness in psychotherapy. *American Psychologist,* 1970, *25,* 727-737.

Gallon, S. L. and Jones, R. R. Systematic therapeutic intervention: An outline of a family treatment program. *Oregon Research Institute Research Bulletin,* 1972, *12,* No. 2.

Garfield, S. L. Idiographic and nomothetic approaches—Implications for psychotherapy. Paper presented as part of a Symposium, *Complementarity between the Idiographic and Nomothetic Methods in Clinical Psychology,* at the meeting of the American Psychological Association, Honolulu, September 1972.

Gentile, J. R., Roden, A. H., and Klein, R. D. An analysis-of-variance model for the intrasubject replication design. *Journal of Applied Behavior Analysis,* 1972, *5,* 193-198.

Gruber, R. P. Behavior therapy: Problems in generalization. *Behavior Therapy,* 1971, *2,* 361-368.

Harris, C. W. (Ed.). *Problems in measuring change.* Madison: University of Wisconsin Press, 1963.

Holtzman, W. H. Statistical models for the study of change in the single case. In C. W. Harris (Ed.), *Problems in measuring change.* Madison: University of Wisconsin Press, 1963.

Hops, H., and Cobb, J. A. Survival behaviors in the educational setting: Their implications for research and intervention. Report No. 13, June 1972, University of Oregon, Contract No. NPECE-70-005, OEC 0-70-4152(607), Bureau of Educationally Handicapped, U. S. Office of Education.

Jones, R. R., The Peace Corps overseas: Some first steps toward description and evaluation. *Oregon Research Institute Technical Report,* 1968a, *8,* No. 3.

Jones, R. R. The validity of the Full Field background report in Peace Corps selection. *Oregon Research Institute Research Monograph,* 1968b, *8,* No. 1.

Jones, R. R. Peace Corps selection without the Full Field. Peace Corps Division of Research, *Report No. 7,* January 1969a.

Jones, R. R. Previous teaching experience and the overseas performance of Peace Corps volunteers. In J. W. Cotton (Chm.), *Teacher selection, teacher training, and teaching methods in overseas service.* Symposium presented at the meeting of the American Psychological Association, Washington, D. C., September 1969b.

Jones, R. R. Intraindividual stability of behavior observations: Implications for evaluating behavior modification treatment programs. Paper presented at the meeting of the Western Psychological Association, Portland, Oregon, April 1972.

Jones, R. R. and Cobb, J. A. Validity of behavioral scores derived from teachers' ratings vs. naturalistic observations. Paper presented at the meeting of the Western Psychological Association, Anaheim, California, April 1973.

Jones, R. R. and Burns, J. W. Volunteer satisfaction with in-country training for the Peace Corps. *Journal of Applied Psychology,* 1970, *54,* 533-537.

Jones, R. R. and Popper, R. Characteristics of Peace Corps host countries and the behavior of volunteers. *Journal of Cross-Cultural Psychology,* 1972, *3,* 233-245.

Jones, R. R., Vaught, R. S., and Reid, J. B. Time series analysis as a substitute for single subject analysis of variance designs. Paper presented in A. E. Kazdin, (Chm.), *Symposium on Methodological Issues in Applied Behavior Analysis.* American Psychological Association Convention, Montreal, Quebec, Canada, August 1973.

Kahneman, D. Control of spurious association and the reliability of the controlled variable. *Psychological Bulletin,* 1965, *64,* 326-329.

Kanfer, F. G. Self-regulation: Research, issues and speculations. In C. Neuringer and J. L. Michael (Eds.), *Behavior modification in clinical psychology.* New York: Appleton-Century-Crofts, 1970. Pp. 178-220.

Kiesler, D. J. Some myths of psychotherapy research and the search for a paradigm. *Psychological Bulletin,* 1966, *65,* 110-136.

Kuypers, D. S., Becker, W. C., and O'Leary, K. D. How to make a token system fail. *Exceptional Children,* 1969, *35,* 523-529.

Lord, F. M. Further problems in the measurement of growth. *Educational and Psychological Measurement,* 1958, *28,* 437-451.

Meehl, P. E. Nuisance variables and the *ex post facto* design. In M. Radner and S. Winokur (Eds.), *Minnesota studies in the philosophy of science.* Vol. 4. Minneapolis: University of Minnesota Press, 1970.

Mischel, W. *Personality and assessment.* New York: John Wiley and Sons, 1968.

Mischel, W. Towards a cognitive social learning reconceptualization of personality. *Psychological Review,* 1973, in press.

Mahoney, M. J. Research issues in self-management. *Behavior Therapy,* 1972, *3,* 45-63.

O'Leary, K. D. and Drabman, R. Token reinforcement programs in the classroom: A review. *Psychological Bulletin,* 1971, *75,* 379-398.

Patterson, G. R. Reprogramming the families of aggressive boys. In C. Thoresen (Ed.), *Behavior modification in education.* 72nd Yearbook, National Society for the Study of Education, 1972. Pp. 154-192.

Patterson, G. R., Cobb, J. A., and Ray, R. S. A social engineering technology for retraining the families of aggressive boys. In H. E. Adams and I. P. Unikel (Eds.), *Issues and trends in behavior therapy.* Springfield, Illinois: Charles C. Thomas, 1973.

Patterson, G. R. and Reid, J. B. Intervention for families of aggressive boys: A replication study. Submitted to *Behavior Research and Therapy,* 1972.

Pelz, D. C. and Andrews, F. M. Detecting causal priorities in panel study data. *American Sociological Review,* 1964, *29,* 836-848.

Porter, A. Analytic techniques appropriate to quasi-experiments, such as Head Start and Follow-Through. Paper presented at the meeting of the American Psychological Association, Honolulu, September 1972.

Redd, W. H. Generalization of adult's stimulus control of children's behavior. *Journal of Experimental Child Psychology,* 1970, *9,* 286-296.

Rossi, P. H. Observations of the organization of social research. In P. H. Rossi and W. Williams (Eds.), *Evaluating social programs: Theory, practice, and politics.* New York: Seminar Press, 1972.

Shine, L. C., II, and Bower, S. M. A one-way analysis of variance for single subject designs. *Educational and Psychological Measurement,* 1971, *31,* 105-113.

Sidman, M. *Tactics of scientific research: Evaluating experimental data in psychology.* New York: Basic Books, Inc., 1960.

Skindrud, K. Generalization of treatment effects from home to school settings. Unpublished manuscript, Oregon Research Institute, Eugene, 1972.

Wahler, R. G. Setting generality: Some specific and general effects of child behavior therapy. *Journal of Applied Behavior Analysis,* 1969, *2,* 239-246.

Walker, H. M. and Buckley, N. K. Programming generalization and maintenance of treatment effects across time and across settings. *Journal of Applied Behavior Analysis*, 1972, *5*, No. 3, 209-224.

Walker, H. M., Johnson, S., and Hops, H. Generalization and maintenance of classroom treatment effects. Center at Oregon for Research in the Behavioral Education of the Handicapped (CORBEH), Eugene, Oregon, *Report No. 11*, 1972.

Weiss, R. L. and Rein, M. The evaluation of broad-aim programs: A cautionary case and a moral. *Annals of the American Academy of Political and Social Science*, 1969, *385*.

Werts, C. E. and Linn, R. L. Problems with inferring treatment effects from repeated measures. *Educational and Psychological Measurement*, 1971, *31*, 857-866.

Williams, W. and Evans, J. W. The politics of evaluation: The case of Head Start. In P. H. Rossi and W. Williams (Eds.), *Evaluating social programs: Theory, practice, and politics.* New York: Seminar Press, 1972.

Zubin, J. Ecological vs. clinical fallacies in personality research. Paper presented as part of a Symposium, *Complementarity between the Idiographic and Nomothetic Methods in Clinical Psychology*, at the meeting of the American Psychological Association, Honolulu, September 1972.

Who Benefits from the Program? Criteria Selection[1]

2

Siegfried Hiebert

Introduction

Researchers may investigate the effects of therapeutic endeavors in the area of clinical psychology for a number of different reasons. One possible reason is to *gain understanding*, by the use of scientific procedure, of how human behavior can be changed. The research activity aimed at gaining such information is done within the framework of what Kiesler (1971) calls, "the science of behavior modification." The research done within this framework is aimed at providing answers to the question, "Which therapist behaviors produce what changes in which kinds of patients?" (Kiesler, 1971, p. 56). A second possible reason for investigating the effects of therapeutic endeavors is to *evaluate the effectiveness* of a treatment, or more correctly, the relative effectiveness of several treatments, in achieving one or more desirable goals.

In selecting dependent variables for any research investigating the effects of therapeutic endeavors it is important to take into account the aim or aims of the investigation. If the investigator wants to advance the scientific understanding of how human behavior can be changed, he can be expected to select dependent variables in terms of their scientific value. His selection may then be based on theoretical predictions and constructs. If, on the other hand, the investigator's aim (or one of his aims) is to *evaluate* a therapeutic endeavor, dependent variables will have to be selected to measure change in relation to some desired goal(s) of therapy. Unlike research which is aimed only at understanding, research aimed at evaluation requires that desirable goals of treatment be specified, because a treatment can be said to be effective (or ineffective) only in terms of the extent to which it achieves a desirable goal.

The requirement of specifying goals for treatment may present a problem for the researcher because not all of the individuals or groups interested in effective therapy will necessarily have the same goals for therapy. Krause (1969) lists four groups or publics all of which are

33

interested in the effects of therapy but whose goals for any particular case may differ. These four groups are: (1) the persons receiving the therapy (the patients), (2) the persons whose complaints will be remedied by the therapy (the clients), (3) the persons whose planning and material support is responsible for the provisions of the therapy (the sponsors) and (4) the persons who "perform" the therapy (the professionals). Sometimes a number of the categories may refer to the same person but in many cases they will refer to different groups—with different values and goals. The idea that different groups may often have different goals for therapy is supported by an empirical study reported by Polak (1970). Polak found that the levels of agreement between patients, relevant community members, and hospital staff about treatment goals for the 11 patients in his study were generally quite low.

If different individuals and groups hold different goals for treatment, investigators planning evaluative research should consider whose goals for treatment will be used as a basis for selecting dependent variables. In addition, they need to know what treatment goals are held by that individual or group, and then select dependent variables that will indicate change in relation to those goals.

This chapter will consider some of the relevant publics—how their goals for treatment might be discovered and some of the ways of measuring change in relation to some of the expected or known goals of these groups.

The Patient's Point of View

If a researcher wishes to evaluate a treatment endeavor in terms of each patient's own goals for himself, it will be necessary for him to find out what the patient's goals are and then to select dependent variables to measure change in relation to these goals.

While some patients may be unable or unwilling to communicate their goals to the researcher, many will be able and willing to do so. It seems likely that voluntary patients would be particularly able to state goals since they would probably not have volunteered if they had not been aware of something they wanted help with. As Kadushin (1969) says:

> No one just drops by his neighborhood psychia-
> trist to say hello. A special reason, called a
> "problem," is required. In fact, an applicant's

"ticket of admission" to psychotherapy is his
problem....(P. 89)

A possible initial step to finding out the patient's goals for his
own treatment is to ask him to state or indicate them in some manner.
There are at least three different procedures a researcher could use to
allow patients to indicate their goals or the problems they want help
with.

One procedure is simply asking the patient to list the problems
with which he wants help. Battle, Imber, Hoehn-Saric, Stone, Nash, and
Frank (1966), reported a series of studies exploring the practical usefulness of this method. The subjects, who were adults applying for treatment at an outpatient department at a psychiatric clinic, were simply
asked to list the problems with which they wanted help. One disadvantage of this method is that patients may not be able or willing to
immediately list on request all the problems with which they want
help. Two studies illustrating this problem are reported by Battle *et al.*
(1966). In both of these studies target complaints were obtained from
patients both before and after an intensive psychiatric evaluation interview, but in the second study each patient reported his complaints to a
different interviewer after rather than before the psychiatric evaluation.
In both of these studies, patients mentioned more problems during the
second interview. In the first study, there was a 28.5 percent increase in
target complaints; in the second study, 20 percent of the patients made
some important change in their target complaints.

A second possible procedure of finding out exactly what the
patient wants changed is to use a standardized interview. This method
has been used by Shapiro (1961b) in conjunction with his use of the
personal questionnaire. Shapiro suggests that the severest degree to
which each problem (he calls them symptoms) has been recently experienced be recorded in the patient's own words. During the interview the
patient can be helped, by means of questions, to think of and verbalize
important problems that might otherwise have been omitted in the list
of target complaints. The value of the interview procedure will depend,
in part, on the adequacy with which the questions cover the important
content areas. The structured interview suggested by Shapiro (1961b)
covers five categories he considers to be the important content areas:
affect, thinking, thought content, perception, and bodily sensations.
Another way of establishing categories would be to start with the problems stated by a large selection of patients and arranging and rearrang-
ing these until meaningful categories covering all the stated complaints
emerged. This procedure was used by Weiss and Schaie (1964) who

arrived at 35 separate categories. Although they did not use these categories as a basis for constructing questions for a structured interview, their categories could be used for that purpose.

A third possible way of finding out a patient's goals is to present him with a list of possible goals and ask him to indicate which ones represent the goals he has for his own treatment. Perhaps the main disadvantage of this procedure is that the list could not possibly include all the possible specific goals of patients.

After the patient has stated his goals, it may be necessary for the researcher to categorize some as inappropriate. Both Battle *et al.* (1966) and Shapiro (1961b) indicate that not all problems mentioned by the patient are appropriate goals for psychiatric treatment. Battle *et al.* (1966) reports:

> Patients often tended to give complaints which were not an appropriate goal for psychiatric treatment. For instance, one patient said 'I do not make enough money to buy a new house', and another patient stated, 'I would like to have my nose changed'. (P. 189)

Shapiro (1961b) may have encountered a similar problem because his manual includes the stipulation that the problem statements be checked by the patient's psychiatrist "to ensure the clinical relevance of the statements" (p. 10).

If therapy goals are stated in the patient's own words, it may be more likely that the patient understands the statements, but it certainly does not ensure that the researcher will understand. According to Mischel (1968), "Persons may present themselves and their objectives initially in terms of very diffuse, oversimplified, global trait-state labels" (p. 237). When such labels are used the patient's goal statements may allow for several interpretations. If, for example, a patient says he wants to "become less introverted," his statement could be interpreted in at least four ways. It could mean that the patient desires any one of the following:

1.   a highly generalized, total personality reorganization,
2.   a changed score on the introversion dimension of a personality inventory,

36

3. a change in the feelings he experiences in or toward certain social situations, or

4. a change in overt behavior in social situations.

When the patient's goal statements could have several different meanings the researcher can ask for examples and elaborations from the patient until he feels certain he understands the patient's viewpoint well enough to be able to measure the change in relation to the goal as perceived by the patient.

In many cases it may be useful for the researcher to check whether the measurement procedure he wishes to use has face validity as judged by the patient. Of course, face validity alone does not guarantee an adequate measurement procedure but it may ensure that change is in fact measured in terms of the goals *as perceived by the patient* rather than in terms of the patient's goal as *misinterpreted by the researcher.*

After the researcher knows what the patient's goals for treatment are he will have to select dependent variables to measure change in relation to these goals. This chapter will consider three general classes of patient goals and some of the measurement procedures that could be used to measure change in relation to these goals. The first kind of patient goal to be considered is a change in moods or experiences which cannot be directly observed by individuals other than the patient. The second kind of patient goals to be considered is a change in the opinions or subjective experiences of others. For example, a patient may want his spouse or employer to be more satisfied with him. A third kind of goal a patient might have is a change in a behavior or condition observable to others.

In cases where the patient desires changes in subjective phenomena, such as moods or covert responses, which are not observable by others, the measurement procedure will generally involve reports by the patient; but the method and frequency with which the patient records and reports his experiences can vary. The patient could report his subjective experiences orally, in writing, by means of rating scales, or by means of a personal questionnaire (Phillips, 1963; Shapiro, 1961a, 1961b). Changes in subjective experiences could be reported in terms of "global evaluations," or the level and/or frequency of a subjective experience could be recorded by the patient at regular intervals; e.g., hourly. Some subjective experiences, such as compulsive thoughts, could be recorded whenever they occur.

Unfortunately there is probably no adequate method of checking the validity of the patient's reports about his subjective experiences. If the patient expects or receives different consequences for different reports, the report content could be partly determined by the consequences rather than by the stimuli the patient is to report. Another problem is that if subjective experiences or covert responses are recorded by the patient when they occur (so they will not be forgotten) the recording behavior may change the phenomena being recorded (Kanfer, 1970).

In cases where the patient desires change in the subjective feelings or experiences of others the researcher can use the same measurement methods as he would use for measuring the patient's own subjective experiences.

For the third class of patient goals, changes in behavior or conditions observable to others, the possible selection of measurement procedures is much greater.

Many procedures suitable for the measurement of such observable criteria have been discussed in an excellent review article by Lichtenstein (1971). Among the methods mentioned by Lichtenstein are the following:

1. the self-monitoring of observable behavior, e.g., number of cigarettes smoked;
2. information about behavior obtained from informants such as friends or relatives, e.g., information about the drinking behavior of an alcoholic;
3. inferred performance measures, e.g., grade point average or income level;
4. direct observation of the patient in a standardized setting either inside or outside a laboratory, e.g., approach behavior to a feared object;
5. direct observation of the patient in natural settings, e.g., monitoring the frequency of aggressive behavior of a child in a classroom.

Additional methods that could be used to assess the attainment of desirable changes in observable behavior or conditions include the following:

1. physical measurements, e.g., the meaurement of weight;
2. medical tests, if the criterion is the cure of a psychosomatic disorder;
3. automated data collecting apparatus, e.g., a pedometer to record the amount of pacing by an agitated patient;
4. inferred improvement measures, e.g., discharge from hospital.

Clients Other Than the Patient

Often a treatment is performed, at least in part, in the interest of persons other than the patient. For example, if a child is brought to a guidance clinic, it may be the parents rather than the child who want the child to change. As Ullman and Krasner (1969, p. 21) suggest, the behavior of the individual may upset, annoy, anger, or strongly disturb somebody (e.g., employer, teacher, or parent) sufficiently that some action leading to treatment results (e.g., a policeman is called, seeing a psychiatrist is recommended, commitment proceedings are started). When the individuals with whom the person interacts outside of the clinic or hospital have a major say in whether or not he will be given treatment, then, unless the results or the therapeutic endeavor satisfies the criteria of these individuals, the patient may soon be back for more treatment.

If the researcher wishes to evaluate a treatment endeavor in terms of the goals of clients other than the patient, it will be necessary for him to find out what these goals are and then to select dependent variables to measure change in relation to these goals.

The three procedures mentioned above for finding out the patient's goals, namely, asking for a list of goals, a structured interview, and a check list of possible goals, could also be used to discover the goals of clients. (Unless stated otherwise, the word client will be used to refer only to individuals other than the patients whose complaints may be remedied by therapy.)

Who should be included in the categorization of "non-patient clients"? For example, if a child is brought to the clinic by his parents, the parents will be included in the category. But what about the child's school teacher, his grandmother, his leader at the Boy Scouts, his stealing companions, and the owner of the corner store? All of these individuals may have complaints about the boy and an interest in the treatment outcome, but their complaints and goals may vary widely. Conceivably it would be possible to find out the goals of each of these various individuals and evaluate the patient's treatment in relation to their various goals.

The same three classes of goals mentioned above as possible patient goals could also be stated by non-patient clients; and, therefore, the same measurement procedures could be used. First, the client might desire changes in the subjective experience of the patient. For example, Anderson, Polak, Grace, and Lee (1965) mention a patient's wife who wanted him "not to imagine things." Secondly, the client might desire a change in the subjective experience or opinion of a third party. For example, a patient's wife may want his employer to be satisfied with his (the patient's) work. And thirdly, the client may desire a change in some observable behavior (e.g., complaining) or condition (e.g., weight, release from hospital, steady employment, etc.).

Many of the treatment goals mentioned by non-patient clients may be motivated by a desire for the patient's own well-being. However, it has also been assumed by some that members of the patient's family are also interested in their own comfort and economic well-being and that psychiatric hospitals relieve the community of people who would otherwise be a burden. Gore, Jones, Taylor, and Ward (1967), for example, say that discharging patients by administrative decision without any substantial and favorable change having occurred will result in hardship to patients and their families. It seems reasonable to suggest that from the viewpoint of the patient's family and community one criterion for the success of therapeutic endeavors would be that the patient become less of a burden and more of an asset.

An empirical investigation of the hardships caused by psychiatric patients to their families was conducted by Hoenig and Hamilton (1967). They investigated the hardships caused by 273 patients who were treated in a program which emphasized treatment on an outpatient basis and thereby tried to avoid long-term hospitalization. Hoenig and Hamilton realized that the patient's family might not agree with the investigators about whether or not the patient had been a burden. Consequently they said there are two types of burden: objective burden and subjective burden. "Objective burden" was used to refer to the following:

1. a negative effect by the patient or his condition on the family's financial status, health, children, or routine (e.g., interference with social life, with children going to school, etc.);
2. abnormal behavior traits exhibited by the patient and considered by the investigators to constitute a burden to the family. Examples of such behaviors were being noisy or wandering at night; generally restless, noisy or talkative; unresponsive, etc.

"Subjective burden" referred to the extent to which the family subjectively felt they had been carrying a burden.

Hoenig and Hamilton obtained their data for estimating objective and subjective burden by interviewing the patient and a relative, if practicable, four years after the patient was initially seen at the hospital psychiatric units. Data for estimating the patient's burden on the family could also have been obtained by rating scales, questionnaires or inventories. The extent to which the patient is a burden on other members of the community could also be estimated, but it might be more difficult to obtain the relevant data.

Although adequate data was not available for many patients, it was found that at least 55.7 percent of the households had experienced a definite objective burden. For the 179 cases for whom information about both objective and subjective burden were available, the findings were as follows. When no objective burden was judged to be present no subjective burden was present. For those cases where an objective burden was judged to be present more than just occasionally, the reports of subjective burden were as follows: severe burden 19.6 percent, some burden 56.7 percent, and no burden 23.7 percent. Hoenig and Hamilton suggest that the percentage representing the number of families who report no subjective burden despite the presence of an objective burden could be regarded as "a kind of measure of family tolerance toward the psychiatric patient" (p. 625).

The conceptual distinction between objective and subjective burden is an important one, and both can provide useful information. However, as measured by Hoenig and Hamilton, only the subjective burden measures the problem from the family's viewpoint (the objective burden was determined in accord with conditions or behaviors considered *by the investigator* to constitute a burden to the family). In cases where an investigator is interested in evaluating treatment in terms of the family's aim to experience less hardship because of the patient, he will have to obtain reliable and valid methods of measuring the subjective burden experienced by the family. One possible approach would be to find out, perhaps by means of a questionnaire or check list, which behaviors performed by the patient or situations caused by the patient are considered by the family as "a burden." Changes in these behaviors or situations could then be used to assess changes in subjective burden.

Society's Point of View

A third category of individuals who will probably have an interest in the effects of therapeutic endeavors are the sponsors—the persons whose planning and material support is responsible for the provision of the endeavor. In Canada, psychological therapy not sponsored by the patient is usually sponsored by the various levels of government which in turn represent all of society.

If a researcher wished to find out society's goals in the area of "mental illness and health," he could attempt to elicit goal statements from the various governmental policy makers, examine current laws and available policy statements, examine government spending policy, or use a combination of these methods, e.g., question policy makers about their goals with regard to projects the government is supporting financially. An alternative approach to finding the goals of society would be to use a survey method to elicit goal statements from a random sample of the population.

Measurement procedures appropriate for the evaluation of therapeutic endeavors in relation to societal goals will vary with the various goals that might be discovered. In this paper three possible (probable) societal goals will be considered: (1) the desire for protection, (2) humanitarian goals related to the patient and his family, and (3) economic goals.

Society's concern with the protection of life and property is shown by the criminal code, the laws permitting a person thought to be dangerous to be committed to a psychiatric hospital against his will (Canadian Mental Health Association, 1964) and the law enforcement and penal systems. Therapeutic endeavors in the area of clinical psychology might involve evaluation or treatment of delinquents, remands, parolees, and persons not suspected of any crime but thought to be dangerous to self and others. In terms of society's goal of protection, such endeavors could be evaluated in terms of how much they decrease the danger to life and property. If the psychologist's endeavor, whether it involves diagnosis or therapy, results in a decreased danger to society, his endeavor can be considered to be beneficial.

What measuring procedures could be used to assess the level of danger to society? One possible method would be using police or court records to compute rates of various kinds of crimes committed by comparable groups of treated and non-treated subjects.

It is suggested that society's humanitarian concern includes a desire to minimize the hardships and sufferings experienced by the patients and their families. Since the rehabilitation of psychiatric patients may satisfy both society's economic and humanitarian goals, the existence of the latter is more clearly shown by the care provided to patients who will probably never be an economic asset to society, e.g., geriatric psychotic patients with no estate.

What dependent variables would be suitable for the evaluation of society's humanitarian goals? Subjective experiences of sufferings could be reported by patients and family members orally, in writing, via rating scales, or by means of personal questionnaire technique. Levels of hardship and suffering could also be estimated from data concerning events, conditions, or test scores that are known or thought to be predictors of subjective suffering. In evaluating the effect of a therapeutic endeavor on the suffering of patients or family, it is important to consider long-term as well as short-term suffering. For example, a treatment procedure in which a child who is engaged in behavior harmful to himself is given some electric shocks may temporarily increase the child's suffering but may also result in a decrease in long-term suffering.

When considering society's concern about the cost of therapeutic endeavors, it is helpful to distinguish between direct costs, indirect costs, and total cost. The distinction between direct costs and indirect costs as they relate to the field of mental illness is clearly stated by Fein (1958):

> By direct costs, we mean the actual dollar expenditures on mental illness. We include the amount spent by government (local, state, and federal), by philanthropic organizations, and by individuals on the care, cure and prevention of mental illness....
>
> The concept of indirect costs is a somewhat vague one. By *indirect* costs of mental illness, we mean the economic loss in dollars (or in work years) that society incurs because a part of society is suffering from mental illness. Thus, we are concerned with a 'what would have been' approach—e.g., what would the individuals suffering from mental illness have added and contributed to our economy if they had not been ill? (Pp. 10-11)

The term "total costs" is used to refer to direct costs plus indirect costs.

Direct costs, which are easier to estimate than indirect or total costs, are important for establishing the relative value of treatments even when non-economic goals, e.g., protection or decreased suffering, are being considered. Since governments always operate on limited budgets, society's humanitarian concern would demand that the available resources be used to the best advantage. Fox and Kuldau (1968) explain how alternative programs can be compared on a pair-wise basis to determine if some should be eliminated because there are alternative programs that cost no more and are more effective or cost less and are not less effective. The method suggested by Fox and Kuldau (1968) can be illustrated with the data presented by Marks, Sonoda, and Schalock (1968). Marks *et al.* compared the effects of reinforcement and relationship therapy on 22 chronic schizophrenic inpatients. The dependent measures used included ratings on social behavior, work competence, and conceptual and communication skills; and tests of mental efficiency, "associative looseness," work set, social skills and self-concept. It was found that both therapies improved functioning and that there were no systematic differences between them. However, it was also mentioned that the relationship therapy was much more expensive because more staff time was required. The application of the method outlined by Fox and Kuldau could result in discounting relationship therapy as an efficient alternative for the treatment of chronic schizophrenics.

In cases where a more effective treatment is also more expensive the cost information is still important. In view of limited financial resources it will have to be decided whether the increased benefits of the more effective treatment outweigh its additional cost. Fox and Kuldau suggest that the choice between these "efficient alternatives" should be made by a "decision maker," such as a political figure. While it is true that the choice between "efficient alternatives" requires a value judgment, the more information the "decision maker" is given the easier it will be for him to make wise choices. This information should include not only all known benefits of the various "efficient alternatives" but also what further information can and cannot be obtained, and at what cost.

Now let us consider how therapeutic endeavors could be evaluated strictly in terms of how much they advance society's economic goals. It is suggested that society's economic aim in regard to psychiatric problems is a minimization of total costs. But it must be remembered that, for society, the costs of mental illness include both the direct and indirect costs. Fein, in his book *Economics of Mental Illness*, writes:

> Once it is clear that we must deal with total cost, it is also clear that costs (in this sense) cannot be eliminated. Surely we all agree that direct costs can be decreased in a variety of ways, e.g., elimination of existent programs or even the obscuring of problems. This, however, does not eliminate total costs and may not (indeed, probably does not) reduce them. (1958), p. 128)

Therefore, comparing treatments in terms of how much they advance society's economic goals would require an estimate of how their effects would influence society's total cost for mental illness. In terms of this criterion, some treatments that would be recommended for young, highly trained individuals would not be recommended for the elderly or untrained.

The Therapist's Point of View

The fourth category of individuals, mentioned by Krause, having an interest in the effects of therapeutic endeavors is the professionals who "perform" the treatments. Therapist's goals for patients could be investigated in regard to individual patients or patients in general by means of the same procedures used to discover patient's goals, e.g., asking the therapist to list goals he considers desirable, using a standardized interview, or using a check list of goals.

It could be argued that therapists have an obligation to take seriously the goals of the other three groups mentioned previously. Krause (1969) describes this obligation when he says, "As responsible venders, they [the therapists] should subscribe to the values of their sponsors; as honest contractors, to the values of their clients; and, as humanitarians, to the values of their patients" (p. 525). However, we can expect that therapists will also have an opinion of their own about the nature of the problem and what the goals of therapy should be. Urban and Ford (1971) argue that a therapist's perception of the problem and his opinion about appropriate goals of therapy will be influenced by his conceptual or theoretical viewpoint. To illustrate how therapists' opinions about appropriate treatment goals may be expected to vary with their theoretical positions, it may be helpful to review a few of the currently accepted theoretical positions.

Eysenck (1960) points out the important distinction between those who view neurotic behaviors as symptoms of a more basic difficulty and those who view the neurotic behaviors as unadaptive conditioned responses. Mischel (1971) also emphasizes the distinction between theories that consider deviant behavior as a symptom and those that focus on the disturbed behaviors themselves. He says that, "Perhaps the most important theoretical issue [in current conceptions of psychological disorder] has to do with whether one views the individual's abnormal behavior merely as a *symptom* (sign) of an underlying disorder or focuses on the deviant *behavior* itself" (1971, p. 431).

Mischel (1971) describes three current theories that consider deviant (disturbed) behaviors to be symptoms of underlying disorders. The first is the biological view in which disturbed behaviors are considered to be symptoms of organic pathology.

The second and the third theories he mentions both consider the disturbed behaviors to be symptomatic, not of an underlying physical pathology, but of an underlying personality or psychological problem. One of these approaches regards personality in terms of traits and therefore describes the patient's problem in terms of mental disease or trait categories. Mischel says:

> ...the disease view is still widely used as an analogy of conceptualizing psychological problems even when no physical disease has been implicated. In this quasi-disease approach the person is seen as a 'patient' whose deviant behaviors are considered 'symptoms' of his underlying *mental* or emotional pathology comparable to a physical disease like influenza or cancer. The patient's disturbed behavior is not the focus of interest because it is seen as merely symptomatic of his underlying pathology.
>
> Note that the concept of deviant behaviors as symptoms of underlying mental pathology is similar to the trait theory assumption that behaviors are 'indicators' (signs) from which the person's underlying traits (mental pre-dispositions) have been inferred.... The mental disease view of abnormal personality thus is another example of the trait approach to behavior, in this instance, abnormal behavior. (P. 432)

The third theory mentioned by Mischel differs from the second in that the patient's basic psychological disorder is not thought of in terms of undesirable traits or mental diseases, but in terms of internal emotional conflicts and other psychodynamic processes. Mischel says:

> Guided by psychodynamic theory rather than by descriptive psychiatry, many clinicians doubt the value of formal psychiatric diagnosis and reject the concept of distinct mental

diseases. Instead, these clinicians, in accord with psychodynamic theory, seek to infer the person's unconscious conflicts, his defence structure, problems in his psychosexual development, and the symbolic meaning and functions of his behavior.

The psychodynamic approach to disordered personality thus does not search for underlying physical pathology; it does, however, maintain the disease-approach distinction between symptom and underlying problem. It views the individual's disturbed behavior as symptomatic (rather than of main interest in its own right) and searches for the possible causes of these symptoms by making inferences about his personality dynamics. (Pp. 435-436)

Mischel presents social behavior theory as being basically different from the previous three theories because it considers the disturbed behavior itself to be the basic problem.

For therapists who accept one of the three theories which consider the disturbed or deviant behavior to be symptoms of an underlying disorder the appropriate goal of treatment would be an improvement in the hypothesized underlying disorder. Some possible ways in which improvement in the hypothesized underlying disorders could be measured will now be considered.

If the basic problem is thought to be organic pathology, the aims of treatment will be to cure or arrest the disease process and/or reduce the unpleasant results of the disease process. The dependent variables for evaluating treatment would be selected along the same principles as when evaluating treatment for other physical illnesses. Malan, Bacal, Heath, and Balfour (1968) point out that these dependent variables will differ according to our ability to understand the pathology.

...three stages of a continuum can be recognized:
1.   We may be unable to make a diagnosis, in which case there is no question of understanding the pathology, and we can do no more than say that all known symptoms and signs must disappear.

2. We may be able to make a diagnosis of an illness whose pathology is little understood. Although this is unsatisfactory, it may enable us to make use of empirical knowledge (e.g., about the relation between various symptoms or signs and the ultimate outcome) for distinguishing between those signs of *apparent* recovery that are reliable indicators of *true* recovery and those that are not.

3. We may be able to make a diagnosis that represents a true *explanatory hypothesis* about the pathology of the illness. Here we are much more likely to be able to look beyond the mere disappearance of symptoms and signs for indication of true recovery. This is especially true in those illnesses that easily become "latent", such as pulmonary tuberculosis or syphilis, where there is no way of recognizing recovery without the aid of special methods of investigation such as X-rays or blood tests. (Malan *et al.*, 1968)

For most patients with disturbed behavior no explanatory organic pathology can be identified, and, therefore, treatment would have to be evaluated in terms of changes in the symptom(s) or symptom syndromes.

If the disturbed behavior is thought to be symptomatic of an underlying psychological problem, the aim of therapy would be to cure, or alleviate the effects of, the underlying psychological problem. The approach which views disturbed behavior as symptomatic of distinct mental diseases or deviant personality traits would presumably aim to cure these psychiatric diseases or reduce the strength of undesirable traits. However, diagnosis according to psychiatric disease categories is usually based on manifest symptoms and Malan *et al.* (1968) suggest that the psychiatric diagnosis, while relatively easy to make (they do not mention the problem of reliability and validity, c.f. Costello, 1970), does not carry with it much knowledge that would help us select appropriate outcome criteria.

The absence of knowledge about the assumed underlying problem may cause some researchers to focus on symptom change as the dependent variable. Battle, Imber, Hoehn-Saric, Stone, Nash, and Frank (1966), for example, say, "In the absence of adequate knowledge of the causes of psychiatric complaints, we assume that psychotherapy has removed the causes if the complaints are permanently relieved, and no new ones are substituted for them" (p. 185). Symptom change may be evaluated by selecting or constructing different instruments for different patients or by using standardized instruments thought to evaluate most of the important symptom areas. However, since changes in overt behaviors may result from changes in environment rather than changes in underlying dispositions, a decrease in disturbed behavior may not always be a valid indicator of changes in the hypothesized underlying problem. Often researchers use personality tests, which were designed to help diagnose psychological disorders or describe personality traits, as dependent measures to evaluate therapeutic endeavors. Although it has been argued (e.g., by Bereiter, 1962) that tests constructed to measure stable traits are not very sensitive to personality changes, such personality tests continue to be used. A review article by Bergin (1971) lists the *MMPI,* the *Eysenck Personality Inventory,* Cattel's *Objective-Analytic Personality Factor Battery* and *Sixteen Personality Factor Questionnaire* and the *TAT* and derivatives thereof among the frequently used outcome measures.

If traits or source traits (Cattel, 1965) are thought to determine overt behavior, personality tests could be thought to measure not symptoms but underlying causes of disturbed behavior.

According to the third theory Mischel mentions, which considers disturbed behavior to by symptomatic of psychodynamic (emotional) conflict, the goal of therapy should be the resolution of the conflict and not just change in the problematic behavior. Malan (1959) outlines a method of assessing change in the psychodynamic conflict. This method aims to differentiate between what he calls true solutions (a resolution of the neurotic conflict) and false solutions (a reduction of symptomatic behavior without a resolution of the neurotic conflict).

The method of evaluation suggested by Malan (1959) includes the following aspects:

1. Before therapy starts, the therapist should make a list of all the disturbances he can discover in the patient's life.
2. The therapist should formulate a psychodynamic hypothesis to explain these disturbances. This hypothesis should not be overly elaborate; it should be the minimum psychodynamic hypothesis required to explain the disturbances.

3. The therapist should state the criteria which, on the basis of his psychodynamic hypothesis, would indicate the occurrence of a "true resolution." These criteria should be described as far as possible before treatment starts.
4. Data needs to be gathered concerning changes in behavior relevant to the stated criteria. At present this data is usually based on information provided by the patient during an interview, but it could also be obtained by other methods.
5. The results are judged qualitatively in psychodynamic terms on the basis of the stated criteria. In making the qualitative judgements about the results, the behavior of the patient outside of therapy should be the main consideration, but changes in therapy and evidence from tests are not ignored.

The qualitative judgement about results allows one to estimate the amount of "resolution" that seems to have occurred, e.g., he presents cases to illustrate considerable, moderate, limited, and no resolution.

The use of Malan's (1959) procedure of assessing change in the psychodynamic conflict has been illustrated by a study of untreated neurotic patients conducted by Malan *et al.* (1968). They found that 51 percent of the patients were symptomatically "improved" or "recovered" but for between one-third and one-half of these the recovery was psychodynamically suspect.

It is obvious that the strategy a researcher would use to assess change in hypothesized underlying disorders may be quite different from the strategy he would use to assess improvement in terms of the goals advocated by patients, clients, or society. When the researcher wishes to evaluate therapeutic endeavors in terms of therapist goals, it will be necessary to measure change in relation to whatever the therapist's goals are. It needs to be stressed, however, that measurement procedures used to evaluate change in hypothesized underlying disorders cannot be assumed to indicate change in relation to the goals advocated by patients, clients, or society *unless they have been empirically shown to do so.*

For therapists who consider the deviant or disturbed behavior to be the basic problem rather than just a symptom of a more basic difficulty, the aim of therapy will be to remove the disturbed or disturbing behavior and perhaps increase the occurrence of more desirable behaviors. The dependent variables used to evaluate therapeutic endeavors will then have to be measures of these behaviors. As Lichtenstein (1971) says, "For the behaviorist, the behavior speaks for itself; it is viewed primarily as a sample and the major issue is the representativeness of the behavior sample for the goals of psychotherapy" (pp. 3-4).

Measurement methods congruent with this viewpoint include situational behavior sampling by trained observers, self-reports of behavior, and physiological measures (Mischel, 1971).

Since therapists accepting social behavior theory may be more likely than some other therapists to try to discover and accept the patient's or client's goals for therapy (Mischel, 1968) the same dependent variables acceptable to therapists of this theoretical viewpoint may often be acceptable to patients or clients as well. However, this will not always be the case. Since social behavior theorists advocate defining patients' problems in terms of publicly observable behaviors, they may sometimes neglect a patient's concern about change in subjective experiences.

Conclusion

To evaluate a therapeutic endeavor it is necessary to measure change in relation to the desired goals of therapy. Since different individuals and groups (publics) interested in effective therapy will often hold different goals for therapy, investigators planning evaluative research should consider whose goals for therapy will be used as a basis for selecting dependent variables. This paper has suggested some methods of discovering the goals of patients, clients, sponsors and therapists and has discussed some procedures for measuring change in relation to the expected or known goals of these groups.

The application of such a rational approach to the selection of dependent measures for the evaluation of therapeutic endeavors involves both costs and benefits. Among the costs are the necessity of investigating the goals of the public(s) for which the evaluation is intended and the necessity of developing or improving procedures to obtain valid measurements of change in relation to those goals. Among the benefits is the increased likelihood that the results of the evaluative research will be accepted and acted upon by the public(s) for which it is intended.

Footnotes

1. The author wishes to express appreciation to Dr. P. O. Davidson for his critical comments and suggestions on an earlier draft of this paper.

References

Anderson, M. L., Polak, P. R., Grace, D., and Lee, A. Treatment goals for patients from patients, their families, and staff. *Journal of the Fort Logan Mental Health Centre,* 1965, *3,* 101-115.

Battle, C. C., Imber, S. D., Hoehn-Saric, R., Stone, A. R., Nash, E. R., and Frank, J. D. Target complaints as criteria of improvement. *American Journal of Psychotherapy,* 1966, *20,* 184-192.

Bereiter, C. Using tests to measure change. *Personnel and Guidance Journal,* 1962, *41,* 6-11.

Bergin, A. E. The evaluation of therapeutic outcome. In A. E. Bergin, and S. L. Garfield (Eds.), *Handbook of psychotherapy and behavior change.* Toronto: John Wiley & Sons, 1971. Pp. 217-270.

Canadian Mental Health Association. *The law and mental disorder; One: Hospitals and patient care.* Toronto: Canadian Mental Health Association, 1964.

Cattel, R. B. *The scientific analysis of personality.* Baltimore: Penguin Books, 1965.

Costello, C. G. Classification and psychopathology. In C. G. Costello (Ed.), *Symptoms of psychopathology: A handbook.* Toronto: John Wiley and Sons, 1970.

Eysenck, H. J. Learning theory and behavior therapy. In H. J. Eysenck (Ed.), *Behavior therapy and the neuroses.* Toronto: Pergamon Press, 1960.

Fein, R. *Economics of mental illness.* New York: Basic Books, 1958.

Fox, P. D. and Kuldau, J. M. Expanding the framework for mental health program evaluation. *Archives of General Psychiatry,* 1968, *19,* 538-544.

Gore, C. P., Jones, K., Taylor, W., and Ward, B. Needs and beds: A regional consensus of psychiatric hospital patients. In H. Freeman and J. Farndale (Eds.), *New aspects of the mental health services.* Toronto: Pergamon Press, 1967. Pp. 409-418.

Hoenig, J. and Hamilton, M. W. The burden on the household in an extramural psychiatric services. In H. Freeman, and J. Farndale (Eds.), *New aspects of the mental health services.* Toronto: Pergamon Press, 1967. Pp. 612-635.

Kadushin, C. *Why people go to psychiatrists.* New York: Atherton Press, 1969.

Kanfer, F. H. Self-monitoring: Methodological limitations and clinical applications. *Journal of Consulting and Clinical Psychology,* 1970, *35,* 148-152.

Kiesler, D. J. Experimental designs in psychotherapy research. In A. E. Bergin, and S. L. Garfield (Eds.). *Handbook of psychotherapy and behavior change.* Toronto: John Wiley and Sons, 1971. Pp. 36-74.

Krause, M. S. Construct validity for the evaluation of therapy outcomes. *Journal of Abnormal Psychology,* 1969, *74,* 524-530.

Lichtenstein, E. Techniques for assessing outcomes of psychotherapy. In P. McReynolds (Ed.), *Advances in psychological assessment: Volume II.* Palo Alto, California: Science and Behavior Books, 1971.

Malan, D. H. On assessing the results of psychotherapy. *British Journal of Medical Psychology,* 1959, *32,* 86-105.

Malan, D. H., Bacal, H. A., Heath, E. S., and Balfour, F. H. G. A study of psychodynamic changes in untreated neurotic patients: Improvements that are questionable on dynamic criteria. *British Journal of Psychiatry,* 1968, *114,* 525-551.

Marks, J., Sonoda, B., and Schalock, R. Reinforcement versus relationship therapy for schizophrenics. *Journal of Abnormal Psychology*, 1968, *73*, 397-402.

Mischel, W. *Personality and assessment.* New York: John Wiley and Sons, 1968.

Mischel, W. *Introduction to personality.* Toronto: Holt, Rinehart and Winston, 1971.

Phillips, J. P. N. Scaling and personal questionnaires. *Nature*, 1963, *200*, 1347-1348.

Polak, P. Patterns of discord. *Archives of General Psychiatry*, 1970, *23*, 277-283.

Shapiro, M. B. A method of measuring psychological changes specific to the individual psychiatric patient. *British Journal of Medical Psychology*, 1961a, *34*, 151-155.

Shapiro, M. B. The personal questionnaire—An abbreviated manual. London: Institute of Psychiatry, 1961b.

Ullmann, L. P. and Krasner, L. *A psychological approach to abnormal behavior.* Englewood Cliffs, New Jersey: Prentice-Hall, Inc., 1969.

Urban, H. B. and Ford, D. H. Some historical and conceptual prospectives on psychotherapy and behavior change. In A. E. Bergin and S. L. Garfield (Eds.), *Handbook of psychotherapy and behavior change.* Toronto: John Wiley and Sons, 1971. Pp. 3-35.

Weiss, J. M. A. and Schaie, K. W. The psychiatric evaluation index. *American Journal of Psychotherapy*, 1964, *18*, 3-14.

Process Control: A Guide to Planning

Bryan C. Smith

Introduction

It is very popular today to be a part of programmatic thrusts in various fields. Coming from the field of Health Education I am exposed to an endless variety: poverty programs, drug abuse programs, venereal disease programs, immunization programs, air pollution abatement programs, and so on. Whenever program is mentioned, it conjures up the image of a carefully organized effort moving toward the achievement of an objective which society has agreed upon as worthy of being attained. The elimination of accidents, leukemia, and sickle cell anemia are worthy program objectives, but are they achievable? It's axiomatic that when there isn't a realistic objective, there is usually no meaningful program.

Once a program goal is established, a plan or blueprint is developed to accomplish it. It is built to conform to the parameters of time and cost restraints that it will take to achieve the performance level stated in the objective. Once the plan is established, the program moves into an operational phase by producing the activities that are expected to lead to the objective. As tasks are accomplished, there is a need to evaluate progress to see how well the actual work is going in terms of how it was planned to go. Evaluation in this sense is what management refers to as *process control* as opposed to concerns about the quality of the end product.

A System

The word *system* is the identification of all parts working to accomplish previously specified objectives. For example, our educational responsibility relates to a system, the school system, where many parts are working toward a specific outcome. This system requires a number of subsystems with an administrator who acts as system manager. It is his job to coordinate the efforts and see that the educational mission is met.

A system is not computers, television, projectors, or other hardware. These are only tools and techniques used as solutions to problems.

The system approach is the application of system analysis and system synthesis to determine the necessary activities to help assure that goals will be met. By using this approach, the best or alternate methods can be selected for solving problems. There is nothing in the system approach which stifles creativity or demands automation.

System Approach

The system approach carries no preconceived solution with it. It applies the tools and steps of logical problem solving to the problems of the organization. This allows the workers to design a system on the basis of meeting their needs with the best solutions in the most relevant and practical manner possible.

The fragmentation of the production of complex products into sequences of simple repetitive operations has created specialists to the point where many workers have become machine-like. Living for some has been postponed until after work hours. Creativity has been sacrificed for productivity, worthwhile living for an increased standard of living.

The system approach can be humanistic by allowing the individual to belong to a group in which responsibilities are assigned. The autonomy of each individual is determined and agreed upon by group action, usually improving his efficiency and effectiveness. Argyris (1970) found that in industrial settings a reduction in supervision helped workers to internalize their own need to become responsible. As the workers assumed greater responsibility and ownership over what they were doing, attitudes improved and so did the quality of their work.

In a system model, the traditional hierarchial ladder is de-emphasized (sometimes disappears), participation and worker initiative are maximized by creating organizational quality through group process. In seeking initiative, there must be an atmosphere in which there is freedom to make mistakes, to communicate, to make new approaches, to learn, to grow and to develop without someone in management anticipating failure. The growth and development of the individual are the primary goals. Hawthorne Effect occurs, improving the organization and the product it produces.

The following example may help to demonstrate this important point. Picture seven people, each located at his own station in front of a conveyor belt on an assembly line. Each will do his part in a machine-like manner to create an electronic instrument. *A* picks up a printed circuit, reaches over to a bin, picks up an output transformer and attaches it. He then places it back on the belt. It moves to *B* and *C* who both add three diodes. On to *D* and *E* who add transistors. *F* tests it and *G* mounts it to the instrument chasis and returns it to the belt. This process repeats itself for eight hours a day, five days a week.

What is being proposed here is that a group of people should be assigned to a group of operations and they should decide among themselves how to create the instrument. The series of operations accepted by the group should be visibly interrelated in the product. Each member has a responsibility and his contribution can be seen by each of the others. Their work takes on meaning in relation to other work, and they have a place with respect to the other people who share the same purpose.

Imagine 50 of these stations with seven people assigned to each. That amounts to 350 people. Assume also that there is a supervisor for every 20 people. The supervisor plus 20 people would constitute one group which would have to organize itself into three teams of seven persons each to turn out subassemblies.

They could form the teams in any way they wanted and divide up the tasks in any way they desired. Under these conditions, the work takes on new meaning, increased challenge and greater reward. Each person would have a clearly defined part in decisions relevant to his work. Thus, humanizing work occurs.

This concept can be applied to research, education, and community service. Draw your own analogies with these examples: one educator teaches five classes of fourth-grade science for five separate 50-minute periods each day. What is on the conveyor belt? Research projects which can be broken into six components but yield only one finished project. What is on the conveyor belt? Suppose an agency has an annual report of seven chapters, each written by a different person. What is on the conveyor belt?

System Analysis

Before starting this type of restructuring it is important that a *Need Assessment* be conducted to determine the need for action. In this phase, an attempt is made to survey needs, placing priorities on each so the most urgent can be identified. A need can be defined as a discrepancy between what we have and what we require. Much of what is done in a bureaucracy is based upon needs which no longer exist. Much of the action is not responsive to the current needs of the people served.

Once the needs have been assessed and the top priority need has been identified, then the action to be taken must be found. Many organizations start off with solutions and find problems which fit them. Team teaching and individualized instruction are solutions used in education. But what are the problems for which these may or may not be valid or efficient?

A clear definition of purpose known as a *Mission Analysis* should be agreed upon. It points out exactly what has to be done, identifies the performance requirements and constraints and sets the limits or ground rules under which people must operate. A *Mission Profile* which lists all of the functions which have to be accomplished to perform, meet, or reduce the need can be drawn up. This profile shows the order and sequence of the required functions.

What has emerged is a preliminary management plan. Preliminary because all the functions listed in the mission profile need to be analyzed into constituent sub-functions so that *what* must be done to get each function can be identified. This analysis of function is appropriately termed a *Functional Analysis* and usually takes the form of a flow block diagram.

Sometimes it is valuable to break these functions down into smaller units of performance known as tasks in a process identified as *Task Analysis.*

In summary, *System Analysis* is the process of breaking things down. It is expressed as the requirements and factors needed to perform the mission. It provides management with the input of all of what is involved in solving the problem. In essence, it is simulating the problem solution on paper, brainstorming, and studying to see if it is feasible before implementation. This approach creates a communication tool and a communication referent while helping to guide the organization in the steps of logical problem solving.

The payoff of simulation comes in the form of revision. The system approach model has a *Closed Loop* built into it. A closed loop means that there is a constant feedback on how all the elements are performing. These data are used to upgrade and improve the system. In revision, the performance data are used to improve what went on before. Thus, the members of the organization are learning from experience by evaluating performance against measurable objectives and using the resulting data to revise the system.

Network Based Systems

The two most popular network-based management systems are the Program Evaluation and Review Technique (*PERT*) and the Critical Path Method (CPM). While each of these has some unique characteristics, they have enough similarities that both can be discussed under the general concept of *network techniques.*

The implementation of a network based system for a program or project can be subdivided into: *planning* and *control*. Operationally, they are interdependent and go on concurrently.

The first step in planning is to break down the work in order to achieve program objectives. This process known as establishing a *Work Breakdown Structure* is a top-down activity. The primary objectives at the top are broken down into successively smaller units until a point is reached at which there is no value in breaking down the tasks any further. The final unit is a *Work Package.* It is at this point that the work breakdown process and the mission profile derived from systems analysis become integrated. Once the analysis program has been carried through the task analysis stage, the work breakdown structure required for network planning should be well established.

The network is a graphical representation of a plan which shows the logical sequence and interdependency of work from beginning to completion. Individual tasks to be accomplished which consume time are called *activities*. They are represented on the network by a straight line with flow moving from left to right. *Events* are found at the start and completion of every activity. These are milestones which do not consume time. They are represented on the network by a circle in which there is an identifying code number.

The network serves many functions but the most important are: (a) its value to work groups and administration as a communication tool, (b) a graphical representation of the program plan, and (c) a basis for supervisory and managerial control.

A time frame needs to be established for these functions to be performed. Three time estimates (minimum, best and maximum) are secured from the work group which owns the work package contained in each activity. These estimates are made assuming resources are planned or available in the five-day work week. Three estimates are used to help deal with the uncertainty problem which characterizes much developmental work. An average time estimate is obtained by the

Figure 1   Simple Network

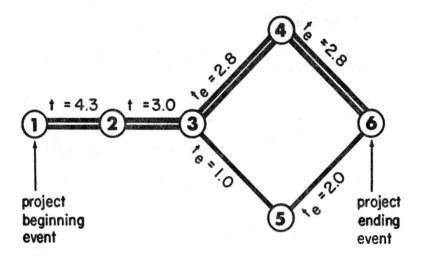

Critical path = 1-2-3-4-6
= 1 2.9 work weeks
or 64 ½ days

application of the following formula:

$$t_e = \frac{a + 4m + b}{6}$$

in which a is minimum time; b is maximum time; and m is the best time estimate. The uncertainty of the estimate is expressed by the variance $= \frac{b-a}{6}$ for the activity. If the uncertainty is small, the variance will also be small.

After the average time estimate (t_e) is secured for each activity they are summed along every activity path. The one set of activities which is the most time consuming is identified as the *Critical Path*. It is critical because it determines the earliest completion time from the beginning event to the ending event of the project. Along the other pathways there will be a certain amount of slack time. Slack is the difference between the earliest time an event can take place and the longest allowable time it can occur without jeopardizing the project completion.

Figure 2 The Network is rewritten to reduce the time on the critical path.

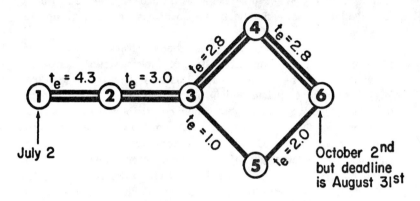

Critical path = 12.9 work weeks

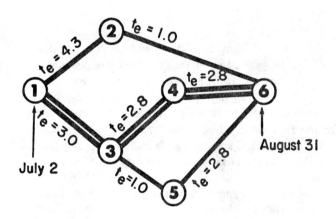

Critical path = 1-3-4-6
= 8.6 work weeks
or 43 days

Once the time frame is established, schedule dates are set for start and finish of work. Often one or both of these are fixed, thereby creating a deadline. The amount of time it takes to move along the critical path will determine how realistic the time estimates are. If the deadline cannot be met then the time estimates must be recalculated. Usually recalculating those with the greatest variance can tighten up the schedule.

Once the schedule has been established and agreed upon, work on the project can begin. The second stage of implementation, control, is initiated. Periodic reports of the actual status of the program schedules regarding work completed and in progress are presented to management by the work groups. Reports should contain only the most serious problems, i.e., deviation of performance from the work package. Solutions by management may require additional resources, redefining or eliminating tasks, or paralleling activities which were originally in linear order. Management action in the form of group decision-making can revise or make changes in the network. Work continues until the next reporting period or until the final event is completed.

Conclusion

The employment of systems analysis and synthesis procedures offers a challenge and an opportunity to improve planning efforts. These techniques force organizations to face up to the question of what exactly it is they want from people and how it can be harmoniously accomplished. The specification of the objective and its analysis help to identify the functions and tasks required to reach the goal. They are derived in a highly logical and visible manner.

Once the analysis is made, the operations necessary to accomplish the objectives have to be initiated and carried out. This requires a selection and employment of a management system, assuming that the plan is accomplished in a humanistic way and within the time/cost/performance constraints imposed. Group processing should prevail and process control should be continuous. The highly successful network-based systems provide a viable means of meeting this end. They allow simulation and revision. Evaluation is ongoing. Staff time can be allocated rationally, budgets estimated more precisely, bottlenecks can be spotted and eliminated, and most importantly objectives can be met.

References

Archibald, R. D. and Villoria, R. L. *Network-based management systems.* New York: John Wiley and Sons, 1967.

Argyris, C. *Integrating the individual and the organization.* Homewood, Illinois: Dorsey Press, 1970.

Boulanger, D. G. Program evaluation and review technique. *Advanced Management,* 1961, 16-23.

Cook, D. L. PERT: Applications in education. Cooperative Research Monograph No. 17, U. S. Office of Education, 1966.

Cook, D. L. *Better project planning through system analysis and management techniques.* Educational Research Management Center. College of Education, The Ohio State University, 1967.

Granger, C. H. The hierarchy of objectives. *The Harvard Business Review,* 1964, *42,* 63-74.

Head, R. Management information systems: A critical appraisal. *Datamation,* 1967, 22-27.

Paige, H. How to plan and control with PERT. *The Harvard Business Review,* 1963, *41,* 87-95.

Smith, B. C. Ongoing program education. In P. C. Browning (Ed.), *Evaluation of short term training in rehabilitation.* University of Oregon Press, 1970.

Considerations in the Implementation of Program Evaluations[1]

4

Aldred H. Neufeldt[2]

Across North America it has become quite fashionable to talk about the *need* for program evaluation. Indeed "program evaluation" has become an ostensible objective, if not reality, of program planners and implementers in health settings from general medicine through psychiatry, in educational settings from elementary school through university, in welfare settings, manpower training and placement settings, etc., etc., etc. Virtually every sphere of government activity today, along with many programs in the private domain, give evidence of this drive toward total evaluation of programs. In large part this drive is spurred by the anticipation of tremendous advantages (usually fiscal, though the altruist might anticipate social advantage as well) which might accrue as sound information is fed back into the planning, implementation and evaluation cycle. Yet, it has been the conclusion of a sizeable number of observers that despite all the rhetoric about the desirability of conducting "program evaluations," no substantial improvements have been made in the introduction of program evaluations. Decisions with respect to changes in program direction today would seem to be based on scant more knowledge of program efficacy than those made a decade ago.

Despite the apparent problem of implementing program evaluations, interest continues to grow at least on an intellectual level. Of interest to an operations researcher such as this observer, is the apparent fact that the enthusiasm for "program evaluation" is not limited to any one sphere of the human service field, or to a single professional group. The Fifth Banff International Conference on Behavior Modification illustrated this observation in that the participants ranged from the psychologist concerned with the effectiveness of a very specific interventive technique on a single "subject" (N = 1 research) to the economist concerned with relative effectiveness and efficiency of large-scale program changes (N = great research). All participated in a conference on "behavior modification" for the purpose of dealing with "program evaluation." However, it also was apparent that the definition of what, in fact, the term "program evaluation" means tended to vary considerably from individual to individual.

Thus, it would seem that we have two inter-related problems: that of overcoming resistances and problems related to introducing program evaluations so that decision-making can be made on a more knowledgeable basis; and, that of eliminating much of the "noise" with respect to the definition of program evaluation. The primary purpose of this chapter is to deal with the former, the underlying problems seeming to be more intransigent than the latter. Indeed, viewed from a systems perspective the differences between the various kinds of approaches are not as great as they might seem. The "N = 1 researcher" can be viewed as an evaluator of *micro-systems,* the "N = great researcher" as an evaluator of *macro-systems.* While the specification of problems to be dealt with and consequent evaluation techniques will differ from system level to system level (cf. Katz and Kahn, 1966; Miller, 1971), the fundamental factors effecting the success and failures of program evaluations tend to remain reasonably constant.

The purpose of this chapter, then, is to present some of the underlying commonalities of problems that exist in the implementation of "program evaluations," whatever the frame-of-reference of the program evaluator. In particular, a distinction will be made between what might be termed *instrumental* as opposed to *expressive elements* of evaluation. Within these an overview of technological as distinct from *value aspects* of evaluation will be made.

Problem Sources

To help sharpen the focus on the nature of the dimensions we are dealing with, two examples of evaluative programs are sketched briefly for the purpose of highlighting the kinds of problems needing to be dealt with in implementing program evaluations.

Example 1

A new psychiatric center was being planned for a region of our province previously served only by a small out-patient clinic and by distant inpatient psychiatric facilities. The planning of this center offered the opportunity of conducting a before-and-after study of the effect of opening such a center on a previously grossly under-serviced region (Neufeldt, 1971; Neufeldt, Berrien and Smith, 1972). The evaluation involved an appropriate quasi-experimental design, and the use of a somewhat innovative definition of concepts such as "subject" and "treatment conditions." Given the availability of an invaluable data source in the form of a case and event-monitoring record system (Neufeldt, 1969), we were able to introduce a program evaluation schema with a minimum of fuss, and with reasonable success.

An inherent problem of this project, however, was that of determining appropriate criterion variables to evaluate the program. How do you measure program effectiveness? Indeed, how do you measure efficiency? In the ultimate sense, efficacy would have to be determined in terms of treatment effectiveness on individual patients. Yet, the research literature is replete with unsuccessful attempts at finding a broadly accepted definition of effective outcomes. Given that there was some need for haste to get our project off the ground (program evaluators almost always seem to become aware of changes somewhat late), and having concluded that we would not be able to improve on the previously unsuccessful attempts without some major input, we simply adopted the rationale used by Ullman (1967), limiting our criterion variables to those most characteristic of system functioning; i.e., admissions and discharges to inpatient care, the amount of outpatient contact, etc.

Example 2

Over the years, beginning with the work of Ayllon (1962), we have had various experiences with introducing behavior modification programs. The introduction of these inevitably seems to give rise to a series of problems. The most recent such "behavior-mod" program was introduced in one of our major mental health settings; indeed, it still is in the process of being introduced!

Approximately one year ago, psychologists at the center decided that a behavior modification scheme could profitably be introduced to assist in the rehabilitation of chronically hospitalized patients. Since such approaches have been fairly successful in the past, and since the methodology, definition of relevant variables, etc. is reasonably clear-cut, this seemed to be a relatively straight-forward task. A fair amount of background work was conducted, including the gaining of various types of approval from medical and non-medical staff. Commencing in the fall, concrete planning activities were undertaken, this including an in-service education program on the nature of behavior modification programs. It looked as if "all systems were go." Then, just as subjects were about to be selected for admission into the program, resistances started to appear. Some of the medical staff commenced blocking the introduction of the behavior-modification program. The immediate reason for blocking was perfectly legitimate. An elementary mistake had been made by the psychologists. They had failed to clear the process of selecting candidates for the program with medical officers in charge on the assumption that earlier permissions were sufficient. Nevertheless, this failure to seek the desired final approvals was seized upon as the rationale for stopping a complete program that had been long in the planning. While it may yet get underway, the program currently is at a standstill.

Dimensions of Implementing Program Evaluations

These two examples outline the bare bones of the problem sources we face in implementing program evaluations. On the one hand, we have those that might be called "technological" and "instrumental" in nature— problems of methodology and measurement often held to be the essence of science; the "science of science." On the other hand, we have those which are very much of a human sort—expressive components of human interaction, essentially problems in the "art of science." In terms of the relative sophistication of the program evaluations, the second example given had the methodological aspects well taken care of. Sound methodologies were available, as were appropriate and relatively clear criterion variables. The problem most definitely lay in the expressive, or human dimensions—the "art" of program implementation. This situation was reversed in the first example. No great problems were encountered from the human side; however, considerable problems of a technological-instrumental nature posed themselves—specifically, the definition of criterion variables.

Conclusion number one, then, is that there are two important "Elements" to be considered in undertaking program evaluations— "instrumental" and "expressive." While all of us have some awareness of this dimension, a large portion of would-be researchers fail to distinguish clearly between the two. The facts of the matter are that most researchers tend to consider only those Elements of an "instrumental" nature in planning their research, and give relatively little attention to the "expressive" side of things.

A second conclusion that might be derived relates to the distinction between "technological" and "value" aspects of research. The key word, when we talk about program evaluation, is not so much the word "program" as the word "evaluation." Dictionaries variously define this word as "to place a value on," "find the amount of," or "to examine and judge." Throughout, the cue is the word *value*. Using this definition, published usages of the word evaluation, as well as the actual practices, can be divided into those in which "value" means: (a) a number-value; or (b) a value-value. The former indicates some empirical worth, a number that has some absolute (or at least relative) worth. The latter implies a more subjective judgement—that of preciousness, excellence, worth or desirability (cf. Weckworth, 1969). There is a tendency for researchers to consider the *instrumental* Elements of evaluation to involve only problems of a *technological* nature, and for them to dismiss the *expressive* problems as simply differences in *value* systems. Yet, if we examine the way in which any Element (in the sense described above) is selected for number-value measurement, it becomes apparent that such selection arises from the selector's priorities. That is, the number-value, in essence, is the outcome of a decision involving someone's value-value system. At the same time very real technologies might be applied to overcoming problems of an *expressive* nature.

Implications for Implementing Program Evaluations

The two dimensions here described in terms of evaluation Elements (Instrumental and Expressive), and Aspects (Technological and Value), might be cross-classified as in **Figure 1**. The remainder of this chapter will offer a number of observations of the outcomes and implications derived therefrom.

Instrumental Elements

Instrumental elements typically are those to which greatest attention is given in academic training. For instance, courses in research design and statistics long have been a central part of graduate training in all of the social sciences. Despite this heavy emphasis, graduates in the past have shown relatively little transfer of the learned skills from laboratory to practical settings. In part at least this is a function of the fact that most classes in methodology stereotypically have confined themselves, and the world of "science," to those mini-problems that could be dealt with

Figure 1　　"Element" and "Aspect" Dimensions of
Program Evaluations

	Elements	
	Instrumental	Expressive
Technological	Range of: —research designs; —operationally defined independent and dependent variables; —statistical techniques of analysis.	Proven methods and techniques of: —introducing evaluation schema; —data collection; and —ensuring future co-operation.
Value	Considerations that lead to: —choice of given criterion variables; —numbering systems chosen; —type of analyses conducted.	Considerations leading to: —decision to conduct program evaluation; —type of evaluation undertaken; —actions taken following evaluation.

A
S
P
E
C
T
S

in a neat way in laboratory sessions using introductory-psychology students or the pervasive white rodent. Obviously, the realm of program evaluation is not for those faculty and students whose personal dispositions allow for little deviation from equal-N, multivariate designs. Problems to be tackled within the program-evaluation sphere simply cannot always be fitted within those constraints. Since a sizeable amount of literature has been published dealing with instrumental Elements of research, the comments that follow simply are summative in nature.

Value Aspects. In a previous section reference has been made to the fact that personal value systems come into play in the very selection of problems for research, methodologies, criterion variables, and so on. It should be recognized, however, that even more fundamental value-related problems exist which tend to increase the difficulty of conducting evaluations.

The most commonly accepted operational definition of evaluation is: to compare accomplishment with stated objectives. This is a relatively straightforward definition, in that it is goal-oriented. If the operational definition is so simple, why then is evaluation so difficult? Some clue can be found if we look at the operational definition in some detail. In it, five assumptions are made:

(a) that the objectives are stated;
(b) in measurable terms;
(c) that accomplishments or outcomes are documentable;
(d) in the same measurable terms as the objectives; and
(e) that one knows what the word "compare" means—that is, we know what needs to be done both in the process of implementing and conducting the evaluation, as well as with the final observations.

Each one of these assumptions contains the seeds of difficulty. First, objectives very often are not stated. Too often no differentiation is made between the term "goal" as opposed to the term "objectives." Indeed, there seems to be a not inconsiderable degree of confusion; hence, little distinction between objectives and goals. Our goal may be to assess the efficacy of some new form of therapeutic intervention. However, this statement is insufficient in that it does not determine those intermediate states (objectives) that will allow for the goal to be reached. The goal of the Wright brothers was to fly. To attain that goal, a wide range of intermediate objectives had to be reached—the appropriate shape of wings to provide loft, the attainment of balance and control, the shape of propellers for proper power ratios, etc. While we may hear of purposes, of goals, of statements extolling motherhood and country, it regretfully is still a rare commodity to determine objectives. This simple step, in and of itself, would vastly increase both qualitative and quantitative successes in program evaluation.

Even if objectives are stated, many are not independent. In fact, they often are in conflict with one another and rarely would their summation add to the ultimate program goals. For example, the goal of our mental hospital theoretically has been to cure people. Yet, many of the objectives inherent to operating the institution— maintain patient and staff stability, encourage efficient operations, etc.—have been inimical to other objectives more in concert with the goal.

In addition, the "state of the art" of evaluation is such that we have not developed the means of measuring most of our value system objectives. Unfortunately, there seems to be an inverse relationship between what is really important in life and what is easily measurable. Thus our measurement ineptness reflects both our ignorance and our errors.

Even if objectives can be stated, and appropriate measures made, very frequently there is difficulty in documenting accomplishment. In the even more rare event that accomplishment can be documented, commonly nobody knows what to do with it! Or, if in fact someone knows, the comparison will still depend entirely on the judgement of whoever has the right to decide what to do with it. And so we start and conclude with "values"—values in terms of the choice of goals and objectives; choice of measurements and ultimately choice of actions to be taken if and when outcomes are determined.

Technological Aspects. A plethora of books have been published dealing with the technology of implementing instrumental research. In particular, much has been written about the logic of the scientific method, and the technologies associated with experimental designs. At the same time, many researchers (particularly a large number of psychologists) have missed the fact that the "scientific method" applies to program evaluation in general, not only to specific forms of research endeavours. The "true" experimental design, with all variables except the critical independent variable controlled for, may be ideal; however, it is not the only legitimate approach to evaluation. The "scientific method" is not limited to this, or any other method. Quasi-experimental designs, while being vulnerable to certain internal threats (cf. Campbell and Stanley, 1966) and external threats (cf. Bracht and Glass, 1968) to validity, often are much more practicable and of greater utility. Indeed our increase in knowledge has not come about so much from use of the so-called "true" experimental design as from the use of even more "primitive" methods of enquiry, all of which should be considered fair game in the conduct of evaluations.

On the other hand, many seemingly intractable problems in fact could legitimately be examined by means of "true" experimental and "quasi"-experimental designs. What often has prevented this from happening has been a misperception or, at least, a limited perception of what a "subject" is (to use psychological jargon), and, therefore, what consequent "behaviors" legitimately are available for observation. In many settings the "subject," as traditionally defined, is most appropriate as the single unit of observation. That is, we observe the behaviors of individual organisms. However, this unit of observation can also be altered to be some combined behavior of a group of organisms—as, for instance, in the circumstance where a new teaching technique is tried on a number of classrooms, there being equivalent classrooms receiving some control condition. In such a situation, entire classrooms can be treated as "subjects," or the units of observation. Indeed, as has been discussed in some detail elsewhere (Neufeldt, Berrien and Smith, 1972), the unit of observation might be yet larger. Obviously, as the unit of observation changes, so do the possibilities of types of "behaviors" that might be observed.

Expressive Elements

While there exists a vast array of problems to be solved on the Instrumental side of the research coin, one at least is comforted by the feeling that they are potentially solvable. Typically, much less comfort is felt with respect to those problems essentially involving the perversity of our fellow man. Yet, this dimension too is potentially solvable. Certainly there are a number of program evaluators (alas, all too few) who have achieved a creditable track record at implementing program evaluations. Thus, there must be a certain technological aspect, as well as value aspect, to such successful implementations.

Value Aspects. Road blocks, run-arounds and sabotage are not an uncommon part of the diet of program evaluators. In trying to determine the "Why's" of this fare, it would seem that at least three value-laden aspects contribute—*credibility* of the concept of program evaluation; *confidence* (or, lack of it) in program evaluators, and the *consequences* associated with participating. Each will be considered in turn.

While endorsements of evaluation are given about as readily as a kind word for apple pie, the endorsers are not always so ready to open themselves to having their own programs evaluated. Thus, while program evaluations publicly are touted, in private they lack in credibility. As observed elsewhere, "no one enjoys being policed; moreover, most of us exhibit greater energy in contemplating the future than in mulling over the past. Thus, when evaluation is looked upon as little more than a search for past failures, it is not surprising that little enthusiasm is generated, especially among those whose wrists may get slapped in the process" (Reinke, 1972, p. 44). Such sceptical views of program evaluation and program evaluators are all too common. The air of the "efficiency expert" is still around. Regretfully, these attitudes are prevalent among administrators and planners, as well as among front-line workers.

In large part this would seem to be the result of a failure to understand two important roles that evaluation offers to the administrative planner: (1) to provide a means for continuing self-study, and (2) to offer periodic external review. Thus, "when the notion of continuing self-study is recognized to connote current and private surveillance designed to keep an individual or an agency in line with objectives—or perhaps to help explain why this is impossible to do—then the merits of evaluation begin to be appreciated. Further, when the review of accomplishments is designed for future improvement as well as past assessment, evaluation is likely to become still more palatable" (Reinke, 1972, p. 44). Reinke (1972) and others suggest that evaluation procedures become more credible, not only to the extent that the instrumental tools to be employed enjoy reasonable validity and reliability (perhaps the single most frequent disclaimer used against implementation of evaluations), but also as the role of evaluation is perceived to alter from simply examining what *has been* done, to what *can be* done." The ultimate goal and *raison d' etre,* then, is of utmost importance in establishing the credibility of program evaluations.

The second critical concern that the evaluator needs to give some thought to is the degree of confidence evaluatees have in him. Reference already has been made to the fact that a certain element of "fear" is aroused in evaluatees at the very mention of an evaluation. In part, at least, such lack of confidence is justified. Too often, in fact, evaluatees are instructed to participate in a so-called evaluation, only to find that the outcomes of the study either are nonsensical (hence, the participation a waste of time) or are used against them. In game-theory terms, evaluation has been experienced as a zero-sum game similar to others in which he was *told* to play, but where he had no chance to win. Obviously, some very real value decisions have to be made if an element of confidence or "trust" is to be established. In particular, careful thought has to be given to the type of contract that is established between evaluator and evaluatee.

Finally, value-decisions have to be made with respect to what actions will be undertaken consequent to completion of the evaluation, these decisions preferably being made prior to implementing the program evaluations. It is safe to say that planning without implementation leads to nothing, and that implementation without evaluation could conceivably make matters even worse. However, the degree to which evaluation findings are translated into revised plans and thence to improved performance is, at least in part, as much the responsibility of the evaluator, as it is of a program planner or implementer. In the process of achieving such a translation, the very real political implications of evaluation and planning, as described by Campbell (1969) and Hall (1972), will need to be considered. A failure to do so leads to an emasculated form of evaluation, usually too late in conception and too light on consequence.

Technological Aspects. Since the Expressive Element is so central to the implementation and success of program evaluations, consideration will be given to ways (technologies) of meeting the value-related concerns parallel to the order in which they were raised in the previous section.

1. Credibility. Several tactics are of considerable importance to establishing credibility in the eyes of planners and administrators. The chief of these is that the ultimate goals, as well as the intermediate objectives, need to relate directly to interests of the program leaders. Without such a direct and strong correlation, hopes of conducting an evaluation on a program of any significant degree of appropriateness or adequacy[3] are minimal. Once the interests of administrators have been determined, there is some utility in demonstrating that evaluators do indeed have and can fulfill an important service role to the administrators. In part this can be achieved through such devices as measuring achievement through existing standards and targets; however, additional attention should be given to whether original goals and objectives in fact were appropriate, whether resource development (facilities, manpower, etc.) is actually moving in the direction most suited to given conditions, whether the data gathering system is producing useful information, etc. Thus, credibility will be achieved if:

(a) Evaluation is forward looking; and
(b) Evaluation exhibits concern for the *relationship between ends and means.*

2. Confidence. Confidence, or "trust," is somewhat of an ephemeral property that constantly needs bolstering in program leaders, as well as rank-and-file workers, for many of the reasons already cited. Given the fears that workers have of "zero-sum games," consideration should be given to renegotiating from an apparent zero-sum game to one that is non-zero-sum. That is, evaluatee as well as evaluator should legitimately be able to expect some positive and real profits or pay-offs (at least, no losses) to arise out of participation. In a recent, rather splendid article, Weinstein (1972) has critically examined the experimental games literature, as well as literature on source credibility in communication and research into inter-personal trust and friendship, distilling a number of findings on ways and means of establishing and maintaining such confidences. The technologies so determined, might be summarized as follows:

(a) From experimental-games research it has been found that co-operation between various parties, in games involving mixed motives (as in non-zero-sum games), improves when: each player is able to find a sensible pattern in the behavior of the other—that is, that such responses of behaviors are predictable, and that they can be reliably anticipated; maximum co-operation only occurs when there are evident positive returns for all parties (mutual trust does not tend to develop in situations where pay-offs are so arranged that one party is strongly tempted to defect—to act so as to harm the other); contracts are established to maintain a stable, co-operative degree of dependence (indeed, one might assume that contract negotiation process itself will help to build trust) and provide the necessary history of co-operation for subsequent evaluation to be successful; and, communications between players are frequent, as well as open.

These findings lead to the following guidelines for evaluation to succeed:

    i.   Spell out the rules of the game—in particular, whether the "game" is zero-sum or non-zero-sum with respect to the evaluatee.[4]

    ii.   Negotiate a "contract," in Pratt's (1966) terms, in which the needs of both evaluator and evaluatee are clearly outlined, and in which the rules of action are summarized, preferably in written form. Allow for flexibility in revision of the contract.

    iii.   Use obviously confidential mechanisms for collecting data, since such a visible apparency has a reassuring effect on evaluatees that data will not be used against them individually.

iv. Provide an adequate amount of feedback on performance to evaluatees, usually presenting grouped data.

v. Establish the "humanness" of the evaluator through face-to-face discussions, using written communications for follow-up purposes only.

vi. Provide adequate opportunity for communication so that evaluatees are kept informed of every phase of the evaluation process.

vii. Make certain that there has been a history of cooperation before entering a high-threat area, such as feedback of performance, making certain that this perception is held by evaluatees as well as evaluators.

(b) Work on "source credibility" suggests that essentially five characteristics determine the credibility and trustworthiness of a speaker—his perceived expertness, his reliability, his apparent intentions, his dynamism, and his personal attractiveness. The importance of a speaker's expertness will be readily apparent to anyone with any experience at all in negotiating the development of program evaluations. Technical knowledge of statistics and methodology of such evaluation are important, but not nearly sufficient. Indeed, if this is the only apparent knowledge of the evaluator, then he is likely to be readily dismissed as an "ivory tower ideologue." Consequently, it is vital that the evaluator either knows a good deal about the program being evaluated, as well as about program evaluation itself; or lets someone speak for him who does. The evaluator's intentions, as well as his reliability, will be conveyed through the delivery. One that is clear and logical is important. In addition, the choosing of a presenter who is perceived to be dynamic (i.e., has the quality of being more active than passive in the course of communication) seems to lead to greater trust. It may be, as Weinstein (1972) suggests, that such behavior indicates greater commitment by the speaker. Finally, the personal attractiveness of the speaker to the listener, while definitely an intangible, is vital. This suggests that trust might be especially difficult to develop when the evaluator represents a totally different milieu than that he wishes to evaluate.

From these observations, the following additional guidelines might be added.

> viii. Choose a person who is knowledgeable about the program, as well as the instrumental technology of evaluation, to initiate and conduct the "negotiation" in establishing the program evaluation contract. If he already is a trusted person within the program, so much the better.
>
> ix. Choose an active, dynamic negotiator, rather than one who is passive, since the former is likely to be more persuasive.
>
> x. Do not choose a negotiator who is totally unattractive to evaluatees, this decision being based on criteria of attractiveness among evaluatees, not evaluators.

(c) Finally, research into interpersonal trust also lends itself to certain conclusions. In particular, it provides some utility in determining the general level of trust that a group of "listeners" or "evaluatees" might have prior to approaching them. For instance, higher levels of trust tend to be found in individuals who feel less alienated and more in control of their lives, come from slightly higher socio-economic classes, etc. These, and other observations, provide the basis for several additional suggestions:

> xi. Consider the personality and demographic characteristics of evaluatees before approaching them about the conduct of an evaluation. Extra caution will have to be used in those cases where individuals within a program are especially alienated.
>
> xii. Consider the "trustworthiness" of the person introducing the notion of program evaluation, both in terms of the occupational group he is perceived to represent, and in terms of the group to be approached.

To these observations might be added the one that one of the most intractable obstacles to change is the innate human conviction that what everyone is used to doing must be right. Normal human pride of involvement leads to an almost uncontrollable subjective bias. Innovation requires both a willingness to give up even the most sacrosanct culturally accepted ways of doing things and an openness to the new. Thus, the need for objectivity in evaluation should be self-evident. Not only must the evaluator guard against the subjective involvement that leads to selective misperceptions, he must also be trustworthy.

3. Consequences. Little will be said about the concern for what happens at the conclusion of a project, other than already has been said. From the previous observations, it will be obvious that this writer feels it imperative that an evaluator become involved in seeing to it that the implications of his findings are translated into recommendations of plan changes and altered performances. This conclusion has been reached, partly because of the observation that research reports all too often become more efficient at gathering "dust" than fingerprints; partly, because program planners frequently do not understand the technological jargon that tends to be inherent in evaluation reports; and, partly, because it will provide the evaluator with a better grasp of the practical considerations to be faced in implementing future evaluations and program changes.

Summary and Concluding Remarks

The implementation of program evaluations is by no means the easiest of tasks. The purpose of this chapter has been to explore some of the issues related to this difficulty so as to more clearly ascertain the nature of these problems and to elucidate ways in which they might be overcome. The first observation was that research methodology, as traditionally taught in our university classes, typically has concentrated on the Instrumental Elements associated with such evaluation. Indeed, they usually have been restricted to those Instrumental Elements of a technological nature and ignored the value aspects. Observation two was that, while instrumental elements are important, an equally, and sometimes much more important element is the Expressive one. That is, problems of human relations very often are as important as problems of methodology. Thus, the technological and value aspects of this dimension, too, were explored in some detail, it being felt quite possible to radically improve the way in which our evaluations are implemented. The sum and substance of the entire chapter is that in the preparation for a program evaluation, both Elements have to be considered simultaneously. There is no sense working out a detailed research design when, in fact, it will not be acceptable to the people being evaluated. At the same time, if a good receptivity is achieved, it may be quite possible to develop a more rigorous and far-reaching research design than initially had been envisaged.

Footnotes

1.   Based on a paper presented at the Fifth Banff International Conference on Behavior Modification, March, 1973. The helpful comments by Mr. A. A. MacKinnon and Dr. J. C. K. Silzer are gratefully acknowledged.

2.   Formerly Director of Operations Research, Psychiatric Services Branch, Saskatchewan Department of Health. Presently, Western Regional Representative, National Institute on Mental Retardation, Saskatoon, Canada.

3.   "Appropriateness" might be defined as tackling a problem of some importance as opposed to one that is of mere parochial interest. "Adequacy" might be defined as whether a mountain is to be removed through the use of teaspoons or bulldozers.

4.   "Evaluatee" is used in a broad sense, meaning the variety of "players" in the game from front-line workers to senior administrators.

References

Ayllon, T. and Haughton, E. Control of the behavior of schizophenic patients by food. *Journal of Experimental Analysis of Behavior*, 1962, *5,* 343-352.

Bracht, G. H. and Glass, G. V. The external validity of experiments. *American Educational Research Journal,* 1968, *6,* 437-474.

Campbell, D. T. Reforms as experiments. *American Psychologist,* 1969, *24,* 409-429.

Campbell, D. T. and Stanley, J. C. *Experimental and quasi-experimental designs for research.* Chicago: Rand McNally and Co., 1966.

Hall, T. L. The political aspects of health planning. In W. A. Reinke, (Ed.), *Health planning: Qualitative aspects and quantative techniques.* Baltimore: Waverly Press, Inc., 1972. Pp. 73-95.

Katz, D. and Kahn, R. L. *The social psychology of organizations.* New York: John Wiley and Sons, 1966.

Miller, J. G. The nature of living systems, and Living Systems: The group. *Behavioral Science,* 1971, *16,* 227-398.

Neufeldt, A. H. A province-wide EDP system for community-based psychiatric services. *Canadian Psychiatric Association Journal,* 1969, *14,* 135-141.

Neufeldt, A. H. Planning for comprehensive mental health programs. *Canada's Mental Health,* March-April, 1971, Mongraph Supplement No. 67.

Neufeldt, A. H., Berrien, V., and Smith, L. *The developing community mental health centre: A study of referral and treatment patterns before and after the opening of a modern 'total care' psychiatric facility.* Saskatoon: Marcotte Research Centre, Saskatoon Department of Health publication, 1972.

Pratt, S. and Tooley, J. Human actualization teams: The perspective of contract psychology. *American Journal of Orthopsychiatry,* 1966, *XXXVI,* No. 5, 881-895.

Reinke, W. A. Methods and measurements in evaluation. In W. A. Reinke (Ed.), *Health planning: Qualitative aspects and quantitative techniques.* Baltimore: Waverly Press, Inc., 1972. Pp. 44-52.

Ullman, L. P. *Institution and outcome: A comparative study of psychiatric hospitals.* Toronto: Pergamon Press, 1967.

Weckworth, V. E. A conceptual model versus the real world of health care service delivery. In C. E. Hopkins (Ed.), *Outcomes conference: Methodology of identifying, measuring and evaluating outcomes of health service programs, systems and subsystems.* Rockville, Maryland: Office of Scientific and Technical Information, NCHSRD, 1969. Pp. 39-62.

Weinstein, M. S. The role of trust in program evaluation: Some guidelines for the perplexed administrator. *Canadian Psychologist,* 1972, *13,* No. 3, 239-251.

Evaluating Community-Based Psychiatric Services

5

Peter D. McLean

The vast majority of psychiatrists in North America work in private practice. Since the psychiatrist in private practice is typically paid by a prepaid health insurance plan administered either by the government (Canada) or private carriers (United States) and since his practice is not restricted to a geographical catchment area, he is in many ways more responsible to the specific health plan than he is to the patient who is insured by the plan. Patients as clients, on the other hand, are in the strange position of paying for a service the quality of which is not directly under their control. The private-practice model's sole criterion for payment to psychiatrists is number of people seen in what context (e.g., individual therapy, group therapy, consultation, etc.). The individual private practitioner decides what patients are seen, how frequently and for how long. Documentation of the psychiatrist's decision processes which determine the type of therapy the patient is to receive, how improvement is assessed and whether a follow-up check was made is left entirely to the preference of the individual psychiatrist. It is for these reasons that private-practice psychiatry remains an art form in which the codification of decision-making remains implicit and unexamined, and evaluation of treatment results is almost impossible. One cannot expect private-practice psychiatrists to contribute time to standard evaluations of patient progress if they are not paid for doing so. In effect, the conscientious private-practice psychiatrist is caught in a conflict—if he chooses to spend time carefully evaluating the effectiveness of his treatment procedures he does so at the expense of revenue. Oddly enough, we seem to expect psychiatrists to be morally accountable by virtue of their certification oath and not respond to a financial incentive system which is divorced from any demonstrable results of treatment efficacy.

These two characteristics of private-practice psychiatry, the method of payment and the lack of geographical responsibility, have profound implications in the evaluation of community-based psychiatric services.

Contemporary Evaluation of Private-Practice Psychiatry in the Community

The only method of evaluating private-practice psychiatry currently employed by some, but not all, prepaid health insurance plans is that of *peer review*. In this method, various features of an individual psychiatrist's practice are compared to the average "pattern of practice profile" of all those psychiatrists billing through a particular health plan. These profiles contain such information as, the ratio of people seen in therapy compared to consultation, the number of billings (i.e., psychiatrist-patient contacts) per case, the number of patients under any one psychiatrist's care, appointment frequency, the relative number of patients under care but not referred by a medical source, etc. A board of peers then compares the profile of individual psychiatric practitioners to mean provincial profiles to detect discrepancies in patterns of practice. This policy of peer review is intended to monitor private-practice in order to detect gross deviations in patterns of practice and does not reflect quality of care. Peer review is a form of structure evaluation which reduces the possibility of exploitation of a prepaid plan and provides information about the logistics of contact between patients and psychiatrists. What happens when patients and psychiatrists are together (process evaluation) and whether it makes any difference in the long run (follow-up evaluation) remain largely unknown.

Beyond this simple form of structure evaluation, community psychiatry in the private sector is not routinely evaluated. The following factors can be considered to be largely responsible for the lack of evaluation procedures in the private-practice sector of community psychiatry.

1. The fee-for-service payment structure of prepaid health insurance plans is incompatible with the concept of evaluation.
2. Neither patients nor practitioners are restricted to specific catchment areas. Accordingly, patient variables cannot be controlled between practitioners, and no conclusions can be drawn about treatment efficacy.
3. There is not sufficient agreement among practitioners on how to measure treatment effects, and the diverse theoretical

orientations of practitioners reflect discrepant treatment goals (e.g., symptomatic relief vs. changes in global functioning).

4. There is a general resistance to evaluation inasmuch as evaluation is often viewed as a threat to professional rewards and runs the risk of negative peer judgement. It is difficult to convince many private practitioners that there is no base line of comparison and that what is to be evaluated are relationships between patients, disorder variables, reaction to specific treatment combinations, costs, etc., and not the competence of any one practitioner.

5. Definitions of the goals of community psychiatry very often portray ideals which are far removed from practice and preclude accountability.

The increasing trend toward the deployment of community psychiatric services away from the private-practice sector to an integrated community mental health center system is probably the only real hope for the evaluation of community psychiatry for several reasons: (1) funding for evaluation is increasingly written into the operating budgets of such centers, (2) geographically defined catchment areas can be delineated, and (3) there is an increasing demand on the part of consumer movements and funding sources alike for accountability.

Given the circumstances, it is questionable whether the evaluation of private-practice psychiatry in the community should be pursued. Instead, work directed toward the development of evaluation guidelines for community mental health *programs* appears to be the best investment at this time.

The Shift from the Private-Practice to Community Mental Health Model

The marked shift away from the one-to-one private-practice delivery model to a community mental health program model requires new evaluation procedures and is largely the result of the following six factors.

Reduction of hospital in-patient care. It is generally accepted that acute and, particularly, chronic hospital care can be reduced by increasing comprehensive social services and treatment facilities at the local level. For example, the work of Holmes and Masuda (1970) and Langsley *et al.* (1968, 1971) in life stress situations and crises management has shown that there is greater social adaptation as a result of crisis training which emphasizes coping techniques than there is as a result of hospitalization, for a variety of patients.

Social engineering vs. psychotherapy. Psychotherapy is no longer considered the priority treatment for all "human suffering" (Goldberg, 1972; Small, 1971). The therapeutic focus is increasingly moving away from a preoccupation with intrapsychic events to interpersonal events and social skills. The object is practical therapeutic change with the smallest possible intervention. This state of affairs has been prompted largely by the influence of behavior modification and the profession of social work, which has recognized the potential of social engineering in altering mental health problems.

An increased use of geographically defined service areas. Defined catchment areas work to ensure greater continuity of care in mental health and social services, which is a measurable process (Bass and Windle, 1972). Continuity of care is a particularly important concept to community mental health because it is oriented toward the individual client rather than the overall service system.

Increased use of nonprofessional manpower. The demand for mental health services greatly exceeds the availability of professionals. Universities have been attempting to provide degree or certificate level programs involving two to four years of training in order to meet the personnel demand, but the largest potential clearly rests with the utilization of the nonprofessional labour force (Matarazzo, 1971). Many imaginative training programs, such as Rioch's (1967) "second careers" for women, have been reported (see Roen, 1971, for review).

From institutional to consumer regulation of services. The evidence that severe psychiatric disorder is greatest in the lowest socioeconomic class is unambiguous (Fried, 1969). Because of the extreme shortage of minority group professionals and the question of relevance of conventional service institutions to the changing needs of communities, some service centers are being confronted by effective and articulate citizens' groups. A number of models for developing a working alliance between consumer and provider have been suggested (e.g., Tischler, 1970). Others warn that local participation is a fad based on the assumption that anything at the local level is automatically virtuous (Martin, 1972). Parker (1970) has demonstrated, however, that, with training, community representatives can contribute effectively to program regulation in the role of policy advisors.

Put simply, the effect of the consumer movement is increasingly strong and does not afford us the opportunity to agree whether we'll let "them" help us decide what we will do to "them" with their money.

A greater investment in prevention. The concept of prevention is derived from physical medicine and reflects a belief that the application of presently available therapy at an early stage of the problem development will curtail its further development. What is assumed, though, is a known effective therapy (Hutchinson, 1969). Community mental health programs view prevention as their ultimate goal; however, the most effective preventive program efforts to date have been in the areas of crisis intervention (see Roen, 1971, for review) and school adjustment.

Evaluation of Community Mental Health Programs and Organizations

With few exceptions the literature in evaluation of community mental health is theoretical. That is, models of organization and assessment are proposed, few of which have been running long enough to be accompanied by results. Nonetheless, a number of antecedent factors which can affect the outcome of evaluation on studies can be identified and should be considered in the design phase of an evaluation program as preliminary requirements.

First among these preliminary requirements is the feeling that *evaluation is punitive.* Since there has been a tradition of non-evaluation in mental health, those now engaging in it are often doing so at some risk if the continued funding of their program is contingent upon the demonstration of positive results. If the program administrators are at all adaptive, they will engage in impression management by discriminating between various forms of evaluation and selecting the one most complimentary to their program. It is unlikely that the quality of evaluation studies will improve until the threat evaluation implies is removed. There are several ways of reducing the resistance to evaluation studies. One is to place more emphasis and reward on the evaluative procedure of a program and relatively less emphasis on the result of the evaluation. Another is to support the evaluation of programs which compare alternate intervention procedures.

The second preliminary requirement is to specify the objectives of a program such that program status can be monitored and compared with these pre-determined objectives at various times. Community mental health centers with programs overly committed to broad consultive services and poorly defined goals which represent basic assumptions about human nature such as people's right to be happy, simply cannot be evaluated. A related issue involves the desirability of establishing agreement among all levels of program personnel, administration and consumers as to what the specific program objectives are to be, how they will be evaluated, what the possible outcomes are and what the implications for subsequent decision-making are for each outcome, before the programs start.

The third preliminary requirement is to ensure that the evaluation of community mental health programs is population-based. Programs and centers which do not deal with a defined population or catchment area are not able to interpret their data without the problem of a biased or unknown population sample. Many major teaching centers are not able to contribute to evaluation research for this reason (Gruenberg and Brandon, 1964).

Regard for the above three requirements will go a long way to provide a basis for program evaluation and will work to avoid the shaky practice of retrospective or salvage research.

Evaluation Strategies

The literature on mental health program evaluation is now extensive, but, as noted earlier, largely theoretical. Consequently, proposed evaluation criterion, methodologies and concepts often compete when programs are designed, simply because they have no operational history by which to organize their utility. The recent literature indicates five main approaches to evaluation: evaluation of program structure, process, outcome, cost analysis, and systems analysis. Historically, psychiatry has been preoccupied with the process-type of evaluation (i.e., number of beds available, quality audits, case studies, etc.) to the relative neglect of other evaluation approaches, particularly cost analysis and outcome evaluation. The ubiquitous plea for accountability, however, has forced serious consideration of alternative evaluation models.

Evaluation of Program Structure

This form of evaluation might also be called administrative, since it is concerned with the allocation of program resources. It is a "housekeeping" type of evaluation of the setting in which the program operates. Indices of resources include staff-patient ratios, magnitude of case load and frequency of contact, quality of physical facilities, etc. "Accreditation requirements for health care facilities are frequently stated in terms of such measures" (Fox and Rappaport, 1972). The advantage of a structure evaluation approach is that concrete information is routinely available (Donabedian, 1966). The disadvantage is that structure evaluation is frequently regarded as the most oblique and least important measure of quality (Zusman and Ross, 1969) because it provides absolutely no information about how well the intervention objectives of the program are being met.

Evaluation of Program Process

Depending on the objective of the intervention program, "process" can involve everything from individual clinical treatment, on the one hand, to prevention through the development of social and employment opportunities which are incompatible with isolation and unemployment within a community, on the other. Program process evaluation typically has not been used to evaluate the efficacy of treatment or intervention procedures. The efficacy has been assumed—a phenomenon which accounts for the dearth of outcome studies. Instead, the job here is to evaluate how well appropriately applied procedures are deployed. That is, assuming the intervention procedures work, are they being distributed responsibly? Indices for evaluation of program process include continuity of treatment, comprehensiveness of treatment, quality audits by independent parties, analysis of case studies and treatment failures, etc. (see Fox and Rappaport, 1972, for review). Information from process evaluation studies allows judgements or inferences to be made about the quality of service and its effectiveness. There have been attempts to measure process events more objectively by the use of quantitative techniques to measure standards. Zusman and Slawson (1972) developed ordinal scales for nine areas considered to be important in evaluating mental health services. The nine factors, such as staff and training qualifications, physical environment, relative cost, etc., combine to form the Service Quality Profile. The scales are non-additive and, therefore, individual factors can only serve as a basis of comparison between service programs, while global comparisons remain impressionistic. This work is particularly interesting, however, because it attempts a comprehensive assessment of program process and introduces the issue of patient satisfaction and short-term outcome into its format. Other attempts to scale critical factors in order to provide a profile of the mental health process, such as the Community-Oriented Programs Environmental Scale (COPES) (Moos and Otto, 1972), depend upon staff and client ratings of relatively nebulous constructs (e.g., autonomy, spontaneity) and, accordingly, are difficult to interpret. A disadvantage with process evaluation is that traditional approaches are favored and innovative ones are penalized (Zusman and Ross, 1969).

Evaluation by Outcome

Outcome information is generally regarded as the most fundamental and significant kind of evaluation data. It is the "proof-in-the-pudding" of all mental health programs. Yet, outcome studies have proven so laborious and often inconclusive that the tendency is to fall back on structure and process forms of evaluation. The problem in outcome evaluation has been what to ask for, how to ask it, and when to ask it. The 'what to ask for' element in follow-up is a conceptual problem since there are many ways a client/patient can be considered "better." Should client satisfaction, global functioning, alleviation of symptoms, prevention of readmission, or psychiatric traits and status be used as measures of outcome? With the exception of 'prevention of readmission,' which is easily documented, the strongest case can be made for 'client satisfaction' and 'alleviation of symptoms' (i.e., problems) to serve as the basis for follow-up evaluation.

Mental health workers are often in the position of having to devise an intervention program for a client and since the client is paying the bill, directly or indirectly, there is considerable face validity in the notion of client satisfaction measures. Such measures would, ideally, reflect in detail the respective dimensions of service in order that specific information would not be lost in global evaluations. Market research has developed a highly specialized multivariate technology for measuring client satisfaction, a technology from which mental health professionals could benefit tremendously.

Psychotherapy, with its emphasis on the whole person, his life style and overall functioning, has encouraged the use of global measures of adjustment in evaluation practices. Similarly evasive in terms of specific measures is the continued use of diagnostic terminology in evaluation (e.g., "five out of seven patients indicated no schizophrenic symptomatology after treatment"). The diagnostic bottleneck adds variance, or noise, to the evaluation system since there are few diagnostic categories at the symptom level which enjoy widespread agreement between practitioners. Most patients receive service from community mental health facilities for specific problems. Therefore, there are probably more advantages to using specific, problem-oriented criteria rather than to using measures of global functioning or diagnostic categories.

Since Kanfer and Saslow (1965) detailed the conceptual and methodological problems of global concepts of psychiatric classification, many others (e.g., Moss and Boren, 1971) have asked that specific behavioral criteria be used to determine therapeutic change. Strupp (1971) has subsequently suggested that these criteria should be tailored to individual clients. The problem-oriented medical record approach, originally promoted by Weed (1968), serves this purpose and has been widely adopted in medical settings. Essentially, the approach organizes a patient's problems into a problem index according to treatment priority. Each problem is then described by means of an explicit data base and treatment goals are specified for each individual problem. The extension of the problem-oriented record approach to follow-up evaluation permits changes on individual, specific problems to be rated by the client or others at various times. Clients/patients appear to prefer this personal approach to follow-up compared to the global, rather lengthy questionnaires or interviews, and accordingly, the attrition rate in follow-up is lower. The problem-oriented approach to community mental health problems provides a "natural" and parsimonious basis for follow-up. In this respect it is antithical to global adjustment ratings. One of the most recent and interesting applications of the problem-oriented approach to evaluation is the use of a goal-oriented progress note (Ellis and Wilson, 1973) which lends itself ideally to follow-up.

Historically, relatives and the client himself have not been utilized as data resources, even though they are in the best position to monitor changes in problematic behavior. When the correlation between relative-professional ratings and relative-patient ratings have been weak, the assumption has been that the intrinsic defect in objectivity rests with the relative (Hogarty, 1970). Increasingly, however, empirical evidence suggests that this assumption is unfounded and that relative ratings and predictions of community adjustment are more accurate than the professional's ratings (Michaux et al., 1969; Angrist, 1968; Freeman and Simmons, 1963; Ellsworth et al., 1968). The crucial factor in client and relative rating scales is the objectivity and specification of the items being rated. Spitzer (1966), in assessing the relationship between patient and relative reports on similar scales at different times disclosed intercorrelations as high as .78 on observed social behaviors, but lower intercorrelations on variables requiring more subjective responses. The problematic behavior approach has the advantages of specificity, client involvement, and economy, as well as being a promising means of routinely monitoring treatment effectiveness.

Having decided what criteria are to be used, the program evaluator has a variety of techniques available for evaluating treatment efficacy. These techniques include peer ratings, self ratings, factor-analytic assessment batteries, mood scales, behavior assessment, self-concept measures, personality inventories, and assessment interviews. The relative merits of these techniques are reasonably well known and it is therefore possible to discriminate among them and select those techniques which will answer the questions being posed by the evaluation.

Bergin (1971) recently reviewed over 60 selected follow-up studies and concluded that "future progress will be more assured by reducing the complexity of therapeutic practices to more specific operations...," which "will require a departure from gross tests of the effects of therapy." These two issues, therapeutic complexity and the use of gross tests of therapeutic effect, probably influence the determination of outcome more than treatment itself. Most psychiatric facilities use a combination of treatments in the hope that a therapeutic effect will result. For example, in the treatment of depression it is common to receive concurrently medication, supportive individual psychotherapy, group therapy, and occasionally E.C.T. This practice prohibits the identification of specific treatment effects. The use of gross tests of therapeutic effect in follow-up evaluation is often self-defeating. If a client receives treatment for one or several specific problems and is then evaluated in terms of his overall functioning, the success of the treatment may not be demonstrated due to the overinclusiveness of the evaluation test.

The final question is: When should follow-up evaluation be done? A six-month follow-up period is considered minimal, but more often a two-year follow-up period is advocated. Considering the complexity of outcome determinants, it seems likely that treatment or intervention effects are of themselves relatively minimal. **Figure 1** notes some of the major factors which interact to determine outcome. Of the six factors noted, the treatment factor alone has received almost exclusive attention by psychiatry, regardless of much evidence indicating that

Figure 1 Sources of Variance That Can Influence Evaluation of Therapy Outcome

$$\text{THERAPY OUTCOME} = f \begin{pmatrix} \text{CLIENT/PATIENT} \\ \text{VARIABLES} \end{pmatrix} \times \begin{pmatrix} \text{PSYCHOLOGICAL} \\ \text{VARIABLES} \end{pmatrix} \times \begin{pmatrix} \text{PROBLEM} \\ \text{VARIABLES} \end{pmatrix} \times \begin{pmatrix} \text{TREATMENT} \\ \text{VARIABLES} \end{pmatrix} \times \begin{pmatrix} \text{THERAPIST} \\ \text{VARIABLES} \end{pmatrix} \times \begin{pmatrix} \text{ENVIRONMENTAL} \\ \text{VARIABLES} \end{pmatrix}$$

1 CLIENT/PATIENT VARIABLES	2 PSYCHOLOGICAL VARIABLES	3 PROBLEM VARIABLES	4 TREATMENT VARIABLES	5 THERAPIST VARIABLES	6 ENVIRONMENTAL VARIABLES
e.g.	e.g.	e.g.	e.g.	e.g.	e.g.
– sex	– Client's expectancies and perception of therapy	– ability to self control	– type of intervention	– interpersonal skills	– marital/family status
– age	– Client's motivation	– articulation of problem(s)	– intensity and duration of intervention	– sex	– living accommodations
– other biological factors		– problem history such as previous therapy contact, chronicity etc.			– work status
					– range of friends and frequency of contact

PROGRAM STATUS:

record	influence/monitor	record	influence	influence	influence/monitor

93

therapist variables often outweigh treatment factors in determining out-come (Truax and Mitchell, 1971). Given these complex interactions, as well as the effect of unknown intervening influences which occur after the client/patient has left therapy, three- to eight-month follow-up is surely the maximum length of time during which any changes can be ascribed to treatment effects. Of course many clients/patients may maintain an original improvement according to whatever criteria were used to determine treatment efficacy. The question remains: Does this maintained or continued improvement have anything to do with a treat-ment program which took place a year or more ago? Research-oriented follow-up programs are in a position to extend the follow-up period beyond the three- to eight-month period advisable for routine service programs. In this case, the program can record, monitor, or directly influence the variables which determine therapeutic outcome (see bottom of Figure 1). With the accumulation of this kind of data, the nature of the interaction between these variables should eventually become more clear.

Cost-Effectiveness Analysis

Mental health costs have traditionally not been the concern of the therapist, many of whom have felt it rather gauche to derive costs for treatment when human happiness is at stake. Based on data for the year 1966, Conley, Conwell and Arrill (1967) estimated the comprehensive cost of mental illness in the United States for that year to be $20 billion. Such economic realities have encouraged alternative mental health programs to be compared on the basis of costs as well as the traditional clinical criteria. The result has been cost-effectiveness as a model in program evaluation.

The two major sources of financial cost in mental health are direct program cost and indirect costs because of decreased product-ivity, lost income and expenses of homemaking services. In the past, the cost of mental health services involved only program costs which were usually expressed in terms of per diem rates. Cost per case treated (average length of stay X average per diem cost) is a more meaningful index of cost-efficiency but does not reflect cost-effectiveness. Cost-effectiveness is dependent on a reasonable measure of therapeutic efficacy, which in turn is dependent upon follow-up information. Cost-effectiveness data on mental health programs provide more information and is therefore of cardinal importance in allocating funds and priorities to programs.

Fox and Kuldau (1968) have illustrated the dependency of cost and treatment effectiveness in determining cost-effectiveness by plotting one against the other (**Figure 2**). In this case, Programs 1 and 2

Figure 2   Cost-Effectiveness Schedule*

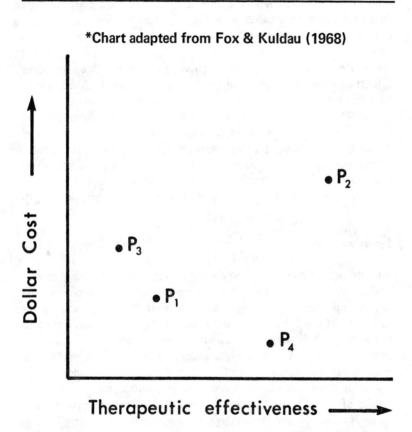

*Chart adapted from Fox & Kuldau (1968)

Dollar Cost

• P₃

• P₂

• P₁

• P₄

Therapeutic effectiveness ⟶

(P$_1$ and P$_2$) reinforce the adage, "you get what you pay for." Program 3 represents a high cost-effectiveness ratio and should be phased out in favor of Program 4. The principle to be followed is that if the therapeutic results are at least equal, then whichever alternative program can produce them at the lowest cost will be regarded as the most effective (McCaffree, 1966). Program 4 is inexpensive compared to Program 2, but not quite as effective. The decision to be made is whether the additional effectiveness of Program 2 warrants its additional costs.

Cost-accounting methodology allows the costs of particular problems, disorders, and syndromes to be determined as a function of time. That is, the cost follows the individual, and the "social cost" of particular disorders can be predicted from pooled estimates of individual cumulative costs. Information on program effectiveness, combined with costs, allows administrators to discriminate between programs and to select the most pragmatic program when funds are a consideration. Given the importance of cost-effectiveness as an index of evaluation, it can be expected that mental health programs which include cost-effectivness data will be considered more important than those that don't. An interesting example is a recent report by Chien and Cole (1973) in which the relative merits of a landlord-supervised cooperative apartment program, "as a new type of community residential treatment modality" for psychotic patients, were compared to those of more conventional settings such as halfway houses, nursing homes, etc. Although the authors did not present cost-effectiveness data as such, they reported program costs, patient satisfaction ratings and patient adjustment data. With this information, the various residential settings could be clearly evaluated from a cost-effectiveness point of view.

Systems Analysis

The planning and evaluation of municipal, regional and national mental health delivery systems faces concerns unknown to less complex mental health organizations. The dynamic nature of large population areas makes it difficult for unaided human skills to relate resources and needs in mental health systems. Computer assistance in the areas of modeling and simulation can optimize the allocation of resources, predict the effect of specific decisions, and simulate the effects of changes in elements of the system by systematically varying the range of possible results of the changes. Operational research has been applied in many areas of health (World Health Organization, 1971), particularly in comprehensive planning.

Structure, process and outcome approaches to evaluation attempt to specify objectives and evaluate program change in terms of the progress made toward these objectives, within a predetermined time period. In contrast, the systems model evaluates the degree to which an organization reaches its goal, given a set of specified conditions (Schulberg and Baker, 1968). Provided with quantitative measures of value, the systems approach can optimize the best strategy for balancing resources and needs within a mental health system. Only recently, through the use of cumulative psychiatric case registers, has the data been available for modeling service needs. The State of New York, for example, has recently proposed a balanced service system model for maximizing its allocation of service resources which was developed by a systems analysis approach (Miles and Gerhard, 1972). In Canada, studies of comprehensive service needs for the City of Saskatoon (Neufeldt, 1969) and a study of the utilization of services by a cohort of specific patients (Cassell et al., 1968) were based on information available from the Saskatchewan Register.

The multivariate analysis and continuous sampling procedures of systems analysis allows an arbitrary currency for estimating the cost of social change to be developed in order to assist decision-making at the policy level. As cumulative psychiatric case registers become more widespread in use, actual costs of mental health services can be estimated. The unique advantage of systems analysis is that it promises to contribute tremendously to the field of psychopathology by evaluating the interaction pattern between all the variables which determine outcome—an otherwise impossible task. Because of the cost of systems analysis, typically only those with large financial resources at stake, such as regional governments, have made routine use of this approach to planning. Like other forms of evaluation, a large part of the costs, utility and potential of the systems analysis approach to evaluation depends upon the availability of "grass roots" data.

The Choice of Evaluation Procedure

An American Psychiatric Association task force on the research aspects of community mental health centers (Klerman et al., 1971) reported two years ago that, "our current knowledge of the nature, causes and treatment of mental illness, while significantly advanced over previous decades, is still inadequate to validate comprehensive programs of prevention and treatment." The task force report says further that, "program assessment techniques are not sufficiently advanced to allow global program evaluation." These two opinions are reiterated throughout the literature and should serve as cautions against under-investment in evaluation planning. The selection of an evaluation procedure is part of program design and depends upon a balanced consideration of (1) detailed program objectives, (2) the range and nature of possible program outcomes, (3) how these outcomes will be measured, and (4) the cost of the evaluation procedure itself. Since evaluation itself is often as expensive as the treatment procedure being assessed, it is advisable to consider evaluation procedures in terms of cost-yield ratios. The yield of information, or value, of any evaluation depends upon (1) the quality of information requested (e.g., follow-up data is more relevant than structure evaluation data when determining treatment efficacy) and (2) how well-defined and specific the evaluation data is. The *cost-yield ratio* of evaluation programs is as important a concept in evaluation as treatment program cost is in determining treatment efficacy.

The "least possible" evaluation in community mental health is detailed program description, which includes minimum standardized information about both client and program characteristics. Beyond program description, the selection of evaluation procedures depends upon the program's objectives and pragmatic consideration of the procedure's cost-yield ratio. Particularly promising is (1) the cost-effectiveness method of evaluation, and (2) the possibility of wider adoption of the cumulative psychiatric case register, therefore enabling clients to be traced through the mental health and social service system by a systems analysis approach to the evaluation of comprehensive services. As a final note, it must be emphasized that the impact of *all* programs, no matter how small or modest, can be constructively evaluated.

References

Angrist, S. S. *et al. Women after treatment: A comparison of former mental patients with their neighbors.* New York: Appleton-Century-Crofts, 1968.

Bass, R. D. and Windle, C. Continuity of care: An approach to measurement. *American Journal of Psychiatry,* 1972, *129,* No. 2, August, 110-115.

Bergin, A. E. The evaluation of therapeutic outcomes. In A. E. Bergin and S. L. Garfield (Eds.), *Handbook of psychotherapy and behavior change: An empirical analysis.* New York: John Wiley and Sons, 1971.

Cassell, W. A., Grunberg, F., and Fraser, H. N. The discharged chronic patient's utilization of health resources. *Canadian Psychiatric Association Journal,* 1968, *13,* February.

Chien, C. and Cole, J. O. Landlord-supervised cooperative apartments: A new modality for community-based treatment. *American Journal of Psychiatry,* 1973, *130,* No. 2, February, 156-159.

Conley, R. W., Conwell, M., and Arrill, M. B. An approach to measuring the cost of mental illness. *American Journal of Psychiatry,* 1967, *124,* No. 6, 63-70.

Donabedian, A. Evaluating the quality of medical care. *Milbank Memorial Fund Quarterly,* 1966, *44,* 166-203.

Ellis, R. H. and Wilson, N. C. Z. Evaluating treatment effectiveness using a goal-oriented automated progress note. *Evaluation,* 1973, Special Monograph No. 1.

Ellsworth, R. B. *et al.* Hospital and community adjustment as perceived by psychiatric patients, their families and staff. *Journal of Consulting and Clinical Psychiatry,* 1968, Monograph (whole part) *32,* No. 5.

Fox, P. D. and Kuldau, J. M. Expanding the framework for mental health program evaluation. *Archives of General Psychiatry,* 1968, *19,* November, 538-544.

Fox, P. D. and Rappaport, M. Some approaches to evaluating community mental health services. *Archives of General Psychiatry,* 1972, *26,* February, 172-178.

Freeman, H. E. and Simmons, D. G. *The mental patient comes home.* New York: John Wiley and Sons, 1963.

Fried, M. Social differences in mental health. In J. Kosa, A. Antonovosky, and I. K. Zola, *Poverty and health: A sociologic analysis.* Cambridge, Massachusetts: Harvard University Press, 1969.

Goldberg, C. A community is more than a psyche: The concept of community mental health. *Canada's Mental Health,* 1972, *20,* Nos. 3 and 4.

Gruenberg, E. M. and Brandon, S. Evaluating community treatment programs. *Mental Hospitals,* November, 1964.

Hogarty, G. E. Selected measures of community adjustment following outpatient psychotherapy: Ratings from significant others. Prepared for NIMH Psychotherapy Outcome Measurements Project, 1970.

Holmes, T. H. and Masuda, M. Life changes and illness suscepti-bility. Unpublished research paper, presented as part of a "Symposium on Separation and Depression: Clinical and Research Aspects" at the annual meeting of the American Association for the Advancement of Science, Chicago, Illinois, December 26-30, 1970.

Hutchison, G. B. Evaluation of preventive services. In H. C. Schul-berg, A. Sheldon and F. Baker (Eds.), *Program evaluation in the health fields.* New York: Behavioral Publications, 1969.

Kanfer, F. H. and Saslow, G. Behavioral analysis: An alternative to diagnostic classification. *Archives of General Psychiatry,* 1965, *12,* 529-538.

Klerman, G. L. *et al.* Research aspects of community mental health centers: Report of the APA Task Force. *American Journal of Psychiatry,* 1971, *127.*

Langsley, D. G., Pittman, F. S., Machotka, P. *et al.* Family crisis therapy—Results and implications. *Family Process,* 1968, *7,* No. 2, 145-158.

Langsley, D. G., Machotka, P. and Flomenhaft, K. Avoiding mental hospital admission: A follow-up study. *American Journal of Psychiatry,* 1971, *127,* No. 10, 1391-1394.

Martin, M. Community mental health centres: Coming to grips with big ideas. *American Journal of Psychiatry,* 1972, *129,* 211-213.

Matarazzo, J. D. Some national developments in the utilization of non-traditional mental health manpower. *American Psychologist,* 1971, *26,* No. 4, 363-372.

McCaffree, K. M. The cost of mental health care under changing treatment methods. *American Journal of Public Health,* 1966, *56,* 1013-1025.

Michaux, W. W. *et al. The first year out: Mental patients after hospitalization.* Baltimore: Johns Hopkins Press, 1969.

Miles, D. G. and Gerhard, R. A balanced community-based mental health service system. New York State Department of Mental Hygiene, 1972.

Moos, R. and Otto, J. The community-oriented programs environment scale: A methodology for the facilitation and evaluation of social change. *Community Mental Health Journal,* 1972, *8,* No. 1, 28-37.

Moss, G. R. and Boren, J. J. Specifying criterion for completion of psychiatric care. *Archives of General Psychiatry,* 1971, *24,* 441-447.

Neufeldt, A. H. *Comprehensive psychiatric care: A study of the psychiatric service needs of a medium-sized urban centre.* A report to the Saskatoon Hospital Council, 1969.

Parker, A. W. The consumer as policy-maker—Issues of training. *American Journal of Public Health,* 1970, *60,* No. 11, 2139-2153.

Rioch, M. J. Pilot projects in training mental health counselors. In E. L. Cowen, E. A. Gardner, and M. Zax (Eds.), *Emergent approaches to mental health problems.* New York: Appleton-Century-Crofts, 1967. Pp. 110-127.

Roen, S. R. Evaluative research and community mental health. In A. E. Bergin and S. L. Garfield (Eds.), *Handbook of psychotherapy and behavior change: An empirical analysis.* New York: John Wiley and Sons, 1971.

Schulberg, H. C. and Baker, F. Program evaluation models and the implementation of research findings. *American Journal of Public Health,* 1968, *48,* No. 7, 1248-1255.

Small, L. *The briefer psychotherapies.* New York: Brunner-Mazel, 1971.

Spitzer, R. L. Evaluation of psychiatric status and history. Progress report. New York: Biometrics Research, State Department Mental Hygiene, 1966.

Strupp, H. H. Comments on the evaluation of outcome in psychotherapy. Paper presented at the annual meeting of the Society for

Psychotherapy Research, Saddlebrook, New Jersey, 1971.

Tischler, G. L. The effects of consumer control on the delivery of services. *American Journal of Orthopsychiatry,* 1971, *41,* No. 3, 501-505.

Truax, C. B. and Mitchell, K. M. Research on certain therapist interpersonal skills in relation to process and outcome. In A. E. Bergin and S. L. Garfield (Eds.), *Handbook of psychotherapy and behavior change: An empirical analysis.* New York: John Wiley and Sons, 1971.

Weed, L. L. Medical records that guide and teach. *New England Journal of Medicine,* 1968, *278,* 593-600.

World Health Organization. Health operational research. A report on a seminar convened by the Regional Office for Europe of the World Health Organization. Copenhagen: Regional Office for Europe, W. H. O., 1971.

Zusman, J. and Ross, E. R. Evaluation of the quality of mental health services. *Archives of General Psychiatry,* 1969, *20,* March, 352-357.

Zusman, J. and Slawson, M. R. Service quality profile: Development of a technique for measuring quality of mental health services. *Archives of General Psychiatry,* 1972, *27,* November, 692-698.

Behavioral Measurement in a Community Mental Health Center[1]

Robert Paul Liberman[2], William J. DeRisi, Larry W. King, Thad A. Eckman, and David D. Wood

Over a decade ago, the Joint Commission on Mental Illness and Health documented its contention that the delivery of mental health services in this country was woefully inadequate. In *Action for Mental Health* (1961), the Commission recommended a vast new program of social intervention, funded by federal and state governments. Ideally such a massive effort would move American psychiatry out of the custodial era of warehousing patients in large institutions, where the Social Breakdown Syndrome (Gruenberg, 1967) was fostered, into the bright new horizons of early, active, and brief treatment in small mental health centers located near patients' homes. Recommendations included an emphasis on prevention of disorders by consultation with community agents, schools and parents who were seen as the mediators of mental hygiene principles. One outcome of the Commission's report was the legislative and public impetus leading to Congress' passage of the Community Mental Health Centers Act in 1963. The NIMH had its national mission greatly enlarged with a mandate and funds to administer and stimulate the development of community-based mental health services (Beisser, 1972). The mid-1960's and early 1970's have seen the rapid development of the Community Mental Health Center (CMHC) concept, with close to 400 centers, out of a projected 2,000 currently in operation.

In the rush to meet the legislative mandates and compete for federal and state funds, little effort was expended on devising new techniques and therapeutic approaches that would meet the challenges of an effective mental health program for the masses. Old methods, largely adapted from the medical and psychoanalytic models, were dressed up in new community treatment settings (Liberman, 1973). As the initial enthusiasm for the CMHC movement wanes, hard questions are now being asked concerning its demonstrated effectiveness (Chu and Trotter, 1972; Panzetta, 1971; Schwartz, 1972). The report by Nader's group (Chu and Trotter, 1972) on the NIMH reflects a growing disenchantment with the community mental health scene as do the severe cutbacks in funding now becoming a reality at the federal level. The Nader report continues:

> In retrospect, the community mental health centers program was vastly oversold, the original goals quickly perverted....NIMH feebly communicated the original intent of the program to state and local officials; failed to coordinate the location of the centers with other HEW health and social welfare efforts; avoided funding centers outside the narrow confines of the medical model; did not engage consumers in the planning or operation of centers; and made only the most piddling evaluation of the program's performance. As a result, community mental health centers tend to be only a renaming of conventional psychiatry, a collection of traditional clinical services that are in most cases not responsive to the needs of large segments of the community.

In California, local county mental health programs will be required to evaluate their services by 1974 to continue receiving funds from the state government (California State Legislature, 1971). The requests for hard data on program evaluation will most likely escalate during the coming years.

The behavioral or social learning model offers mental health workers an educational approach to the delivery of services, principles upon which new and effective techniques can be created, and an adherence to measurement which makes program evaluation an integral part of treatment. Pinpointing and measuring behavioral problems and goals and implementing a variety of behavior modification techniques promises to increase the effectiveness of direct and indirect services. The behavioral approach to clinical problems also sensitizes the mental health consultant to the critical importance of operationalizing *continuity of care* and *evaluation* of service programs. The present chapter describes the use of behavioral observations and procedures to evaluate treatment programs in a typical, comprehensive, community mental health center.

Mental Health Setting

The Community Mental Health Center is located in the downtown area of Oxnard, a city of 80,000 people, of which 30 per cent are Mexican-Americans. Oxnard, the largest city in Ventura County, is situated in the middle of a fertile agricultural basin 50 miles northwest of Los Angeles.

The material that follows is based on work done in the partial hospitalization or day treatment program of the Center. This program is one of four direct services that the CMHC provides. The other three are out-patient, in-patient, and emergency services. The Mental Health Center in Oxnard is one of three satellite centers serving catchment areas of approximately 140,000 each in Ventura County. Each satellite Center is supported by an NIMH staffing grant as well as by the 90-10 percent formula of State-County funds known as the Short-Doyle program in California. There are also fees collected from patients on an ability-to-pay basis. It should be understood that the programs described in this chapter derive from an intact, ongoing CMHC in a rural area uninfluenced by university politics and status. There was no selection of staff, patients, or setting. The Center has been in existence for six years, and some of the staff have been with the Center since its inception.

Staff Training

The staff of the partial hospitalization unit is composed of two occupational therapists, three psychiatric nurses, four mental health technicians, two mental health workers (Chicanos, indigenous to the community), and one half-time psychiatrist. The psychiatrist is also the principal investigator of the research project. Most of the staff had their training in on-site programs at the nearby Camarillo State Hospital and moved to the Mental Health Center when the community program opened in Oxnard. The research team, which consists of a psychiatrist, two clinical psychologists, and four research assistants, has been at the Center by invitation only. All new innovations in program and evaluation of services are negotiated between the research and clinical staff. The lever for changing staff behavior has been social reinforcement established by the close working relationship between the research and clinical personnel. Greater efficiency may be achieved in developing and evaluating a mental health program by having administrative control of the operations, but this would seriously limit the applicability of the findings to other community mental health programs.

The adoption of a behavioral approach to patient care in a community mental health center requires retraining of both staff and patients. Wholesale change in the way the treatment center is operated is likely to produce discomfort in both groups. The resistances to be overcome are remarkably similar and have been enumerated by Liberman, King, and DeRisi (1972).

1. Both must be convinced that the new techniques are effective despite their apparent simplicity.

2. Both must learn to rely less on psychoactive drugs, supportive relationships that reinforce the status quo, and a psychiatric diagnosis.

3. Both must learn to rely more on data and an empirical approach to problem behaviors.

4. Patients as well as staff must learn to rely less on vague, general statements of improvement or satisfaction and more on data-based assessment of the progress or lack of progress.

5. Both groups must learn to set short-term, objective, attainable goals for themselves rather than goals that are long-range, subjective, and idealistic.

6. Both patients and staff must acquire as reinforcers the more frequent attainment of very small but measurable increments in performance.

Few of these learning tasks are likely to come easily to traditionally trained staff or to patients who have expectations of traditional treatment. The discomfort associated with these changes was reduced in the Oxnard Mental Health Center during an 18-month period of gradual but continuous innovation prior to the start of the BAM Research project (Behavior Analysis and Modification). During this time the first author introduced many of the current methods of behavior therapy to staff and patients. He demonstrated the use of a token economy (coupon-incentive system) for day care patients, as well as assertive training, systematic desensitization, covert sensitization, shame aversion therapy, implosive therapy and contingency contracting in the actual treatment of patients.

During this period the first author became established as an important source of social reinforcement to staff and patients, an effect that made it possible to initiate significant changes in the day-to-day operation of the Center. Being part of an innovative, experimental program and having successful experiences with new methods opened another area of reinforcement for the Center's staff—attendance at professional workshops, seminars and conferences. Almost all staff members have participated in at least one of these meetings and some have assisted in making presentations to other professionals in the field. Several other non-budgeted events are currently reinforcing staff involvement in the change process:

Visitors frequently tour the program and need staff guides.

A nurse and three mental health technicians have been included as co-authors of published articles arising from their work.

Five staff members have been paid as consultants by the Center for Training in Community Psychiatry of the California Department of Mental Hygiene.

Patients

The average daily census at the day treatment program is 20 with another 30 individuals receiving services each week in the evening. At any one time, approximately 40 patients are on the active list, with some of them coming to the program on a part-time basis. The patients come from all walks of life since there are few alternative mental health services in Oxnard and little in the way of private psychotherapy. Most of the patients are lower to lower-middle class in socio-economic status and approximately 10 percent are Black and 25 percent Chicano. These minority groups attend the day treatment program in roughly the same proportion as they comprise the general population.

The patients vary in age from 15 to 75 with a majority in the 22-45 age range. Over half are acutely or chronically psychotic and on maintenance phenothiazine or lithium medication. Narcotic addicts are treated in another part of the County's mental health program but other types of drug abusers and some alcoholics are accepted into the day treatment program.

Behavioral Measurement

The behavioral measures to be reported in this chapter derive from two major sources. One is the Behavioral Progress Record which is kept on a weekly basis for each patient by his therapist. The second is the Behavior Observation Instrument, which is a time-sampling of patients' behaviors recorded by research assistants during selected periods of time. Both measures contribute information, on different levels, concerning the impact of a behavior modification program on the behavior of patients in the Mental Health Center.

The essential question is double-edged: Could we develop a convenient, reliable and usable behavioral record-keeping system on a clinical level that could also generate research data? Used by clinicians, the Behavioral Progress Record provides information on the movement of patients toward their therapeutic goals. The individualized Behavioral Progress Record, used in conjunction with experimental designs that call for specified interventions, reversals, and multiple baselines, permits us to determine the functional relationship between patients' behavioral change and their treatment program.

The second question of interest in evaluating the Center's program was whether the introduction of behavior modification produced changes in broad categories of patient activity, such as social participation, work and task involvement, and social isolation. We were also interested in comparing the activity spectrum of patients in the behaviorally-oriented day program at Oxnard with that of patients in other settings such as boarding homes for ex-mental patients, the state hospital wards, and another day treatment center that used more conventional milieu therapy methods. The Behavior Observation Instrument was developed to assess this level of patients' activity in different environments.

Behavioral Progress Record

In the transition from a medical model to a behavioral model, one of the first tasks is to train the staff to translate presenting complaints into observable, measurable behaviors. Given a staff that had many years of training and experience in traditional clinical settings, this was a large task that required a systematic training program (Liberman *et al.,* 1972).

A basic innovation in the operation of the day treatment center is focused on the patient's chart, heretofore an unwieldy manila folder, buried in a file cabinet and exacting considerable response-cost for its use. The chart is still kept, but all information necessary to a patient's program for the current week is displayed on a single page. It consists of the Behavioral Progress Record which is on a clipboard hanging in the nurses' station, a location that is almost impossible to avoid. Goals are set and reviewed on a weekly basis. The staff-therapist meets daily with each of the patients on his caseload. He gathers data, holds individual treatment sessions and dispenses reinforcers. All data gathered are placed on the Progress Record and displayed on the clipboard. Only after a new Record is made is the old Record filed in the "chart." The probability of relevant data being recorded is enhanced in this manner.

The emphasis in setting goals is on observable, measurable goals. A typical Behavioral Progress Record is shown in **Table 1**. As can be seen in the Record, a criterion was attached to each goal in order to assess its degree of attainment. For example, attendance is defined by the criterion of being present at the clinic five out of five possible days; whereas promptness is defined as being at the clinic by 9:00 a.m. A job application in hand is proof enough of attainment of that goal.

As a check to determine the extent to which observable, measurable goals were being written by the staff of the Oxnard Day Treatment Center, on one unannounced day the clipboards were removed, and independent raters categorized the goals as countable, observable or non-countable, non-observable. The results showed that 97 percent of the goals were countable and observable. The percentage of agreement between the raters was 98.5.

Experimental Designs for Individual Patients

One question to be considered is whether the goals established for the patients are attained as a function of the treatment program. In order to determine this, every sixth patient that comes into the day program is designated as an experimental case, and an attempt is made to demonstrate experimental control over a targeted behavior. Two such cases will be presented to convey the kinds of problems and interventions used.

Beverly was a 39-year-old housewife who had a long history of psychiatric treatment and many diagnoses as a schizoaffective psychotic. She had received traditional psychotherapy for a period of eight years. When she first came to the clinic she was manic and delusional in her speech. Beverly's behavior had become so disturbing that her husband transferred her from home to a residential board-and-care facility. It was impossible to engage Beverly in a rational conversation lasting more than one minute.

109

Table 1   Behavioral Progress Record

Total Therapy Sessions This Week: _____

Name: _____John Smith_____   Individual: __4__

Therapist: __Nancy Sanders__   Family: __1__

Week Ending: __3-9-73__   Collateral: __0__

Behavioral Goals (Countable)	Mon.	Tues.	Wed.	Thurs.	Fri.	Sat.	Sun.
1. Attendance: 5 of 5 days							
2. Promptness: At Clinic by 9:00 A.M. each day							
3. Perform four of the seven chores designated in John's contract.							
4. Secure one job application							
5. Attend and practice one scene in the P.E.T. Workshop on Tuesday and Friday.							

Medication: Chlorpromazine 200 mg h.s.	Notes: Check with Board and Care Operator each day to see if John performed chores.

One of the targeted goals for Beverly was for her to engage in appropriate conversation with her therapist each day. The criterion was established as 15 minutes of appropriate speech each day. Throughout the experiment, the therapist recorded duration of appropriate speech by the use of a stopwatch held in her lap underneath a table. Periodically, an independent observer attended the conversation between Beverly and her therapist and performed a reliability check on the duration of rational speech to onset of delusional talk. Eleven reliability checks were made, and the average agreement between rater and therapist was 82 percent. The therapist and rater were said to have agreed if their records of the time duration of appropriate speech were within five seconds of each other.

The experimental design called for a baseline period in which the therapist listened and attended to everything Beverly said. Following baseline, contingent attention was introduced for appropriate speech. As long as Beverly was speaking appropriately, her therapist would listen attentively. Whenever Beverly became inappropriate, the therapist would get up and leave the room. After 20 sessions of contingent attention, there was a return to baseline for five sessions, then a return to contingent attention for five sessions. The results of the procedures are shown in **Figure 1.**

Figure 1   Effects of Contingent Attention on the Duration of Appropriate Speech of a 39-Year-Old Psychotic Female

---

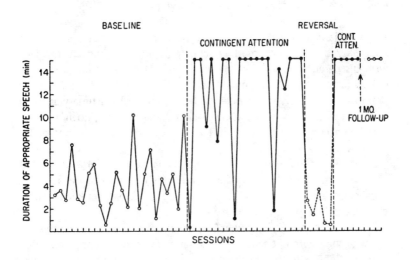

It is evident that the introduction of contingent attention increased the duration of appropriate speech in most sessions to the maximum allowed time of 15 minutes. When the contingent attention was withdrawn, there was a rapid decrease in the duration of appropriate speech. Conversely, when the contingency was reintroduced, the duration of appropriate speech increased to the maximum 15 minutes and remained there for the next four. sessions. One month later, three interviews were conducted and in all three Beverly's speech was appropriate for the full 15 minutes.

Observations by Beverly's therapist and other clinic staff were congruent with the experimental data. Beverly demonstrated marked improvement during her stay at the Center, not only in her speech but in other targeted behaviors as well, such as completion of home chores and occupational therapy projects. Five months later, Beverly was back home with her family. Reports from the couple and from observers sent by the Center indicated that she was functioning well as a mother and wife and was attending college courses at night.

These procedures and results demonstrate that the verbal behavior of a patient in a day treatment center can be brought under reinforcement control. This result is significant because verbal behaviors are important indicators of social deviance and an individual may be excluded from his community because of an inappropriate verbal repertoire.

Another behavior that is frequently seen in a day treatment center is social withdrawal. The second case will describe an attempt to exert experimental control over this behavior.

William was an extremely withdrawn, 27-year-old, single and unemployed man, diagnosed as schizophrenic, who had always lived with his parents, except for one brief hospitalization. William was not only socially withdrawn, but he actively removed himself from the presence of others. At his parents' home, most of his time was spent isolated in his room with the doors closed. He reported no friends, no social contacts, and he only left the house in the company of his parents.

When he first came to the clinic, William spent a large amount of his time outside of the area of the clinic in which most of the activities took place. Not only did he stand in the hall, but William kept his eyes closed, and his fingers stuck in his ears.

The first targeted behavior for William was his presence in the day room of the treatment center. A time sampling recording procedure was used whereby William's therapist observed him ten times during the day and recorded whether William was in the targeted area or not. A reversal design was planned to demonstrate experimental control over this behavior. **Figure 2** depicts the contingencies used and the results of this experiment.

Figure 2   Reduction in Social Isolation of a Young Male Psychotic by Contingency Management. Conditions Are A = Baseline, B = Coupons as Reinforcers, C = Coupons to Buy Time Away From Clinic, D = Response Cost + Coupons to Buy Time Away From Clinic

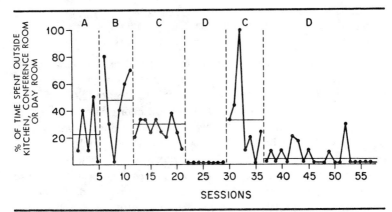

The figure shows that conditions A, B, and C are all essentially baseline conditions since there was no consistent reduction in the 25 percent of time that William spent outside the main area of the day treatment center. The procedures were as follows: For condition A, the therapist was simply to observe William on the predetermined schedule. This condition was the designated baseline phase. In condition B, William was paid coupons for being in the targeted area. The coupons were part of a regular, ongoing token economy at the center. The back-up reinforcers for the coupons were lunch, coffee, snacks, and excursions. In condition C, William was paid coupons but allowed to buy time off from the clinic with the coupons at the rate of one coupon for five minutes away. He could earn two coupons per observation or a maximum possible of 20 per day.

The procedural change in condition D was to combine response cost with reinforcement. For each of the times William was observed outside of the targeted area, he was to relinquish two coupons. The reinforcement contingency was continued with William receiving two coupons with which he could buy time off from the clinic if he was in the day room. With the introduction of condition D, the percent of observations of William outside the targeted area decreased to zero and remained there for eight days. At this point, the response cost procedure was removed; that is, condition C was reinstated. The effect was to increase the percent of observations away from people. With the reinstatement of response cost, condition D, there was a gradual decrease and elimination of social isolation.

Reliability measures were taken throughout the experiment. For six reliability checks, the average percentage of agreement was 98 percent. Reliability was computed for each behavior using the fomula:

$$\text{Percent agreement} = \frac{\text{number of agreements}}{\text{number of agreements} + \text{number of disagreements}} \times 100$$

The results of the experiment are informative on several points. First, again experimental control was demonstrated over a targeted problem behavior of a patient in a day treatment center. Secondly, the results demonstrate the empirical evaluation of a treatment program. The first two interventions that were used, conditions B and C, produced no change in William's behavior. It was only with the introduction of the third contingency that a desirable change was produced. In treatment settings many contingencies have to be tried before one is found to be effective. Thirdly, the results demonstrated improvement in one target behavior, but did not show any changes in other behaviors, such as the amount of time William had his eyes open and the amount of time spent in social conversation. It appears that response generalization must be programmed.

Behavior Observation Instrument

One established and economical method for securing reliable data in behavioral research is the time sampling technique. This procedure involves making observations at prearranged intervals over a specified period of time. Once a notation system is devised and relevant behaviors are operationally defined, observers can be taught to collect data. Nonprofessional staff can be trained to make observations with a high degree of reliability.

The initial phase in the development of an observation system is the creation of a measurement system which standardizes and quantifies behaviors. The instrument used in the present study was derived from a system developed by Schaefer and Martin (1969) for assessing activity vs. apathy in mental patients.

The Behavior Observation Instrument (BOI) is a device that can be used to systematically classify and record behavior in a variety of clinical settings. The BOI can be used to assess staff behavior as well as patient behavior. The BOI possesses flexibility in its categories so that particular behaviors, defined operationally, can be recorded in concordance with the goals of any clinical or research program. The BOI consists of two basic types of behavioral categories: *mutually exclusive behaviors* and *concomitant behaviors.* All behaviors which can be observed at the facility are classified into one of the mutually exclusive behaviors, which may be emitted in conjunction with one or more of the concomitant behaviors. In addition to recording the two types of behaviors, observers also indicate the location within the facility where the behavior was emitted.

The numerical codes and operational definitions for the BOI are as follows:

Mutually Exclusive Behaviors

1. Walking
2. Running
3. Standing (lack of motion from the torso down, but excludes a momentary pause in walking)
4. Sitting
   a. apparently awake (eyes are open)
   b. apparently asleep (eyes are closed or not visible)
5. Lying down
   a. apparently awake (eyes are open)
   b. apparently asleep (eyes are closed or not visible)

Concomitant Behaviors

6. Drinking (holding cup in hand, pouring liquid into cup, bottle in hand, but does not include having cup or bottle in front of target patient)
7. Smoking (touching cigarette, cigar, or pipe, whether or not it is lit)
8. Eating
   a. meals
   b. other than meals
9. Chewing (gum or nails)
10. Grooming (hair, make-up, shaving, etc.)

a. oneself (merely holding comb in hand is not grooming)

b. another person

11. Reading/writing/leafing through magazine or newspaper

12. Recreational activities

a. Group activities (cards, bingo, board games, ping pong, playing guitar for a group, singing along, etc.)

b. Solitary recreation (drawing, guitar, knitting, solitaire)

13. Conversation with another patient

V. Target patient (TP) is talking or reading to another patient

NV. TP is listening to another patient; there must be some gestural indication that TP is attending to the conversation, i.e., nodding, eye contact, etc.

14. Conversation with a staff member

V. TP is talking to the other person

NV. TP is listening; there must be some gestural indication that TP is attending to the conversation.

15. Cleaning or tidying up environment (ashtrays, kitchen table, bird cage)

16. Helping to prepare lunch / plan lunch / helping with groceries / making coffee / away buying groceries.

17. Working on occupational therapy (OT) project or receiving instructions for it; there must be some indication that TP is listening to the instructions or actually working on the project. *Note:* an activity (such as knitting, may be counted as recreation or OT work, depending upon the context in which the behavior occurred; for example, knitting in the day room is recorded as recreation, but knitting in the OT room is recorded as working on an OT project).

18. Individual therapy (the interaction must be a formal therapy session and not an informal conversation with a staff member)

19. Away on a field trip

20. Group meeting

a. Participating in role playing, discussion, etc.

b. Passive participation, alert and listening; TP's eyes are open and there is some indication that he is attending.

c. Apparent inattention (eyes are closed or there is other indication that TP is not attending, e.g., reading a book during the meeting)

21. Not present (verify absence with staff member)

Locations

DA   Day Room
OT   Occupational Therapy Room
K   Kitchen
DI   Dining Room
O   Offices
C   Corridor

Observations are recorded on 4" x 6" index cards. **Figure 3** shows a sample portion of an observation card.

Figure 3   A Sample Data Card Used by Observers Recording With the Behavior Observation Instrument

---

Observer: _____   Date: _____   Time: _____

	TP Name	Code	Comments
1.			
2.			
3.			

In order to maximize the validity and insure the reliability of the behavioral observations undertaken in this study, a formal procedure was established for the training of staff in the proper use of the BOI. A procedures manual was developed (DeRisi, Fabian and Schultz, 1972). Observers studied the manual and memorized the notation system and data collection procedures. Content mastery was tested by means of a paper and pencil proficiency examination which covered situations frequently encountered in a clinical setting. Finally, the observers practiced recording behaviors using the BOI categories until 90 percent or higher reliability was attained. Total time spent in training was approximately four hours.

Procedures

Ten subjects were randomly selected from the clinic's patient roster each day that observations were made. Initially, ten observations per day were taken; however, a comparative analysis between data collected ten times per day and data collected four times per day indicated that there was no significant difference in the percentage of behaviors recorded in the various categories. Thus, it was decided that four observations per day were sufficient for the purpose of this project. The observation periods were 10:00-10:30 a.m., 11:00-11:30 a.m., 1:00-1:30 p.m., and 2:00-2:30 p.m.

Each subject was observed once for five seconds during each observation period. Observations of consecutive subjects were made at regular intervals until all subjects were observed. Two independent observers recorded behaviors simultaneously so that a continuous reliability check could be made. One of the observers signalled the other by tapping his clipboard once with a pencil immediately prior to a five-second observation interval. The observation interval was terminated after five seconds and was signalled by the lead observer who tapped twice. The observers looked at the target patient (TP), coded the behavior, made any additional comments applicable, and observed the next patient precisely 30 seconds after the previous observation.

Observer Reliability

Nonprofessional staff who were blind to the objectives of the research and the hypotheses being investigated were trained in the use of the BOI to observe and record patient and staff behaviors. The raters made their observations independent of one another and were required to remain separated by a minimum distance of five feet during the entire observation session. Reliability was calculated according to act-by-act agreement for 25 percent of the total observations. The percentage of agreement was obtained with the following formula:

$$\text{Percent agreement} = \frac{\text{number of agreements}}{\text{number of agreements} + \text{number of disagreements}} \times 100$$

Observer reliability was consistently high for all observation sessions ranging from 84.6 to 100 percent with a mean rating of 94.9 percent.

BOI Settings

The BOI was developed to provide an objective means for assessing the spectrum of activities of patients in various community care settings and to describe the use of time and work-space by the attending staff. Observations were made in four facilities: male and female wards in a large state hospital, a large residential board-and-care home, a small residential family-care home, and the day treatment centers at Oxnard and in a second, adjacent city.

Observations made at the state hospital and the residential care facilities were for comparison purposes only, as there was no experimental intervention planned for these settings. Serial observations were made at the Oxnard Community Mental Health Center and at Community Mental Health Center II in an adjacent catchment area so that comparisons could be made within and between the two centers both before and after a behavior modification program with an educational format was initiated at the Oxnard Center.

BOI Categories

The spectrum of activities exhibited by patients was obtained by combining specific behavioral acts measured by the BOI into general categories reflecting social participation, nonsocial behavior, and work activities. Table 2 shows the general categories and their component behavioral targets.

While the particular groupings of categories used for the general activities were most relevant to the present investigation, other general classification schemes could be created from the various BOI behavioral categories depending upon the questions being asked of the data. One advantage of the BOI is that it permits considerable flexibility in the organization and retrieval of information.

Results of Group Observation

Data from the state hospital reveals similar levels of social participation for the men's and women's wards but a higher proportion of non-social behavior on the men's ward. The data are shown in Figure 4. The residents of these wards were all considered chronically psychotic. The data reflect the low level of activity characteristically seen on those wards.

Table 2 Components of the BOI General Activity Categories

Social Participation (SP)—Includes any of the mutually exclusive behaviors (1-5) occurring with any of the following concomitant behaviors: 10B, 12A, 13V or 13NV, 14V or 14NV, 18, 20A, or 20B.

Nonsocial Behavior (NS)—Includes any mutually exclusive behavior occurring alone or in conjunction with any of the following concomitant behaviors: 6, 7, 8B, 9, 10A, 11, 12B, 20C. The NS category is intended to indicate a lack of involvement with treatment activities.

Work (W)—Work and NS are mutually exclusive, that is, if a patient is working alone it is recorded as W, but is not considered an NS behavior. Categories 15, 16, and 17 are coded as W.

Other (O)—Includes behaviors which are not relevant to the SP, NS, or W categories and includes 8A, 19, and 21.

Figure 4 Percent of Social Participation, Nonsocial, Work and Other Behaviors (Eating Meals, Away On a Field Trip, Not Here) On Two Wards of a Large State Hospital

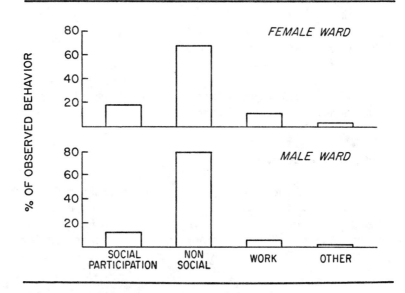

Figure 5 shows that community residential care homes differ little from state hospital wards in these measures. Both facilities house former chronic patients who have been discharged from the state hospital. The large facility has a capacity of 21 and the small, family-style home has six ex-patients. The large residential care facility had 19 male and two female ex-patients, whereas the small facility had only women. In both the hospital and residential care settings women display a slightly greater proportion of social participation than do men. The large facility is of recent construction, pleasant, well-lighted, and scrupulously clean; the smaller facility is a large farm house that is not at all institutional in appearance or atmosphere.

Figure 5   Percent of Social Participation, Nonsocial, Work and Other Behaviors (Eating Meals, Away on a Field Trip, Not Here) In Large and Small Residential Care Homes

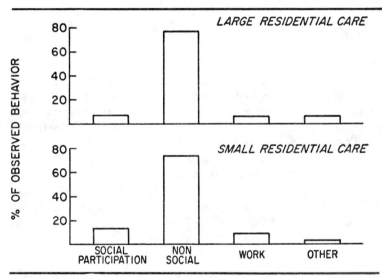

Figure 6 represents the floor plan of the day-hospital portion of the Oxnard Community Mental Health Center, which is housed in a Knights of Columbus building. The floor plan of Day Treatment Center II is shown in Figure 7. This facility is a large, open, pleasant structure of recent construction, incorporating many of the latest concepts in the design of the physical environment of the Community Mental Health Center (Canton, 1972).

Observations taken at Oxnard yielded higher proportions of social participation and lower proportions of non-social behaviors when compared to the state hospital and the residential care facilities.

Figure 6   Floor Plan Oxnard Day Treatment

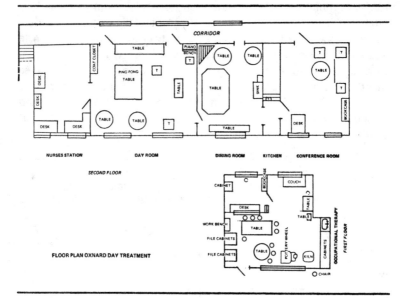

Data collected at Oxnard Day Treatment Center and Day Treatment Center II **(Figures 8 and 9)** revealed significant differences in the social participation, non-social, and "other" behavior categories (test of significance of difference between two proportions). Day Treatment Center II patients were observed to engage in a significantly higher proportion of behaviors coded as social participation than Oxnard patients (37.5 percent vs. 29.2 percent, z = 2.31, p < .01). Oxnard patients were observed to engage in non-social behaviors more often (61.5 percent vs. 32.6 percent, z = 7.73, p < .01). Behaviors coded in the "other" category were observed more often at Day Treatment Center II than at Oxnard (21.8 percent vs. 0 percent, z = 12.6, p < .01).

A new Day Treatment Center program was introduced as an experimental intervention at Oxnard. This program was based on an educational model of rehabilitation and designed to train patients for community adjustment. Courses were developed by Oxnard Day Treatment staff, and presented in a manner similar to that of a college. These courses were designed to teach competent behaviors in such areas as grooming, dealing with public agencies, consumerism, conversation skills, recreation and successful social interaction. **Table 3** depicts a typical weekly schedule for workshops at the Oxnard Day Treatment Center.

Figure 7   Floor Plan of Day Treatment Center II

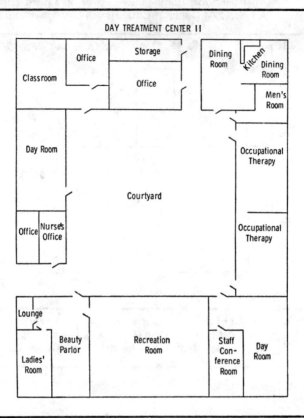

DAY TREATMENT CENTER II

Observations made after the introduction of the educational model at Oxnard showed a significant increase in social participation (29.2 percent vs. 67.7 percent, z = 3.69, p < .01) and a concomitant decrease in non-social behaviors (61.5 percent vs. 17.2 percent, z = 13.84, p < .01). Work behaviors also declined (9.3 percent vs. 7.0 percent) but this difference was non-significant. "Other" behaviors at Oxnard were observed to increase from 0 percent to 8.1 percent, (z = 8.1, p < .01).

Observations taken at Day Treatment Center II showed an increase in social participation, (37.5 percent vs. 52.5 percent, z = 3.19, p < .01), a decrease in work behaviors (8.1 percent vs. .81 percent, z = 15.54, p < .01), and a decrease in other behaviors (21.8 percent vs. 9.3 percent, z = 3.44, p < .01). Non-social behaviors were observed to increase, but not significantly (32.6 percent vs. 36.8 percent).

Figure 8 Percent of Social Participation, Nonsocial, Work and Other Behaviors (Eating Meals, Away on a Field Trip, Not Here) At Oxnard Mental Health Day Treatment Center

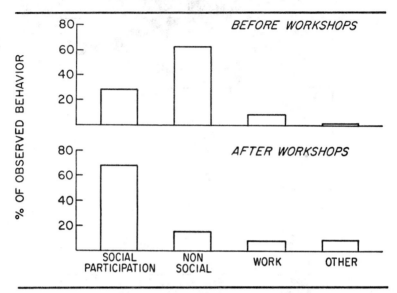

Figure 9 Percent of Social Participation, Nonsocial, Work and Other Behaviors (Eating Meals, Away on a Field Trip, Not Here) at Community Mental Health Center II

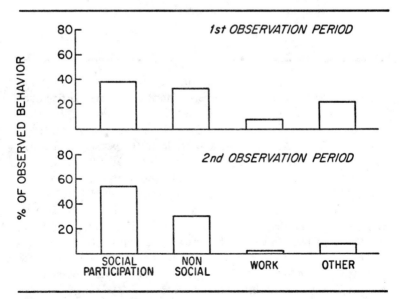

Table 3   Oxnard Day Treatment Center Schedule

Time	Monday	Tuesday	Wednesday	Thursday	Friday
8:30	Program Review	Program Review	Program Review	Program Review	Program Review
9:00					
9:30	Week-End Review		Consumerism Workshop	Personal Finances Workshop	
10:00					
10:30		Personal Effectiveness			Personal Effectiveness
11:00	Current Events Workshop / Cooking Skills Workshop	Training Workshop / Cooking Skills Workshop	Consumerism Lab Shopping	Cooking Skills Workshop	Training Workshop / Cooking Skills Workshop
11:30					
12:00					
12:30	Lunch	Lunch	No Lunch (Close Day Treatment Center at 12:30)	Lunch	Lunch
1:00	Medical and Clinical Consultation				
1:30		Patient/Staff Meeting		Medical and Clinical Consult.	Occupational Therapy Workshop / Anxiety Management Training
2:00			Staff		
2:30	Public Agencies Workshop	Diet Workshop / Occupational Therapy Workshop	Training	Vocational Preparedness Workshop / R.E.S.T. Workshop*	
3:00					
3:30					
4:00	Staff Meeting			Team Meeting	
4:30					
5:00					

* Recreation, Education, Social Activity, and Transportation

Data in **Figure 8** show the effects of the change in Oxnard's program after a series of workshops were introduced to train patients for community adjustment.

Observations of Staff Behavior

Several categories were extracted from the BOI and used for staff observations. Behavioral data relevant for program evaluation in a mental health center should include the proportion of time staff spend in direct contact with patients, with other staff, and in doing administrative tasks. The codes and operational definitions of the behaviors used in the staff observations are given below:

W: Work. Includes office work, telephone conversations, preparing or planning lunch, supervisory meetings with a Supervisor, and conferences with other staff member(s). If the target staff member is in a supervisory meeting or in conference with other staff members, *do not* mark conversations with staff; mark only W. In other instances of Work (e.g., office work, kitchen, food planning, etc.), other behaviors could occur simultaneously and *both* should be coded.

T: Therapy. Includes intake interviews, medication review, individual therapy and group therapy. There should be definite indication that the interaction is structured around some therapeutic operation, such as reviewing goals or graphs, exchanging coupons, or training a patient in some skill. O.T. instruction is considered *therapy* when the staff member is instructing one or more patients but *work* if the staff member is working on some project in the O.T. room by him or herself. Since T implies social interaction, do not code CP or CSP simultaneously with T.

CP: Conversation with a patient(s). The target staff member is talking to or listening to one or more patients.

CS: Conversation with staff. The target staff is talking to or listening to one or more staff with no patients included in the group.

CPS: Conversation with patient and staff. Target staff is talking or listening to two or more people, one of whom is a staff member and the other a patient.

RP: Recreation with a patient. Includes playing games, guitar, singing, ping pong, where participants are patients.

RS: Recreation with staff. Same as RP, with the participants being other staff members without patients being included in the group.

RSP: Recreation with patient and staff. Defined as RP, above, with both staff and patients included in the group.

NA: No activity. None of the above behaviors observed.

Observation Procedures

After each of the four patient observations was completed, the observers located and observed every staff member on duty. Because staff were found to be more active and their behavior more likely to vary than that of patients, an interval method of observation was devised. Each staff member in turn was observed during five intervals of five seconds each, within a two-and-a-half-minute period. The observer located the first staff member on his list, started his stopwatch, and observed the staff member beginning at 0'25" and ending at 0'30". He then recorded his observation and waited until 0'55", at which time he recorded until 1'00". This process was repeated until observations were made in five, five-second intervals. Then the observer located the next staff member on the list and began the process anew. Each staff member was thus observed 20 times each day (five intervals x four observations). Reliability was calculated on an act-by-act basis. Percent agreement, calculated by the same procedure used to calculate reliability with the BOI, averaged 95 percent.

Results

The results of the staff observations made at the two day treatment centers are shown in **Table 4.** The percentage of observations in which staff were observed in direct contact with patients can be calculated by pooling the results found for T, CP, CSP, RP, and RSP. Similarly, the percentage of observations in which staff were observed in contact with other staff members can be calculated by pooling the results found for "conversation with staff" and "recreation with staff." **Figure 10** summarizes the results of the staff observations at Oxnard and at Day Treatment Center II before and after the experimental intervention. At

Table 4 Percent of Staff Behaviors Observed at Two Day Treatment Centers Before and After An Educational Program Was Introduced Into the Oxnard Center

Behavior Category	Oxnard DTC		DTC II	
	Before	After	Before	After
Work	36.3	19.0	27.7	26.6
Therapy	8.1	56.7	14.9	32.1
Conversation w/ Patient	14.8	7.3	9.6	10.8
Conversation w/ Staff	20.0	14.5	18.0	17.4
Conversation w/ Patient and Staff	3.4	0.4	5.4	2.0
Recreation w/ Patient	1.0	0.5	11.0	4.5
Recreation w/ Staff	0.3	0.0	1.8	0.0
Recreation w/ Patient and Staff	3.1	0.0	4.8	2.9
No Activity	13.0	1.7	6.8	3.6
	100.0	100.0	100.0	100.0

Oxnard, 30.5 percent of staff behaviors recorded during the first set of observations included some direct contact with patients, compared to 45.8 percent at Day Treatment Center II, a statistically significant difference (test of significance of difference between two proportions, $z = 6.71$, $p < .01$, 2-tailed). Following the implementation of educational workshops at the Oxnard Day Treatment Center, staff-patient contact increased to 64.8 percent as compared to 52.3 percent at Day Treatment Center II ($z = 3.80$, $p < .01$). The increase in staff-patient contact at Day Treatment Center II between the before and after observation periods (6.5 percent) is not statistically significant, whereas the pre-post difference at Oxnard (34.8 percent) is statistically significant ($z = 12.89$, $p < .01$). Work at Oxnard was observed much less often during the post-observations, decreasing almost half (36.3 percent vs. 19.0 percent), a statistically significant difference ($z = 6.99$, $p < .01$).

The category contributing most to the variance of the staff-patient contact measure was therapy. After the educational format was introduced at Oxnard, T was observed significantly more frequently at both centers. (Oxnard Pre-Post, $z = 20.78$, $p < .01$, DTC II, $z = 7.18$, $p < .01$.)

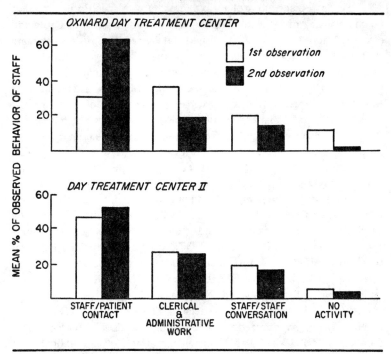

Figure 10 Summary of Results of Staff Observations at Oxnard
Day Treatment Center and Day Treatment Center II
Before and After Experimental Intervention

Discussion

The use of behavioral measurement techniques to assess service programs in community mental health has been demonstrated by these studies. Direct observation of patients' and staff's behaviors in a typical community mental health center is a logical first step in a systematic research and evaluation program. The findings reported in this chapter confront the challenge that "not a single facility exemplifying the community mental health center defined in federal regulations has been subjected to rigorously controlled investigation. In this sense, the community mental health center is an untested entity" (Glasscotte, Sanders, Forstenzer, and Foley, 1969).

While program evaluation in CMHC's can focus on issues such as responsiveness of services to community needs, availability of services, citizen participation, and continuity of care, the present report is concerned with the effects of direct services on patients' behavior. Unless the direct services of a CMHC are first evaluated and demonstrated to beneficially modify clients' behaviors, it seems pointless to expend further effort on more indirect issues of utilization and community support.

Single subject, controlled experiments give specific information on the efficacy of behavior therapy with individual patients. Cause and effect relationships can be established and we can begin to approximate that ideal state when we will be able to predict what intervention will be effective for which type of clinical problem. Targeting specific goals for patients and monitoring their behavioral progress, as is done with the Weekly Progress Record, provides a measure of outcome that is sensitive to each patient's unique problems. Behaviors not relevant to therapeutic goals are excluded from measurement. Treatment planning should accompany evaluation with informational feedback to therapists and administrators having an impact on programs designed for individual and groups of patients.

Reliable measurement of ongoing programs can indicate areas where changes should be made. Observations using the BOI and the Staff Observation Instrument yielded data that showed the need for a thorough overhaul of the Oxnard DTC program. While the BOI was used to "sound out" the behavioral milieu or spectrum of DTC activities by pooling patients' data, it can also be analyzed to evaluate an individual patient's behavior across days.

The significant increase in social participation at DTC II recorded in the post-intervention observations may be due in part to what Saretsky (1972) called the "John Henry effect." "The 'John Henry effect' reflects the impact upon a control group where the experimental group is perceived as competing with and/or threatening to surpass or replace the control group" (Saretsky, 1972, p. 579). In the compact world of a day treatment center, the presence of one or two observers cannot be unobtrusive, nor can observation techniques be unreactive. Observers reported such comments as, "Let's look sharp now," from DTC II staff when the observers appeared. Also, minor changes were made in the DTC II daily schedule when observations were being taken. Group meetings were begun as much as 15 minutes early when the observers were present and staff commented that they now had to "look sharp" because observers were present. Historically, DTC II staff were aware that comparisons between the two centers were being made, although they did not have knowledge of the specific experimental variables being studied.

Although the level of social participation was initially higher at DTC II and non-social behaviors were significantly lower than at Oxnard, the effect of the intervention was so great as to reverse these relationships during the second period of observations. The increase in social participation at the Oxnard DTC as a result of introducing the educational format becomes more strikingly significant in view of the John Henry effect, in which social participation at DTC II increased (significantly) by 15 percent between the first and second observation periods.

To test the hypothesis that the observed increase in social participation at Oxnard was due to regression effects, the proportion of social participation behaviors seen at Oxnard during the second observation session was compared to DTC II's proportion of social participation in the first observation. This procedure takes DTC II's score as the higher estimate of the population mean. The result of this comparison is significant beyond the .01 level (67.7 percent ODTC post minus 37.5 percent DTC II pre = 30.2 percent, z = 7.35, $p < .01$).

Staff observation data showed important differences between the two day treatment centers. Although Oxnard staff were initially observed to be in direct contact with patients less and involved in office-maintenance chores (Work) more than at DTC II, the introduction of a highly structured, education-based program dramatically reversed the initial findings. One consequence of the workshop program was a time savings and the introduction of office hours for each staff member. During certain assigned hours staff were given uninterrupted time to complete paperwork and return phone messages. All telephone messages were intercepted at the receptionist's desk, written down and periodically brought to the nurse's station. This procedure reduced a major source of interruptions of the DTC program.

The application of relatively simple behavior management techniques to community mental health programs can have a beneficial effect on the level of service delivered to the consumer, especially when quality of service is equated with the amount of time trained staff spend in face-to-face contact with patients. In fact, these data serve to demonstrate that some popular conceptions of civil servants are untrue in these two settings: that staff do "nothing," that they sit around drinking coffee or that they are "just goofing off." What might be interpreted as non-productive activity, categories RS, CS and NA, accounted for only 21.0 percent and 16.2 percent of all observations at DTC II and Oxnard DTC respectively during the second observational period.

The BOI has the advantage of gauging the level of activity of residents or clients in a wide range of settings, independent of the theoretical or methodological approaches of the program management or staff. Weaknesses of the BOI include (1) limitations in assessing the rates of low frequency but high amplitude behaviors (e.g., tantrums, aggression) which may powerfully determine the labelling of deviance; (2) lack of evaluation of the content or quality of interactions and behaviors; (3) decreases in sampling reliability as the variety and frequency of behaviors increase; and (4) presence of observer bias and reactivity of measurements.

The planned closing of California's state hospitals by administrative fiat has returned large numbers of institutionalized persons to the community. Their presence imposes a heavy load on local mental health agencies.

If there are no programs to train ex-patients for community living, the closing of large state hospitals means only that we have moved the back wards into a different location. Indeed the popular press already has described residential care facilities as places for ex-patients to vegetate in boredom under chemical restraint (Endicott, Ventura County *Star-Free Press*, 1973). The need for programs that are able to rehabilitate both acute and chronic patients and, concurrently, to prevent rehospitalization has intensified. Local mental health facilities will be judged on their effectiveness in accomplishing these two goals within the economic limits set by the various governmental bodies who fund them.

Maintaining a patient in the community does not prevent him from keeping the behavior patterns of institutionalization. Paul (1969), in his review of studies of chronically hospitalized mental patients, agrees with numerous other authors on the features of institutionalization: dependency, withdrawal, apathy or troublesome behavior, and lack of instrumental role performance. Alteration of the patient's environment may brighten the outlook for the "chronic" mental patient. Indeed, the very buildings in which most mental patients live are often criticized for their socio-fugal characteristics, preventing or discouraging the formulation of stable human relationships such as are found in small, face-to-face groups. By contrast, Paul describes most private dwellings as socio-petal, or fostering social relationships.

Many behavioral efforts have focused on the apathy and withdrawal of chronic patients (Ayllon and Michael, 1959; Schaefer and Martin, 1966; Ayllon and Azrin, 1968; Schaefer and Martin, 1969; Liberman, 1972; Liberman, Wallace, Teigen, and Davis, 1972). No less than 44 studies appear in Morrow's *Behavior Therapy Bibliography* (1971) under the heading "Shyness and Withdrawal," 19 under "Work Habits" and "Work Behaviors"; and "Self Care" behaviors account for an additional 35. Programs designated for the rehabilitation of chronic mental patients can be evaluated on the basis of whether or not they teach and provide practice in social interaction, decrease the rate of bizarre behaviors, and increase the rate of instrumental role behaviors, including self-maintenance, vocational skills, and "housework."

Ittleson, Proshansky and Rivlin (1970) described a large-scale project designed to evaluate and improve the therapeutic effectiveness of the psychiatric facilities of three hospitals through appropriate design. Using a time sampling method of observation, observers recorded 18 classes of behavior and the locations in which they were performed. Roughly speaking, the categories used by these authors measure how many patients are interacting with other people ("social"), interacting with their physical environment ("active"), and not interacting at all. It is evident that these categories include most of the behavioral elements cited by Paul (1969) as important for maintaining a patient in the community.

Observations were made on the psychiatric unit of a private general hospital, a metropolitan hospital's psychiatric service, and a large state hospital. All were teaching hospitals affiliated with medical schools. Act-by-act reliability figures are not given; instead, reliability figures are given by patient, by physical area, and across analytical categories. Agreement between observers is given for these as 83 percent, 84 percent, and 99 percent, respectively.

Changes in behavior were measured in a city hospital solarium as a function of altering the furniture. Before the addition of new furniture, only 15 percent of "social behavior" and 33 percent of "active behavior" took place in the solarium. This rose to 27 percent and 55 percent respectively after the change. While direct observation made with a responsive instrument can detect changes in behavior resulting from changes in environment, it is evident that the wards studied do not emphasize learning of social, task oriented behaviors. Social interactions range from 12.2 percent to 27.9 percent in contrast to nonsocial activities, which range from 36.3 percent to 52.0 percent.

Schaefer and Martin (1966) also used a time-sampling approach to describe the behavior of chronic patients on two psychiatric wards at California's Patton State Hospital. Using an observation instrument later described in their book as the "apathy scale" (Schaefer and Martin, 1969), these authors performed 30 observations of 140 patients each day for two years. "Apathy" was operationally defined as a patient performing one of the five mutually exclusive behaviors on their scale with no other concomitant behaviors. Using 40 patients randomly assigned to experimental and control groups, these authors were able to show a reliable decrease in apathy in the experimental group by differential reinforcement (tokens) of three classes of behaviors—personal hygiene, work behaviors, and social interaction. Controls received a fixed amount of tokens daily.

Risley (1972) has developed the PLA-Check (Planned Activity Check), another behavioral assessment technique that he is presently using to evaluate programs in several community and institutional settings. Observers using the PLA-Check make periodic recordings of the number of persons who are participating in the activity planned for that particular time. By manipulating program elements such as posted schedules, furniture and floor space arrangement, Risley was able to decrease inappropriate and non-productive use of time by both subjects and staff. By designing and posting feeding time schedules in a child day care center, the researchers were able to reduce crying time from 80 percent to 30 percent. Similarly, the researchers increased the amount of child-staff social interaction from 45 percent to 82 percent by making individual staff responsible for carrying out a series of planned, scheduled activities during the day. In another study, Doke and Risley (1972) found that high levels of participation could be maintained by the proper sequencing of activities and by providing sufficient materials for those involved in the activities.

The studies reviewed here provide evidence to show that the behaviors that cause people to be hospitalized fall into a limited number of categories, and that these behaviors can be modified sufficiently to make former or would-be patients acceptable in the community. Social interaction, the presence or absence of bizarre behaviors, and instrumental role performance have been found to be crucial in determining whether a person lives outside a mental hospital (Paul, 1969). Community mental health programs can be evaluated using methods of direct observation to determine their ability to achieve these behavioral goals. The introduction of a structured, educational workshop model at the Oxnard DTC served to enhance the probability that socially important behaviors of both staff and patients would be accelerated.

If community mental health programs need defending, it is up to the administrators of these programs to be able to produce behaviorally based outcome data. Detractors of mental health programs, budget analysts and legislators might not be swayed, but the availability of scientifically acceptable data which describe services rendered should add to the credibility of mental health's protagonists.

Summary

Community mental health centers have not provided data to demonstrate their effectiveness in the delivery of direct services to patients. Because of this deficiency, criticism has been directed at the CMHC. This chapter has been concerned with demonstrating that behavioral measurement can be used to assess direct services to patients.

Behavioral assessment and modification has been introduced into the everyday operations of the Day Treatment Center of the Oxnard, California, Community Mental Health Center. The clinical staff of the Oxnard Day Treatment Center consisted of two occupational therapists, three psychiatric nurses, four mental health technicians, and two mental health workers. Staff was motivated to implement systematic behavioral procedures by the modeling, prompting, and social reinforcement provided by an applied research staff who developed close working ties with the clinicians. Gradually, the research staff faded out its role in the program, continuing a minimal level of supervision with the clinicians.

The interventions included the use of behavioral progress records by the staff, the experimental analysis of treatment effects for randomly selected individual patients, and the use of a time-sampling measure of social interaction by staff and patients, the Behavior Observation Instrument (BOI).

The results of the interventions showed that the staff did set observable, measurable goals for the patients with the use of a weekly, behavioral progress record. Single subject experimental designs demonstrated that contingency management produced a desirable change in the behavior of two randomly-selected patients. An educational workshop model was introduced that included workshops on consumerism, personal finances, use of community agencies, and other topics. Data collected using the BOI showed a doubling of the patients' rates of social interaction at ODTC following the introduction of the workshops. The BOI was also used to assess social interaction rates in state hospital wards and board-and-care facilities. There were essentially no differences in social interaction rates between these two settings. However, the rates at the state hospital wards and board-and-care facilities were much lower than the rates found in either of the two Day Treatment Centers. Data collected at ODTC using a variation of the BOI also showed a statistically significant increase in the proportion of staff time spent in direct contact with patients following the introduction of the educational workshop model. Measures at the second DTC showed a small increase that was not statistically significant.

Mental health service programs in a CMHC can be developed and evaluated through the use of behavioral measurement. The first task of program evaluation should be to demonstrate that programs produce specifiable changes in the behavior of the consumers of services. The use of the Behavioral Progress Record and the BOI can promote reliable program evaluation on a stronger methodological base.

Footnotes

1.   The BAM Project research reported here was supported by the Mental Health Services Development Branch of the NIMH, Grant No. 1R01MH19880-01A1. The authors wish to acknowledge the encouragement and assistance of Dr. Howard Davis and Mr. James Cumiskey of the NIMH, Dr. Rafael Canton, Director of the Ventura County Mental Health Department, and Dr. Stephen Coray, Director of the Ventura County Health Services Agency.

2.   The views expressed here are those of the authors and do not necessarily reflect the official policy of the California Department of Mental Hygiene, the Ventura County Mental Health Department or the Regents of the University of California. The authors are deeply grateful to the clinical staff of the Oxnard Mental Health Center whose eagerness to learn new approaches and therapeutic skill has made this work possible. The data reported here are a result of the labors of a small army of research assistants including Jan Levine, Susan Heyl, Veronica Fabian, Ricnard Schultz, Nancy Austin, Aurora de la Selva, and Paul Gabrinetti.

References

Ayllon, T. and Azrin, N. The token economy: A motivational system for therapy and rehabilitation. New York: Appleton-Century-Crofts, 1968.

Ayllon, T. and Michael, J. The psychiatric nurse as a behavioral engineer. *Journal of the Experimental Analysis of Behavior,* 1959, *2,* 323-334.

Baer, D. M., Wolf, M. M., and Risley, T. R. Some current dimensions of applied behavior analysis. *Journal of Applied Behavior Analysis,* 1968, *1,* 91-97.

Beisser, A. R. *Mental health consultation and education.* Palo Alto: National Press, 1972.

California State Legislature. Sections 5651 and 5656, Assembly Bill No. 2649

Canton, R. The community mental health center team. In A. Beigel and A. I. Levenson (Eds.), *The community mental health center: Strategies and programs.* New York: Basic Books, 1972.

Chu, F. D. and Trotter, S. *The mental health complex. Part I: Community mental health centers.* Center for Study of Responsive Law, Washington, D. C., 1972, P. II, 58-59.

DeRisi, W. J., Fabian, V. and Schultz, R. The behavior observation instrument. Unpublished manuscript, 1972. Available from first author at 620 South "D" Street, Oxnard, California, 93030.

Doke, L. A. and Risley, T. The organization of day care environments: Required vs. optional activities. *Journal of Applied Behavior Analysis,* 1972, *5,* 405-421.

Endicott, W. Post criticizes plans to close state hospitals. *Los Angeles Times,* February 21, 1973. Nelson, H. State to check community mental homes. *Los Angeles Times,* July 21, 1972. Seiler, M. Showdown in board and care controversy. *Los Angeles Times,* February 13, 1973.

Glasscotte, R., Sanders, D., Forstenzer, H. M. and Foley, A. R. *The community mental health center: An analysis of existing models.* Washington, D. C.: American Psychiatric Association and National Association for Mental Health, 1964.

Gruenberg, E. M. The social breakdown syndrome: Some origins. *American Journal of Psychiatry,* 1967, *123,* 12-20.

Ittelson, W., Proshansky, H. M. and Rivlin, L. The environmental psychology of the psychiatric ward. In H. M. Proshansky, W. H.

Ittelson, and L. G. Rivlin (Eds.), *Environmental psychology: Man and his physical setting.* New York: Holt, Rinehart and Winston, 1970.

Ittelson, W., Rivlin, L. and Proshansky, H. M. The use of behavioral maps in environmental psychology. *Environmental psychology: Man and his physical setting.* New York: Holt, Rinehart and Winston, 1970.

Joint Commission on Mental Illness and Health. *Action for mental health.* New York: Basic Books, 1961.

Liberman, R. P., King, L. W., and DeRisi, W. J. Building a behavioral bridge to span continuity of care. *Exchange,* 1972, *1,* 2-27.

Liberman, R. P. Behavior modification with schizophrenics: A review. *NIMH Schizophrenic Bulletin,* 1972, No. 6, 37-48.

Liberman, R. P., Wallace, C., Teigen, J., and Davis, J. Interventions with psychotics. In K. Calhoun, H. Adams, and K. Mitchell (Eds.), *Innovative Treatment Techniques in Psychopathology.* New York: John Wiley and Sons, 1973.

Liberman, R. P. Applying behavioral techniques in a community mental health center. In R. Rubin *et al.* (Eds.), *Advances in behavior therapy.* New York: Academic Press, 1973.

Morrow, W. *Behavior therapy bibliography.* Columbia: University of Missouri Press, 1971.

Panzetta, A. F. *Community mental health: Myth and reality.* Philadelphia: Lea and Febiger, 1971.

Paul, G. Chronic mental patient: Current status—future directions. *Psychological Bulletin,* 1969, *71,* 81-94.

Risley, T. R. Environmental organization: The impersonal control of behavior. Paper presented at the Fourth Annual Southern California Conference in Behavior Modification, Los Angeles, 1972.

Saretsky, G. The OEO performance contract experiment and the John Henry effect. *Phi Delta Kappan,* 1972, *53.*

Schaefer, H. and Martin, P. L. Behavioral therapy for apathy of hospitalized schizophrenics. *Psychological Reports,* 1966, *19,* 1147-1158.

Schaefer, H. and Martin, P. L. *Behavioral therapy.* New York: McGraw-Hill, 1969.

Schwartz, D. A. Community mental health in 1972: An assessment. In H. H. Barten and L. Bellak (Eds.), *Progress in community mental health, Vol. II.* New York: Grune and Stratton, 1972. Pp. 3-34.

_____. Panel Challenges Mental Hospital Shutdown. Ventura County *Star-Free Press.* February 21, 1973.

Methodological Issues and Problems in Evaluating Treatment Outcomes in the Family and School Consultation Project, 1970-1973[1]

7

Srinika Jayaratne, Richard B. Stuart, and Tony Tripodi[2]

There are many methodological problems and issues facing the investigator who conducts treatment outcome research in the natural environment. This chapter discusses the theoretical bases and rationale for methodological decisions, with major emphasis on the practical and reality issues facing the researcher. The research described here represents the activities of the Family and School Consultation Project, whose main thrust has been to develop a set of intervention procedures for use with predelinquent junior high school and senior high school students in their natural environments. An abiding concern of this research has been the development of formats of intervention which could be efficiently implemented and readily taught to other youth workers with varied training and experience.

In seeking to carry out this mission, a multiplicity of operational problems were encountered, many of which were not anticipated. As the program developed, a seemingly endless series of decisions about intervention procedures and experimental design were made through the continuous collaborative efforts of the therapeutic and research staffs. The present chapter is an attempt to chronicle some of these decisions in an effort to portray some of the realities of research in the natural environment following the example of Kershaw (1972). Therefore, this chapter will deviate from the familiar form of papers on evaluative research which deduce a set of experimental practices from a set of research principles, by adding a full description of some of the a posteriori decisions which were essential to the survival of the Project and the achievement of its purposes.

Three sequential and interrelated phases of the program are presented as Study I, Study II, and Study III. Study I employs a design utilizing three time-constrained treatment groups. Study II analyzes a 2x2x2 factorial design, with treatment time again serving as a major variable, and Study III contrasts a time-unlimited treatment group with a qualitatively different treatment group—an "activity-discussion group."

Study Design I (1970-71)

Given the objective of identifying an effective, efficient and explicit intervention program for use with adolescents in the natural community, the first issue was whether to use an untreated control group or factorially delineated contrast groups. In considering the possible use of a classical, untreated control group, it was decided that too many serious problems would be encountered. First, as Fiske, Hunt, Luborsky, Orne, Parloff, Reiser, and Tuma (1970) have observed, "a group not explicitly treated (in some way) as a part of a study is likely to suffer serious attrition or to seek treatment elsewhere" (p. 729). Second, there is reason to believe that the withholding of treatment for a specified period of time, as is common in "wait-list control" designs, could in itself affect treatment outcome by way of changes in the motivations and expectations of the individuals so assigned. Third, it has been suggested (Stuart, 1971b) that research consumers tend to be more interested in the comparative benefits associated with alternative treatments as opposed to the absolute benefits of one. In order to supply information which is more germane to practice, it seems more fruitful to adduce information about the relative effectiveness of differing treatments or different amounts of a single treatment. The fourth and most serious objection to the use of an untreated control group concerned the ethics of this procedure. While the benefits of the experimental procedure are admittedly unknown, the Project staff nevertheless believed that they would be more beneficial than no treatment at all. Thus the withholding of services, in the judgment of the therapists, might seriously contribute to the deterioration of the youth involved. To avoid compromising the rights of clients and to reduce the experimental design problems inherent in the use of untreated controls, therefore, a decision was made to use a contrast group approach.

In general, the experimental literature suggests that both short- and long-term treatments are effective. This finding appears to hold for correctional settings (Adams, 1967), in neuropsychiatric settings (Frank, Gliedman, Imber, Stone, and Nash, 1959), with clients in family service agencies (Reid and Shyne, 1969), and in general clinic settings (Shlien, 1966; Shlien, Mosak, and Dreikurs, 1962). As a general comment, Meltzoff and Kornreich (1970) have concluded: "There is very little good evidence that time in therapy past some undefined point brings commensurate additional benefits" (p. 346). Unfortunately, however, the point at which additional treatment becomes superfluous has remained a mystery. It was perhaps this realization which led

Imber, Frank, Nash, Stone, and Gliedman (1957) to suggest the comparison of amount of therapeutic contact as an alternative to the traditional control group. These findings and recommendations led to the decision to contrast the effects of differing lengths of service rather than whether or not treatment is effective, which is the question answered by the control group designs.

Persuaded by this reasoning, the design used in Study I can best be characterized as a "pre-test/post-test comparison group design." It called for the comparison of behavioral treatment prescribed to terminate in 15, 45 or 90 days, allowing a maximum of 6, 18 or 36 hours of in-person client contact with no limitation on in-person contacts with school personnel. While the designation of treatment periods of 15, 45 and 90 days was essentially arbitrary, the decision was based on two factors. First, the treatment technology which was to be utilized had been successfully implemented by other researchers with populations of subjects having similar descriptive characteristics (Patterson, McNeal, Hawkins, and Phelps, 1967; Tharp and Wetzel, 1969; Stuart, 1971a). And second, the therapists believed that 15 days was the minimum time within which adequate treatment could be provided, and 90 days the maximum time they required.

At the end of the active treatment period, each subject was assigned to a "maintenance" therapist—a trained behavior therapist who was available to provide any further necessary intervention if requested by the family or school. The maintenance feature of the design served several important functions. First, since the minimal length of effective treatment was unknown, the 15-day intervention period may very well have been too short and possibly detrimental. Therefore, it would have been ethically irresponsible not to have made this service available. Second, the post-therapeutic contacts with the family provided an opportunity to gather more precise information about the nature, frequency, and intensity of problems which develop after treatment has ended, as well as data pertaining to the type of help sought and utilized by the families during that time. Finally, we believed that maintenance contacts would facilitate the collection of long-term follow-up data. The fact that 19 percent of the 15-day group and 21 percent in each of the 45- and 90-day groups of the Study I clients received reactivation services during a period of two years more than substantiates the need for maintenance therapists.

Beyond the benefits noted above, the contrast design offers several additional advantages. First, the three-point treatment design utilized in this study enables one to determine whether effectiveness is a linear or curvilinear function. Use of treatment versus no-treatment designs assumes linearity; if this assumption is invalid, differences associated with curvilinear functions may be under- or over-estimated. Linearity is an assumption which cannot be made with confidence at the outset of treatment research. In addition, the results of a time-constrained treatment study might be administratively and economically more beneficial to the consumers of treatment technology, who are interested in the efficiency as well as the effectiveness of service delivery systems. On the other hand, the main disadvantage of the contrast group approach is its inability to answer the question of whether the treatment being offered is better than no treatment at all.

In addition to the three time-constrained treatment groups, two "quasi-control" groups developed as the study unfolded. One group consisted of 15 subjects whose parents were referred for service but refused an initial interview with the Project staff. The second quasi-control group consisted of the total population of one junior high school on whom data were collected for two of the dependent variables (absences and tardies). While these two groups were not randomly selected, they provide some interesting contrasts with the experimental sample.

Design Implementation and Reality Problems

As most applied researchers are aware, it is one thing to design a study and quite another to implement it. Numerous unforeseen and unpredictable problems of reality often stand in the way. Sometimes the design has to be "manipulated" to overcome the problems, thus weakening it. At other times a researcher may accept a problem for what it is and keep the original design, but still end up with a weak product because of the original problem. It is of critical importance that the researcher face these issues and deal with them, especially with research in the natural environment where the reality threats are much more severe than in the laboratory.

In all, Study I received 94 names from the four junior high schools in the catchment area. The referrals were made by school personnel (social workers, counselors, and administrators) for severe social disruption in school and/or poor academic performance. Of the 94 families referred, 79 families accepted service and 15 refused. In the few cases where the families discontinued service after treatment had begun, they were retained in the experimental sample since to eliminate them might have meant the elimination of the less successful cases. The 79 cases were then randomly distributed among ten therapists (who carried from three to 15 cases each, depending on the hours of commitment to the Project). The randomization procedure used guaranteed that approximately equal numbers of subjects would be assigned to each treatment condition throughout the year.

Table 1 reveals that the procedure for subject assignment led to apparently comparable subject populations as determined by chi-square analysis of before-treatment demographic characteristics. In addition,

Table 1   Descriptive Characteristics of Subjects Randomly Assigned to 15-, 45- and 90-Day Treatment Conditions

Characteristics	Treatment Condition			Significance
	15	45	90	
Age				
12	3	2	0	X^2=7.997
13	9	6	6	df =6
14	12	9	15	ns
15+	2	7	4	
Sex				
Male	15	23	16	X^2=5.461
Female	11	4	10	df =2
				ns
Race				X^2=0.666
White	24	23	23	df =2
Black	2	4	3	ns
Income				
< $6,000	6	7	4	X^2=0.881
$6,000–12,000	10	7	8	df ≈6
$12,000–18,000	7	7	6	ns
> $18,000	3	5	6	
Family Composition				
Both parents	13	17	17	X^2=3.109
Mother only	8	6	4	df =6
Stepfather and mother	4	2	3	ns
Adopted or foster	1	2	1	
Child Management Ideology Scale (I-D Scale)				
55-65	8	9	10	X^2=0.999
66-75	17	15	14	df =4
76-85	1	2	1	ns
Parent Evaluation Form				
5-10	8	10	9	X^2=1.499
11-15	16	13	15	df =4
16-20	2	4	2	ns
Jesness SM Scale				
0-10	8	8	8	X^2=1.794
11-20	14	13	11	df =4
21-30	2	5	5	ns
Prior Court Contacts[a]	2	5	6	N/A

[a]Statistical evaluation precluded by small expected frequency values.

the subjects in the "dropout" quasi-control group also roughly corresponded to the treatment sample with no significant differences being observed at the time the sample was assembled. As will be shown in connection with Study III, however, this apparent homogeneity proved to be illusory with respect to at least one important characteristic of the population.

In contrast to the seemingly smooth operation of the subject assignment procedure, Table 2 shows that the duration of treatment varied somewhat from the prescribed conditions, with some 90-day treatments actually having less in-person contact time than some 15-day treatments. On the whole, however, the ascending order of the contact time is commensurate with the intentions of the study. Unfortunately, the overlap in times brought about by the deviations from the prescribed conditions may have contributed to the lack of discrimination between the groups with respect to treatment outcome. In effect, the therapists found it difficult to terminate therapy when they perceived that unresolved problems were still present or when they felt a substantial amount of pressure from the schools to continue intervention with subjects who were acting-out in the schools. At the other extreme, the therapists argued that it might have been detrimental to keep seeing a family for purely research purposes, i.e., attaching importance to secondary problems could have led to the aggravation of

Table 2   Average Observed In-Person Contact Hours and Minutes for Each Treatment Condition

Treatment Condition		Home	School
15 DAY	Average	7:25	2:42
	Range	3:30–15:45	0:10–6:30
	S. D.	2:41	1:41
45 DAY	Average	11:03	3:26
	Range	4:45–20:40	0:00–10:25
	S. D.	4:10	2:47
90 DAY	Average	16:35	7:25
	Range	4:30–37:35	0:00–15:00
	S. D.	10:07	4:48

those problems. Another factor which could have affected treatment outcomes is the concentrated effort it would have taken in those cases where nearly 15 hours of contact were made with the family in a 15-day period. There is reason to believe that a subject who received intensive therapy of that sort would essentially have received qualitatively different therapy from the other subjects in the study. However, it should be recognized that deviations from the research prescriptions were the exceptions rather than the rule. If a researcher is fortunate enough to have a large sample, it may be worthwhile to eliminate these subjects from the experimental sample, treating them perhaps as a special subsample.

The preceding discussion suggests that a major weakness in the study was its inability to control the major variable of experimental interest—time in treatment. Beyond this structural variable, it also appeared that therapists differed greatly in the manner in which they rendered service. (Kiesler [1966] accused much of psychotherapy research as having succumbed to the myth of therapist uniformity, that is, "the selecting of various therapists for a research design on the assumption that these therapists are more alike than different" [p. 112].) Given the fact that ten therapists are bound to differ somewhat in their knowledge of the treatment technology and their techniques of delivery, a special effort was made to obtain an acceptable degree of uniformity among the therapists. First, all therapists at the Project had similar training in behavior modification technology. Second, the treatment procedures were structured so as to insure comparability among the activities of the therapists. Third, each therapist was assigned to all of the treatment conditions, thus eliminating any therapist bias within a given treatment condition. And finally, videotapes and/or audio tapes were made of all interview sessions, and the presentation of these at staff meetings allowed for the continuous training of therapists, the sharpening of therapeutic procedures and the monitoring of service delivery techniques.

Any study which utilizes more than one therapist must face the question of therapist uniformity. While it is possible to standardize treatment procedures, especially in behavioral treatment, via the use of highly structured stepwise procedures, it is much more difficult to standardize the techniques of delivery. "An optimal design would permit statistical evaluation of differences among therapists in their effectiveness" (Kiesler, 1966, p. 130). However, such an investigation would require a factorial design controlling for various therapist variables (Kiesler, 1966; Bergin, 1971). Data from the present study indicate that while the subjects assigned to different therapists did not differ significantly in outcome (Stuart and Lott, 1972a, p. 168), the nonsignificant differences were nonetheless great. To explain these differences, a comprehensive analysis of every aspect of service delivery would be required. In this study, however, only the therapists' handling of behavioral contracts was investigated. This analysis revealed significant differences between the types of contracts which each therapist prepared with clients with respect to the number of privileges, responsibilities, bonuses and sanctions in addition to the number of contracts written with each family (Stuart and Lott, 1972a, p. 166). Therefore, it is evident that despite the efforts made to minimize the likelihood of treatment outcome differences attributable to therapist style, these differences emerged as a very real problem in the present study, accountable for an unknown but possibly large proportion of the variance in results.

Selection of Outcome Variables and Measurement Problems

Whatever the treatment modality, the measurement of treatment outcomes involves three basic issues: (1) *the selection of outcome variables,* (2) *the relevant points of measurement,* and (3) the question of *follow-up.* All of these issues are important and must be thoroughly reviewed prior to initiating a study. Each will be discussed during the course of this chapter, with an emphasis on the problems of implementation.

Four classes of outcome data were collected in Study I: (1) school performance data as measured by attendance, tardiness and grades, and classroom behaviors as rated by teachers on the Pupil Behavior Inventory (Vinter, Sarri, Vorwaller, and Schafer, 1966); (2) social behavior at home, as measured by an original Parent Evaluation Form; (3) behavior in the community, as measured by referral for court services; and (4) attitude changes as measured in the adolescent by the Jesness Social Maladjustment Scale (Jesness, 1962) and in parents by an original Child Management Ideology Scale. In a sense, these categories were preselected for us, since the Project was established to deal with predelinquent and delinquent clients, and these three target areas are generally considered to be suitable parameters for studies in juvenile delinquency. Owing to the belief that therapists could not be expected to render unbiased assessments (Avnet, 1965), all data were supplied by the clients themselves or by salient members in the community such as teachers, counselors, and court officials, as recommended by Fiske (1971a).

148

Once the parameters have been selected, one must be concerned with the selection of the measurement instruments. The critical problem is to find relevant measures. A "valid" evaluative tool may be totally irrelevant for a given population and/or for a given problem. Hence, it is important to find instruments that not only reflect the salient dimensions of outcome but are also sufficiently sensitive to record changes that may occur as a result of intervention.

In the selection of outcome measures, the first decision to be made is whether the instruments used should be global, addressing generalized aspects of behavior, or focal, stressing highly specific target behaviors. The advantages of global measures are that they tend to coincide with the kinds of language which clinicians exchange among themselves, and they may measure dispositions to act which generalize across a range of response classes. They may not, however, adequately assess change in the specific behavioral dimensions which are the targets of the intervention. The advantage of focal measures is their sensitivity to the effects of treatment in particular areas. Their disadvantages, however, are their immunity to what has been termed the "ripple effect" (Kounin and Gump, 1958), a dispersion of either negative or positive changes associated with modification of the target behavior. This possibility of deterioration (Stuart, 1970, Chapter 3; Bergin, 1971, pp. 246-248), coupled with the need to include measures sensitive to the specific behaviors of concern to therapists, would seem to require the inclusion of both global and focal measures.

The second measurement issue to be addressed concerns whether or not the criteria of outcome will be obtrusive (i.e., whether they will be reactive) or nonobtrusive (i.e., nonreactive). Measures such as the Parent Evaluation Form, Child Management Ideology Scale, Jesness, and Pupil Behavior Inventory could be classified as obtrusive. In each instance, parents, adolescents or teachers were cued to some degree about the investigators' expectations and may have been influenced by such response biases as the "guinea-pig" effect, response set, and social desirability (Webb, Campbell, Schwartz, and Sechrest, 1966). Study I also included nonobtrusive measures in the form of student grades, attendance, tardiness and court records. In theory, these parameters would not be readily influenced merely because the subject participated in this phase of the research, but in fact record-keeping errors can have a pointedly adverse effect upon the validity of these measures.

In this type of research, it is almost impossible to avoid reactivity in measurement procedures. As long as these measures of questionable validity are counterbalanced by more unassailable criteria, however, it is believed important that they be included in this type of evaluative research for two reasons. First, they assess dimensions which are of particularly meaningful concern to therapists, clients and salient members of the community. Second, it is by no means certain just how potent the negative impact of repeated application of reactive measurements might be (Goldstein, Heller, and Sechrest, 1966, p. 21).

A third major issue facing the researcher is whether the measures should be individualized or applicable across all experimental subjects. Only group measures were used in Study I for several reasons. First, the research study as it was set up was considered a large-sample study, and therefore it was felt that the measures used should be viable across all experimental subjects. Second, one of the stated purposes of the research program was to develop and test measures suitable for the evaluation of behavioral intervention techniques, which could then be utilized by other researchers and practitioners. Third, since we had reason to expect a large number of referrals and since we were able to assign them randomly to the different groups, we felt that measures could be developed that would be sensitive enough to indicate differences between groups.

It is important, however, to be aware of the value of individualized measures. First, improvement could be indicated by changes in opposite directions for different individuals, which would become evident in individualized measures but not in group measures. Second, if the changes sought for different individuals are different, then standardized measures may be less sensitive than individual measures. And finally, it is clinically desirable, whenever possible, to uniquely determine the treatment criteria for each client (Bergin, 1971). While the individualized approach has a valuable contribution to make, the implementation of such a program of evaluation with a large population is a sobering experience (see Study III).

A final question facing the researcher is whether to use a single measure of outcome or a series of measures. At this time there is no research evidence to support the use of a single instrument to measure change. On the other hand, there appears to be a general consensus among researchers in treatment evaluation (Fiske *et al.,* 1970; Kiesler, 1966; Bergin, 1971) that multifactorial measurement of outcome is desirable. Since we expected multiple changes to occur both within the individual and his environment and within the family structure, it would have been presumptuous to expect one measure to tap all of these different sources of change.

A few of the measures used in this study (such as the Jesness and the Pupil Behavior Inventory) are standardized instruments, a procedure recommended by Fiske *et al.* (1970), while the majority are original questionnaires. In general, it should be noted that all the family measures are subjective and therefore open to the weaknesses of subjective and obtrusive measurements. While most of the school and community measures are objective, they are susceptible to inaccuracy, in that they were obtained from records kept by the schools and the juvenile court. With respect to the school measures, it must be noted that there is a strong tendency for teachers, counselors and others to be influenced by predisposing variables such as the student's social class rather than his or her performance (Garfield, Weiss, and Pollack, 1973), making grades unresponsive to behavioral changes. With respect to court records, it has been shown that inaccuracies as great as 300 percent exist with regard to such tangible variables as the number of days of institutionalization (Huetteman, Briggs, Tripodi, Stuart, Heck, and McConnell, 1970).

When evaluative measures are implemented, a wide range of problems are encountered which deserve attention. Our primary sources of data were the families and schools. We were very successful in obtaining complete data from the families (other than in a few cases where individual members refused), primarily because therapists administered pre- and post-treatment questionnaires during formal sessions—a particular advantage with illiterate or non-English-speaking parents. While some may consider this an invitation to positive response bias and socially acceptable answers, our data indicate that this did not occur.

Data collection in the schools posed a different set of problems. Absences, tardies and grades were obtained from a computer printout at the end of each academic semester. It is possible that Project children were "missed" and reported as absent or tardy more frequently than their "nondeviant" counterparts because the Project students had already earned the "deviant" label and were made more "prominent" in the teachers' view by the presence of the therapists in the schools.

A subsequent analysis revealed a second problem: A positive but very low-correlation of .25 was obtained between the daily and weekly performance grades given to students on daily or weekly "class cards" by teachers and the report card grades given ultimately by teachers. Teachers consistently erred in the direction of being inaccurately positive during the ongoing weeks of intervention, only to right the record after their contact with the students was terminated. Unfortunately, this gave false positive feedback to students and cued parents and therapists to mediate reinforcements at home essentially indiscriminately, i.e., students were as likely to be reinforced for poor work as for good. Additional problems for consistent data collection were continuously created by schedule changes (hence different teachers completed pre-test, post-test and follow-up forms), experimental programs, absent teachers and their substitutes, and various other administrative changes which are inevitable in the schools.

The other two basic issues referred to at the beginning of this section were points of measurement and follow-up. The research design in Study I called for four points of measurement: pre-treatment, post-treatment, 6-month follow-up, and 12-month follow-up. All family data were collected by the therapists, the pre- and post-treatment data being collected during formal sessions, and the follow-up data in the clients' homes. While this was an expensive and time-consuming data collection procedure, it was a highly effective one, with the response rate ranging from a minimum of 78 percent to a maximum of 96 percent after 12 months.

The reality issues of follow-up pose several problems depending on the nature of the research program. First, there may be differential loss from the various experimental groups due to families moving. A second threat is the changing of family composition due to death, divorce, or marriage, all of which could serve as intervening sources of invalidity in attempting to measure the long-term effectiveness of treatment. And third, while it is possible to determine whether the family had other treatment contacts, it would be impossible to evaluate what effects those contacts had. Extra-experimental treatment contact is obviously an important intervening variable on which data should be collected religiously.

In attempting to collect follow-up data from the schools, we were confronted with several new problems. Due to the nature of our data and measures, we were constrained to collect the information during the school semesters. Thus, in a sense, our data collection points were predetermined. An additional problem with which we had to deal, and one over which we had no control, was administrative and policy changes in the school system. Policy changes in grading and attendance procedures could substantially affect the continuity of the data being collected. These data were also naturally affected by adolescents moving from junior high schools to senior high schools, where these policies were different.

Despite these problems, we were able to collect follow-up data with respect to the stability of intervention (see **Table 3**). For example, comparisons between one- and two-parent families yielded significant differences at the 12-month follow-up period on the mother's Child Management Ideology Scale and the Jesness SM Scale. These were also

Table 3   Analysis of Covariance of Changes in the Average Performance of Subjects From One- and Two-Parent Families in the 1970-71 Sample

Outcome Measure	Time of Measurement	One-Parent Families (N=21)	Two-Parent Families (N=61)	F
Grades[a]	Pre $\bar{X}$	5.69	6.44	N/A
	Post	+0.73	−0.01	0.9278
	6 Months	−0.81	−1.24	0.3635
	12 Months	+0.56	+0.33	1.2749
	Net Change, Pre-12 Mo	+0.48	−0.90	2.2332
Absences[b] (Percent)	Pre $\bar{X}$	14.31	11.05	N/A
	Post	−2.13	−5.83	0.7991
	6 Months	+5.84	+0.21	2.1658
	12 Months	+1.61	+0.96	0.2013
	Net Change, Pre-12 Mo	+5.32	−4.66	3.9700*
Mother Parent Evaluation[b]	Pre $\bar{X}$	11.06	10.67	N/A
	Post	+0.21	+0.30	0.1739
	6 Months	+0.22	+0.32	0.3399
	12 Months	+0.60	+0.30	1.7146
	Net Change, Pre-12 Mo	+1.03	+0.92	0.1246
Mother-Client Change[c]		9.36	10.07	N/A
Mother I-D Scale[a]	Pre $\bar{X}$	64.00	66.80	N/A
	Post	+1.45	+2.55	3.8470*
	6 Months	+0.85	+1.06	1.5999
	12 Months	−1.96	+0.70	4.3686*
	Net Change, Pre-12 Mo	+0.34	+4.31	3.9634*
Jesness SM Scale[b]	Pre $\bar{X}$	25.12	23.25	N/A
	Post	+3.34	−0.31	4.1361*
	6 Months	+1.21	+1.27	0.1034
	12 Months	+4.90	+0.72	6.6858*
	Net Change, Pre-12 Mo	+9.45	+1.68	6.8188*
Court Contacts[b] (Percent with one or more)	Pre $\bar{X}$	14.00	8.00	N/A
	Post	−d	−d	
	6 Months	+9.00	−4.00	
	12 Months	0.00	+3.00	
	Net Change, Pre-12 Mo	+9.00	−1.00	
Suspensions[b] (Percent with one or more)	Pre $\bar{X}$	24.00	18.00	N/A
	Post	−d	−d	
	6 Months	−5.00	+6.00	
	12 Months	+15.00	−8.00	
	Net Change, Pre-12 Mo	+10.00	−2.00	

Table 3, continued

[a] With each of these variables, a high score is desirable. In this table, however, arithmetic signs have been corrected for direction of change. Thus, +0.73 in grades means an improvement in school grades.

[b] With each of these variables, a low score is desirable. In this table, however, arithmetic signs have been corrected for direction of change. Thus, −2.13 absences means a decrease (deterioration) in school attendance.

[c] On this item, a lower score shows greater change. Rating made at 12-month follow-up only.

[d] Because the duration of treatment was different for subgroups of subjects, post-treatment measures are omitted because they would be misleading due to the differing amounts of time upon which they would be based.

[*] $p < .05$

found to be significant at the post-test period. In view of the time/ expense issue, do these data vindicate or expunge the necessity for follow-up? Obviously, one study can do neither, but the issue is important enough to be given due consideration in studies of this sort.

Analysis and Conclusions

Four major analyses were conducted with these data. First, since the primary object of the study was to determine whether there were any differences between the three experimental groups (15/45/90), an analysis of covariance was performed on all dependent measures. Fiske (1971b) has challenged the use of pre- and post-test raw scores as the basis for evaluating results. He argues that "under some circumstances, such differences can be expected to correlate as much as -.71 with pre-treatment scores, clients with low pre-treatment scores thus obtaining high 'outcome' or change scores" (Fiske, 1971b, p. 315). This statement has three implications. First, it assumes that indices of outcome will be highly sensitive to the effects of intervention. The correlations between our pre- and post-treatment measures range from lows of .20 and .23 (Pupil Behavior Inventory and Teacher Evaluation Form) to highs of .80 and .88 (mother and father Marital Adjustment Scale of the Parent Evaluation Form). Second, Fiske appears to suggest that "regression toward the mean" will lead to greater change in scores of the more deviant subjects. But as the present research and that of Garfield, Prager, and Bergin (1971) have shown, the fact is that more extreme subjects are likely to show the least amount of change. Finally, the salience of Fiske's argument is obviated through the use of analysis of covariance as a statistical treatment of results (Edwards, 1972, Chapter 18). This method of analysis controls statistically for the likely inequality of subjects randomly assigned to intervention conditions. (For details of the results and conclusions, see Stuart and Tripodi, 1973.)

The second major analysis compared the experimental groups with the "dropout" quasi-control group. Table 4 reveals that the rates of deterioration of school attendance and grades were significantly greater for the "dropout" group. Furthermore, although not statistically significant due to the small number of court contacts after referral to the Project, the quasi-control group subjects were more likely to be referred to the juvenile court than were the experimental subjects (16.7 percent compared to 6.3 percent). These results are particularly relevant in terms of the "value" of treatment, especially since the "dropout" group was equivalent to the experimental group at pre-treatment.

Table 4   Comparison of the Results Experienced by Subjects In the Experimental and "Dropout" Groups[a]

Behavioral Measures	Experimental Group		"Dropout" Group		Significance
Attendance	Mean =	−8.66	Mean =	−34.06	$t = 6.29$
					$df = 70$
	S. D. =	18.32	S. D. =	38.46	$p < .001$
Tardiness	Mean =	−12.20	Mean =	−10.22	$t = 0.2869$
					$df = 61$
	S. D. =	19.79	S. D. =	14.60	ns
Grades	Mean =	−0.19	Mean =	−2.06	$t = 3.01$
					$df = 62$
	S. D. =	1.82	S.D. =	1.42	$p < .01$
Court Contacts After Referral	5 of 79		2 of 12		$X^2 = 1.256$
					$df = 1$
					ns

[a] Determined by subtracting pre-test from post-test score, expressed as improvement (+) or deterioration (−).

The second quasi-control group, the total population of one junior high school on whom attendance data were collected, served as the basis for the third major analysis. These data, represented in **Figure 1**, reveal that the experimental subjects were not only *less deviant* than all the students but in fact *deteriorated less* than the rest of the pupils. As Stuart and Tripodi (1973) point out, "these observations provide some slight vindication for the deterioration...although efforts are obviously necessary to correct this trend in future years of this research" (p. 14).

A final analysis attempted to find out the effect of parental consensus on deviant behavior. Bearing in mind that parental agreement may act as an important mediating variable on changing adolescent behaviors, the responses to the Child Management Ideology Scale and the Parent Evaluation Form were analyzed. In 16 of the 18 possible comparisons, parental consensus increased as a function of treatment. Although not conclusive, these data suggest that parental agreement may serve as a major intermediary variable affecting therapeutic outcome. Support for this is also gained by a pre-test conducted on the Child Management Ideology Scale, which revealed that parents of delinquents and nondelinquents, while having similar averages on the questionnaires (65.4 versus 66.1), differed significantly in the correlations (.12 versus .72—Stuart and Tripodi, 1973).

On the basis of the results summarized here and the methodological problems and issues encountered, the major conclusion reached was that further study of the relationship between time-constrained treatments and outcome was both possible and desirable. It was also concluded that the failure to discriminate between the three time periods (15/45/90 days) was primarily due to (a) overlap in time—resulting in small differences among the three treatment groups, (b) insensitivity of measures—the measures perhaps being too global, and (c) therapist differences—these data were not analyzed but still remained a plausible alternative source of error.

With these factors in mind, Study II was designed essentially as a partial replication of Study I (but with more controls and variables added to eliminate some of the weaknesses observed in the latter). It was hoped that this partial replication would enable us either to discriminate between the effects of time-constrained treatments or to verify the observations of Study I that the outcomes of treatment of different time durations are more homogeneous than disparate.

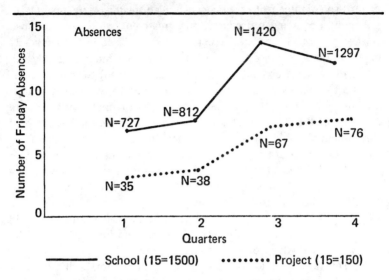

Figure 1 Total Number of Friday Absences and Tardies Per Quarter in One Junior High School for Project-Treated Students Compared To All Students

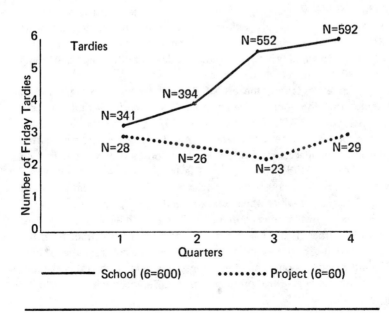

Study Design II (1971-72)

Study II employed a 2x2x2 factorial design which called for the comparison of three factors: time-constrained treatment, treatment with fading or nonfading procedures, and treatment with fixed or open contracts. Two time-constrained groups were utilized in this study—21 days and 60 days. Since the controls for standardization in Study I in terms of hours of contact and duration of treatment were ineffective, an effort was made to obtain greater separation between the two time conditions in Study II. No minimum lengths of treatment time were specified in the first study, and it was felt that the establishment of such minima would enhance the separation of the time conditions. Hence, the range of treatment contact hours for the 21-day condition was set at 4-7 hours and for the 60-day condition at 12-21 hours. The results of Study II indicated that while there was a difference between the 21- and 60-day groups in terms of average hours of family contact (6:13 hours in the 21-day to 12:18 hours in the 60-day), there was still an overlap in the range, with the 21-day ranging from 2:35 to 18:35 hours and the 60-day from 3:00 to 32:10 hours.

The second factor, which had implications for both treatment and contact time, was the use of fading and nonfading procedures. This variable, it was hoped, would discriminate between those cases where there is an abrupt ending of therapy (nonfading) and where there is a gradual disinvolvement by the therapist (fading). Contact during the fading period was only by phone (no post-therapeutic contact being allowed in the nonfading condition) and was limited to 1-2 hours within a period of 15 days for the 21-day condition and 2-4 hours within 30 days for the 60-day condition.

The third factor, the use of fixed and open contracts, was an attempt to bring about some controlled variation in therapist procedures (see Stuart, 1971a; Stuart and Lott, 1972a, 1972b, for descriptions of contracts and contracting procedures). The fixed contract presented alternative privileges, responsibilities, sanctions and bonuses (based on an analysis of Study I contracts). The family negotiated the contract among themselves, and it was kept in force for a minimum period of two weeks, after which renegotiation could take place with therapist involvement. In the open contract condition, there were no alternatives prescribed; the therapist and family negotiated the contract from the very beginning, and they were free to change the contract at any time. If contracting was one area of variability (see below), then this manipulation was expected to produce some differences which would be measurable.

The 2x2x2 factorial design produced eight groups: short fading fixed; short fading open; long fading fixed; long fading open; short nonfading fixed; short nonfading open; long nonfading fixed; and long nonfading open. In addition, the two quasi-control groups—the "dropouts" and the school population from one junior high school— were still available as contrast groups. Some of the main features of Study I were retained in this study: (1) the same therapists were used; (2) the subject population was the same; (3) the same randomization procedures were employed; (4) the maintenance therapists were still available for reactivations; and (5) the same points of measurement were used, namely pre/post/follow-up. Although the data from Study I indicated that pre/post measurement may be sufficient, we decided to collect follow-up data on the Study II clients for two major reasons: First, more focal measures were to be used, and they might have been more sensitive than the measures employed in Study I. Thus, changes which may have occurred but were not measured may become evident in follow-up of the Study II sample. Second, it is important to establish the stability of the treatment before offering it as a viable alternative technology.

Therapist Variation

It has been argued that actual intervention is under the control of the therapist and not the investigator (Krause, 1972). Luborsky, Chandler, Auerbach, Cohen, and Bachrach (1971) assert that therapist variables such as experience, skill, and empathy are important determinants of outcomes in psychotherapy research. Thus, considerable effort went into the examination of the question of therapist variability in Study II, particularly since it was assumed that such differences could have played a significant role in Study I. With this in mind, several investigations were initiated.

The fixed and open contracts were instituted in an attempt to bring about some controlled variation in therapist differences on contract formulation. A fixed contract is one in which the number of privileges, responsibilities, bonuses and sanctions is standardized, with therapists and families negotiating only the details of the agreements. Generally, fixed contracts did appear to offer some advantage in standardizing treatment results across therapists, with three significant differences emerging across therapists in the open contract and none in the fixed contract. In addition, the fixed contract did also appear to be associated with more positive results (see Stuart, Tripodi, and

Jayaratne, 1972).

Beyond efforts to standardize the contract, an effort was made to explore other ways in which therapists differed in the techniques of service delivery. Carter and Levy (1972) first sought to determine the extent to which client actions were instigated (i.e., "the systematic use of specified suggestions and assigned tasks in the patient's daily environment" [Kanfer and Phillips, 1969, p. 452]) by the therapists. Several differences were noted and a decision was made to standardize instigations to be used in association with the fixed contracts in Study III. In addition, Carter and Levy indicated that there were major differences in gross variables such as the degree of directiveness, specificity and positiveness of the therapists and in their selection of targets in verbal exchanges. Thus, our data appeared to agree with Krause (1972) that therapists seem to control their own behavior despite attempts at standardization. The researcher has two alternatives for dealing with the problem of therapist differences. The first is to give up research utilizing more than one therapist, thus literally eliminating differences but making the technology somewhat idiosyncratic. The second is to conduct nomothetic research with more than one therapist, maximizing therapist uniformity and technique delivery and simultaneously studying those standardization attempts as intervening variables. We chose the latter alternative since we were confident that a sufficient degree of standardization could be achieved and since we had already developed methods of measuring some of the intervening variables.

Final Outcome Measures

Twenty-eight outcome measures were employed in Study II—13 relating to school behavior, eight to behavior at home and in the community, and seven to attitude change (note that only seven measures in all were used in Study I). The fourfold increase in measures resulted from the experience of the first year. Although we had no reason to eliminate the parameters used in Study I, for Study II new measures were added and existing ones were modified (for a detailed description of the measures used, see Stuart and Tripodi, 1972).

The intercorrelations between these measures are presented in **Table 5.** These correlational data support the parameters chosen for the study in that the measures cluster around the three major dimensions. That is, out of 110 possible intercorrelations between indices of home behavior, 67 percent reached a level of significance in contrast to 40 percent of 110 possible intercorrelations between indices of school

Table 5 Correlations Among Responses of 1971-72 Subjects at Post-test to All Continuously Scaled Outcome Measures (N=79)[a,b,c]

		1	2	3	4	5	6	7	8	9	10	11	12	13	14	15	16	17	18	19	20	21	22	23	24	25	26	
SCHOOL BEHAVIOR																												
PBI, Scale A	1																											1
PBI, Scale B	2	+	−																									2
PBI, Scale C	3	·	+	−																								3
PBI, Scale D	4	+	·	+	−																							4
PBI, Scale E	5	+	+	·	+	−																						5
Grades	6	+	+	·	·	+	−																					6
Absences	7	·	+	·	+	·	−	·																				7
Numerical Achievement	8	·	+	·	+	·	+	·	−																			8
Language Achievement	9	+	+	·	+	·	·	+	·	−																		9
Counselor Evaluation	10	·	·	+	·	+	·	+	·	·	−																	10
Teacher Evaluation	11	+	+	+	·	+	·	+	·	·	·	−																11
HOME BEHAVIOR																												
Parent Eval., Mo: Mar. Adj.	12	·	·	·	·	·	·	·	·	·	·	·	−															12
Par-Child	13												+	−														13
Total	14			+									+	+	−													14
Change	15												·	+	+	−												15
Parent Eval, Fa: Mar. Adj.	16	+											+	·	+	·	−											16
Par-Child	17												·	+	+	·	+	−										17
Total	18												+	+	+	·	+	+	−									18
Change	19												·	·	·	+	+	·	·	−								19
Client Eval: Punitiveness	20												+	·	+	·	+	+	+	·	−							20
Total	21												+	+	+	·	+	+	+	+	+	−						21
Change	22												·	·	·	+	·	·	·	+	+	+	−					22
ATTITUDE MEASURES																												
I-D Scale, Mother	23	·	·	·	·	·	·	·	·	·	·	·	·	·	·	·	·	·	·	·	·	·	·	−				23
I-D Scale, Father	24			+															+	·		·	+	−	−			24
Client Self-Esteem	25			+					+									+			+	+		·	·	−		25
Jesness SM Scale	26																					·	+	·	+	·	−	26
		1	2	3	4	5	6	7	8	9	10	11	12	13	14	15	16	17	18	19	20	21	22	23	24	25	26	

[a] Number of Ss contributing to each entry is variable due to unobtainability of data, e.g., for absent fathers in one-parent families.

[b] Correlation coefficients corrected for sign.

[c] Plus signs (+) represent correlations with significant levels p .05.

behavior and 33 percent of the six possible intercorrelations between attitude measures (for more detailed analyses, see Stuart and Tripodi, 1972).

In reviewing these data, it is important to note that the clusters of observations may portend the failure of the global intervention methods used in Study II. That is, to the extent that behaviors in home and school settings are under the control of different social contingencies (Bailey, Wolf, and Phillips, 1970; Wahler, 1969), it is as possible that intervention not specifically targeted to both environments will fail as it is possible that a generalized intervention program might succeed. This raises an empirical question which might best be answered by a study designed to measure the effect of home as opposed to school intervention upon home as opposed to school behavior.

Analysis and Conclusions

The analytic procedures followed in Study II adhered to the format described in the previous study. The major analysis was restricted to comparison of the three factors—short (21 day) versus long (60 day), fading versus nonfading, and fixed versus open contracts.

The results of Study II are discussed in detail in the paper by Stuart, Tripodi, and Jayaratne (in press), "The Family and School Treatment Model of Services for Predelinquents." In general, as in Study I, there was a lack of significant findings, but the directional trends were the same, the results indicating again that treatments of different durations are more homogeneous than disparate outcomes. However, it could also be argued that the small number of significant findings occurred by chance, considering the large number of dependent measures. The fading/nonfading conditions showed no significant differences on any of the dependent measures, while the fixed contracts (in contrast to the open contracts) not only helped standardization procedures but also increased parental consensus.

In view of the data from Study I and Study II, it was evident that a new approach was needed for the third year. Two alternatives were available to us. The first was to continue with a similar design by contrasting time-constrained groups but utilizing different measures of change and/or more extreme time differences, e.g., comparing 2-week, 26-week and 52-week treatments. The second alternative, and the one we chose, was harder to accept. We had to defer any further investigation of the optimal length of treatment to a later date and question our original assumption: Is this particular treatment technology effective in its ability to deal with the problems of this client population? Two years of data seemed to indicate that this may not be the case and that our original assumption was wrong. In addition, the Project consultants argued that we really did not have any choice—we must confirm the validity of our approach. In order to do so we needed a somewhat different research design.

Study Design III (1972-73)

In trying to answer the question of whether our treatment is better than no treatment at all, the obvious approach was to compare a treatment group with a no-treatment control group. However, we felt that we could not ethically accommodate a classical control group in the design, nor could we practically have accomplished this due to the many theoretical and reality problems stated earlier. In addition, if we intended to use a control group, we would have to explain to the school system why we were unable to treat clients in our usual fashion, since we had provided immediate service in the past two years. For our purposes, therefore, we had no choice but to find a client population which could be compared with our experimentally treated population.

The selection of an "activity-discussion" group was motivated by several important considerations. First, we needed an intervention condition to which clients could be randomly assigned and which would afford a valid comparison with the experiences of those subjects receiving the focal experimental treatment. Second, this group had to have sufficient appeal to the referring agencies to allow it to be accepted as an alternative to our prime intervention condition. This condition was important not only as a means of ensuring the assignment of a minimum of 30 subjects (which was necessary for our planned statistical analyses) but also to make certain that neither school personnel nor parents would seek treatment elsewhere. Third, this procedure would permit the monitoring of severe problems among untreated adolescents so that in no instance would the withholding of service prove harmful to the subjects.

A major disadvantage in the use of the activity-discussion group was the possibility that the group might indeed have a beneficial impact. Staffed by a group leader experienced with adolescent groups and one of the full-time Project therapists, it was planned that each activity-discussion group would meet once a week for one hour and have from five to eight adolescents. During the one-hour sessions, the major emphasis would be on planned activities such as educational games, handicrafts, etc., with a general discussion of school and/or home problems if requested by the members. In essence, the control group contacts with the Project therapists were both quantitatively and qualitatively different from the contacts the experimental sample had with the therapists. The therapist would see the parents of an activity group adolescent *only* at pre-treatment and post-treatment—when evaluation data are collected. But, through contacts with the therapists and constructive and focused peer interaction, the group experience might have had an unanticipated positive impact upon the participants. This impact, if it exists, would be analogous to the salubrious effects of placebo control conditions in other studies, and therefore it could only operate to make any emerging comparisons with the focal procedure more conservative.

Design Modifications

The problems encountered in this design were somewhat different from those in the two previous designs. First, we had to "sell" the idea of an activity-discussion group to the schools. Not only were the majority of the school counselors and social workers (our major referral sources) generally opposed to the idea of group treatment, but two years of saturation about the values of behavior therapy and family treatment seems to have made some inroads. Second, there was a considerable degree of resistance to the whole idea of an activity-discussion group from the therapists. Although our data did not indicate that the therapists' treatment efforts had any significant effects (as measured by our scales), they argued that much of the verbal feedback they received from the families and school personnel was positive and, further, that there were positive changes which our scales were not recording for whatever reason. Third, a severe threat to the nonbehavioral contact with the activity-discussion group subjects has been brought about by the fact that Project therapists had trained some of the school counselors and social workers in behavioral techniques (such as contracting, contingency management, etc.). Hence, we were in the position of having to control and monitor the possible use of behavioral techniques by school personnel with those adolescents in the activity-discussion group, and there were indications that this sometimes did occur. Fourth, the number of referrals may be reduced simply because the school personnel are unwilling to accept the activity-discussion group as an alternative model of treatment. And finally, we developed a "new" group of clients whom we labeled "political cases." These were clients who were randomly assigned to the activity-discussion group, but since they continued their disruptive behavior in the schools therapists were obliged to intervene at the family level. When this did occur, a political case was created, and we were forced to deviate from our random assignments by removing the adolescent from the activity-discussion group and treating him according to the family model. These families were eliminated from the data analysis, and they comprise a third "contrast" group of subjects. Since these cases are likely to be the most difficult ones, a positive bias may have been created favoring the activity-discussion group, thereby making the intergroup comparison more conservative.

A procedural problem in executing the experimental design of Study III was that of handling the random assignment of subjects to the focal experimental or activity-discussion-group conditions. Data from Study I, which were not available until the end of the Study II intervention year, created the suspicion that the randomization procedure followed in the first two years might have actually been under therapist control—a practice which, if true, might partially explain the lack of significant differences occurring in the outcome of cases assigned to each of these groups. Therefore we decided to select new sets of random numbers for every successive block of six referrals—three for each condition—with referrals being randomly assigned to therapists. The essence of the procedural shift in randomization was to render case assignment virtually immune from therapist assignment.

In addition to the design changes, several modifications were made in the treatment format. One of the major changes involved the prescribed intervention procedures. Since an analysis of the Study II data indicated that significant therapist differences were present, more rigid treatment procedures were instituted in a further attempt to bring about uniformity. The first of these prescribed procedures involved the exclusive use of fixed contracts. As our data indicated, this should bring about more uniformity in types of problems, number of privileges and responsibilities, and total length of contracts (see Stuart and Lott, 1972b; Stuart, Tripodi, and Jayaratne, in press). A second method of increasing uniformity was the introduction of "fixed instigations." These instigations were derived from an analysis of the instigative behavior of therapists with the more "successful" cases in Study II (Carter and Levy, 1973). The fixed instigations prescribed not only what instigations to make, but also the essential verbal format as well as the point in time (in terms of the sequential process of treatment). Finally, the contents of the first four interviews were prescribed, such that all therapists would be required to conduct their interviews according to specified guidelines.

Obviously, these precautions and procedures do not guarantee therapist uniformity, but they do provide more controlled and analyzable data. For example, by examining the contracts negotiated by the therapists, the extent of therapist deviation from the fixed format can be determined. A similar analysis would reveal any trends in the instigative behavior of therapists. While it is possible that this type of "control" may bring about some rigidity in the therapeutic process and perhaps inhibit therapist "spontaneity," it appears to be necessary if we are to have any command over therapist variability.

Measurement Refinements

As indicated before, the instruments used in Studies I and II measure group performance in that they are administered to all cases in both groups, and statistical analyses attempt to differentiate between the two groups. In view of the correlational data from Study II and the nonfindings from some scales across two years of research, only 12 scales were retained for use in Study III. However, it was felt that the addition of an individualized measure was feasible and desirable at this point in time, thus adding a new dimension for statistical analysis.

Since a major referral problem was inappropriate and unacceptable behavior in the classroom, we set up a monitoring system whereby a subsample of the Project adolescents would be observed in their classes. Two academic class hours were randomly selected for each adolescent in the sample. A "classroom observer" then recorded the behaviors of the client along with the rest of the class at 15-second intervals according to a "behavior checklist"; thus each client was compared to his classmates. These data should provide comparative behavioral measures on the classroom activities of Project and non-Project adolescents for a given number of class hours.

The cost and logistical problems associated with this one behavioral measure are enormous (perhaps a reason why such procedures are shunned in large sample studies). First, due to overlap in classes, a number of research assistants are required if these data are to be collected regularly, thus creating problems of cost and observer reliability. Second, due to changing schedules and/or administrative changes, the classrooms observed during the baseline period may not be the same as those observed during treatment—which may lead to inaccurate comparisons. Third, since truancy and tardiness are major problems with those adolescents referred to the Project, the observers quite often find the clients missing from the classroom. Hence, the time period within which the data are being collected may vary from client to client since we are collecting data on an absolute number of class hours. And finally, although the observers are not identified as Project staff, the adolescents not only learned of their identity but often knew who was being observed, causing a major threat to the validity of the observations.

The one other major modification in Study III is related to the points of measurement. Whereas in the previous two years the evaluative measures were administered at pre-treatment and post-treatment, they are now administered at pretreatment, after a period of four months from the beginning of therapy. The four-month point of measurement has been decided upon for several reasons. First, since the design calls for unlimited treatment, a uniform point of data collection is necessary in order to retain some semblance of standardization and to enable statistical analyses. Second, our experience has shown us that four months would provide adequate time for treatment as well as change. And finally, these data would indicate whether further treatment was necessary and what modifications in treatment, if any, are desirable. (For the results of this study, see Stuart, Jayaratne, and Tripodi, 1973).

Recommendations

The three studies discussed in this chapter attempt to measure the effectiveness of a behavioral treatment program in dealing with the problems of junior high school and senior high school adolescents. The lack of differentiation between the time-constrained treatments in Studies I and II resulted in the unlimited-treatment group versus activity-discussion group design of Study III. Each study was presented and discussed in turn, and the emphasis has been on the methodological issues, both practical and theoretical, involved in the design and implementation of treatment outcome research. Out of this three-year program have emerged several tentative recommendations for investigators conducting treatment research in the schools in particular and long-term outcome research in general:

(1) Research design flexibility is a *must* in long-term treatment outcome studies. This flexibility must exist not only within a given design (to deal with unforeseen problems) but also from year to year,

when it may be necessary to consider alternate intervention plans, subject populations, therapist configurations, and the like. The implication is that "formative evaluation" (Weiss, 1972) must take place, such that progress can be examined and modifications made, if necessary.

(2) A second major recommendation is to build on experience and data from previous research and other studies. The results from the first study year should be thoroughly analyzed prior to making any decisions on the second year of study. This recommendation is related to the first in that design flexibility and evaluation is an integral part of building on existing data.

(3) While it is probably impossible to achieve complete uniformity among therapists, substantial control over therapeutic procedures can be gained via the use of a prescribed stepwise format. To the extent that it is feasible, these therapist differences should be controlled and studied as intervening variables.

(4) When a research design calls for time-constrained treatment groups, "maintenance" therapists (or their equivalent) should be available to activate cases if necessary. In addition to being an ethical responsibility, it could prove to be a valuable research "tool" in the collection of follow-up data.

(5) While the "control group" versus "contrast group" debate continues, we feel that it is a moot issue in treatment research in the natural environment, where a no-treatment control group is extremely difficult to obtain. Thus, an investigator conducting treatment outcome research should be well aware of the possibilities of using quasi-control groups as alternatives to nontreated control groups.

(6) The evaluation of treatment outcome requires multiple measurement. Our data indicate that changes took place in school attendance, attitude, and marital relations, among others. While all of these specific areas are relevant to our intervention technology, no one instrument could have measured them all.

(7) Related to the idea of multifactorial measurement is the issue of who does the measuring. We believe that the evaluation should be done by salient members of the community. While it may be interesting to obtain therapist evaluations, the literature indicates that these data have very little validity (Avnet, 1965; Paul, 1969).

(8) While experimental groups may not vary on some common criteria, it is quite possible that individuals within the groups may reveal important changes on these dimensions. Therefore, a strong case can be made for individual case analyses with individualized measures. Although the collection of individualized data is expensive and time-consuming, it would be valuable to conduct a few idiographic studies

(with reversals, multiple baselines, Markovian or time-series analyses, etc.) on a random subsample in a nomothetic study. These data may expose differences overlooked by the group measures.

(9) A much less controversial but costly recommendation is the deployment of subprojects, that is, special evaluative and hypothesis-testing programs within a major study. The studies on interaction (Carter and Levy, 1972) and instigations (Carter and Levy, 1973) were two such subprojects. If utilized effectively, subprojects could serve a useful and important function in the overall program.

(10) The question of follow-up is controversial. While our Study I data indicated that 6-month and 12-month follow-ups may be redundant (in that they show no differences from post-treatment measurement), we are continuing to collect follow-up data for Study II primarily to establish long-term stability of treatment and to validate the findings of Study I. But if the follow-up data from Study II indicate that there are no differences from post to 6-month to 12-month, then indeed we would have to question the cost/benefit value of repeated follow-up assessments. While we are skeptical about the utility of follow-up at this point, we hesitate to make a definite statement until more data have been collected and analyzed.

Footnotes

1.   This research was supported in 1970-71 by a grant of 314(d) funds administered by the State of Michigan Department of Mental Health and in 1971-73 by grant number MH 21452 from the Center for Studies of Crime and Delinquency, National Institute of Mental Health.

2.   The authors wish to acknowledge the valuable contributions of three consultants: Montrose M. Wolf of the University of Kansas, G. R. Patterson of the Oregon Research Institute, and Harold Stevenson of the University of Michigan. Their suggestions invariably improved the research, but they are nonetheless not responsible for our failure to act upon all of their recommendations.

References

Adams, S. Some findings from correctional caseload research. *Federal Probation,* 1967, *31,* 48-57.

Avnet, H. H. How effective is short-term therapy? In L. R. Wolberg (Ed.), *Short-term psychotherapy.* New York: Grune and Stratton, 1965.

Bailey, J. S., Wolf, M. M., and Phillips, E. L. Home-based reinforcement and the modification of predelinquents' classroom behavior. *Journal of Applied Behavior Analysis,* 1970, *3,* 223-233.

Bergin, A. E. The evaluation of therapeutic outcomes. In A. E. Bergin and S. L. Garfield (Eds.), *Handbook of psychotherapy and behavior change: An empirical analysis.* New York: John Wiley and Sons, 1971.

Carter, R. D. and Levy, R. L. Interim report on interaction research. Unpublished manuscript, Family and School Consultation Project, Ann Arbor, Michigan, 1972.

Carter, R. D. and Levy, R. L. Interim report on instigation research. Unpublished manuscript, Family and School Consultation Project, Ann Arbor, Michigan, 1973.

Edwards, A. L. *Experimental design in psychological research.* (4th ed.) New York: Holt, Rinehart and Winston, 1972.

Fiske, D. W. *Measuring the concepts of personality.* Chicago: Aldine, 1971a.

Fiske, D. W. The shaky evidence is slowly put together. *Journal of Consulting and Clinical Psychology,* 1971b, *37,* 314-315.

Fiske, D. W., Hunt, H. F., Luborsky, L., Orne, M. T., Parloff, M. D., Reiser, F., and Tuma, A. H. Planning of research on effectiveness of psychotherapy. *American Psychologist,* 1970, *25,* 727-737.

Frank, J. D., Gliedman, L. H., Imber, S. D., Stone, A. R., and

Nash, E. H. Patients' expectancies and relearning as factors determining improvement in psychotherapy. *American Journal of Psychiatry,* 1959, *115,* 961-968.

Garfield, S. L., Prager, R. A., and Bergin, A. E. Evaluating outcome in psychotherapy: A hardy perennial. *Journal of Consulting and Clinical Psychology,* 1971, *37,* 307-313.

Garfield, J. C., Weiss, S. L., and Pollack, E. A. Effects of the child's social class on school counselor's decision-making. *Journal of Counseling Psychology,* 1973, *20,* 166-168.

Goldstein, A. P., Heller, K., and Sechrest, L. B. *Psychotherapy and the psychology of behavior change.* New York: John Wiley and Sons, 1966.

Huetteman, M. J., Briggs, J., Tripodi, T., Stuart, R. B., Heck, E. T., and McConnell, J. V. A descriptive comparison of three populations of adolescents known to the Washtenaw County Juvenile Court: Those referred for or placed in psychiatric hospitals, those placed in correctional settings, and those released following hearings. Unpublished manuscript, Family and School Consultation Project, Ann Arbor, Michigan, 1970.

Imber, S. D., Frank, J. D., Nash, E. H., Stone, A. R., and Gliedman, L. H. Improvement and amount of therapeutic contact: An alternative to the use of no-treatment controls in psychotherapy. *Journal of Consulting Psychology,* 1957, *21,* 309-315.

Jesness, C. F. *The Jesness Inventory.* Palo Alto, California: Consulting Psychologists Press, 1962.

Kanfer, F. H. and Phillips, J. S. A survey of current behavior therapies and a proposal for classification. In C. M. Franks (Ed.), *Behavior therapy: Appraisal and status.* New York: McGraw-Hill, 1969.

Kershaw, D. N. Issues in income maintenance experimentation. In P. H. Rossi and W. Williams (Eds.), *Evaluating social programs: Theory, practice, and politics.* New York: Seminar Press, 1972.

Kiesler, D. J. Some myths of psychotherapy research and the search for a paradigm. *Psychological Bulletin,* 1966, *65,* 110-136.

Kounin, J. S. and Gump, P. V. The ripple effect in discipline. *Elementary School Journal,* 1958, *59,* 158-162.

Krause, M. S. Experimental control as a sampling problem in counseling and therapy research. *Journal of Counseling Psychology,* 1972, *19,* 340-346.

Luborsky, L., Chandler, M., Auerbach, A. H., Cohen, J., and Bachrach, H. M. Factors influencing the outcome of psychotherapy: A review of quantitative research. *Psychological Bulletin,* 1971, *75,* 145-185.

Meltzoff, J. and Kornreich, M. *Research in psychotherapy.* New York: Atherton Press, 1970.

Patterson, G. R., McNeal, S., Hawkins, N., and Phelps, R. Reprogramming the social environment. *Journal of Child Psychology and Psychiatry,* 1967, *8,* 181-195.

Paul, G. L. Behavior modification research: Design and tactics. In C. M. Franks (Ed.), *Behavior therapy: Appraisal and status.* New York: McGraw-Hill, 1969.

Reid, W. J. and Shyne, A. W. *Brief and extended casework.* New York: Columbia University Press, 1969.

Shlien, J. M. Cross-theoretical criteria for the evaluation of psychotherapy. *American Journal of Psychotherapy,* 1966, *20,* 125-134.

Shlien, J. M., Mosak, H. H., and Dreikurs, R. Effect of time limits: A comparison of two psychotherapies. *Journal of Consulting Psychology,* 1962, *9,* 31-34.

Stuart, R. B. *Trick or treatment.* Champaign, Illinois: Research Press, 1970.

Stuart, R. B. Behavioral contracting within the families of delinquents. *Journal of Behavior Therapy and Experimental Psychiatry,* 1971a, *2,* 1-11.

Stuart, R. B. Research in social work: Social casework and social group work. In R. Morris (Ed.), *Encyclopedia of social work.* New York: National Association of Social Workers, 1971b.

Stuart, R. B., Jayaratne, S., and Tripodi, T. Changing of adolescent deviant behavior through reprogramming the behavior of parents and teachers: An experimental approach. Paper presented at the 84th annual meeting of the American Psychological Association, Montreal, August 1973.

Stuart, R. B. and Lott, L. A., Jr. Behavioral contracting with delinquents: A cautionary note. *Journal of Behavior Therapy and Experimental Psychiatry,* 1972a, *3,* 161-169.

Stuart, R. B. and Lott, L. A., Jr. Fixed behavioral contracts and instigation programs: An initial description. Unpublished manuscript, Family and School Consultation Project, Ann Arbor, 1972b.

Stuart, R. B. and Tripodi, T. Contingency contracting in treatment of delinquents: 1972-73 continuation grant proposal. Behavior Change Laboratories, Ann Arbor, Michigan, 1972.

Stuart, R. B. and Tripodi, T. Experimental evaluation of three time-constrained behavioral treatments for predelinquents and delinquents. In R. D. Rubin, J. P. Brady, and J. D. Henderson (Eds.), *Advances in Behavior Therapy.* Vol. 4. New York: Academic Press, 1973.

Stuart, R. B., Tripodi, T., and Jayaratne, S. The family and school treatment model of services for predelinquents. Journal of Research in Crime and Delinquency. In press.

Tharp, R. G. and Wetzel, R. J. *Behavior modification in the natural environment.* New York: Academic Press, 1969.

Vinter, R. D., Sarri, R. C., Vorwaller, D. J., and Schafer, W. E. *Pupil Behavior Inventory: A manual for administration and scoring.* Ann Arbor, Michigan: Campus Publishers, 1966.

Wahler, R. G. Setting generality: Some specific and general effects of child behavior therapy. *Journal of Applied Behavior Analysis,* 1969, *2,* 239-246.

Webb, E. J., Campbell, D. T., Schwartz, R. D., and Sechrest, L. *Unobtrusive measures: Nonreactive research in the social sciences.* Chicago: Rand McNally, 1966.

Weiss, C. H. *Evaluation research.* Englewood Cliffs, New Jersey: Prentice-Hall, 1972.

Benefit-Cost Analysis and the Evaluation of Mental Retardation Programs

8

William B. Neenan[1]

Introduction

This paper has a double purpose: 1) to present a simplified yet critical discussion of the benefit-cost technique and 2) to explore the applicability of this technique to the evaluation of mental retardation programs. This double task will be accomplished in three stages: 1) a description of benefit-cost analysis; 2) a review of how it has been used to evaluate human investment and, more specifically, mental retardation programs; and 3) a concluding critique of benefit-cost analysis.

Benefit-Cost Analysis

Benefit-cost analysis construed in the narrow sense of quantifying in dollar terms the costs of a project and comparing them with the dollar value of the project's outcome is of comparatively recent origin. The Flood Control Act of the 74th Congress in 1936 stipulated that the U. S. Federal Government should undertake water resource projects "if the benefits to whomsoever they may accrue are in excess of estimated costs." In the intervening years, a growing consensus about technical details to be utilized in evaluating such projects has led to the refinement of technique. In the 1960's, benefit-cost analysis and the related technique, cost-effectiveness analysis, were given prominence when President Johnson endorsed the PPBS (Planning-Programming-Budgeting System), and all federal agencies were required to evaluate their programs in terms of these techniques. At this time notable efforts were made, especially by the Department of Health, Education, and Welfare, to evaluate human investment programs. Most recently, these techniques have been increasingly applied to measure the impact of various activities on environmental quality.

Basic Concept

The basic concept of benefit-cost analysis is simple.[2] It is a systematic attempt to compare the inputs of any action with its outcomes in terms of a commensurable unit, usually monetary. The purpose of such an exercise, of course, is to determine whether the outcome is worth the candle. Harberger concludes a discussion of benefit-cost analysis directed to his fellow economists with this peroration:

> And so, having made my plea, let me salute the profession with what might well have been the title of this paper, with what is certainly the key that points to the solution of most problems in applied welfare economics, with what surely should be the motto of any society that we applied welfare economists might form, and what probably, if only we could learn to pronounce it, should be our password:

Equation 1.

$$\int_{z=0}^{z^*} \sum_i D_i(z) \frac{\delta x_i}{\delta z} dz \qquad 3$$

where D_i = the excess (distortion) of marginal social benefit over marginal social cost per unit level of an outcome i.

x_i = the number of units of outcome i.

z = the policy variable whose effects we wish to measure.

This notation can be clarified, even if not put into pronounceable form, by applying it to a hypothetical mental retardation program. Assume we are evaluating a special education program that provides counseling and vocational guidance to help clients move from high school to unsheltered full employment. First, we need to know the technical relationship between small program changes, say, hiring one more counselor, and the program outcome which can be defined in terms of hours of counseling and vocational guidance but ultimately must be expressed in terms of finding full, unsheltered employment for a student. This technical relationship is expressed by $\frac{\delta x_i}{\delta z}$. The measurement of such an input-output relationship is necessary but not sufficient in itself for benefit-cost analysis. We may know, for example, that eighty placements will result from adding one counselor to a staff for one year but this information alone does not allow us to judge whether the candle, in this instance the placement of eighty students, is worth the resource cost of one counselor for one year. Comparing eighty placements with one teacher is like comparing a partridge with a pear tree. They are in themselves incommensurable.

D_i introduces the common denominator which allows us to evaluate the technical relationship $\left(\frac{\delta x_i}{\delta z}\right)$ in terms of comparable benefits and costs. If we: 1) can estimate the total gains evaluated in dollar terms accruing not only to one student but also to the rest of society because of his placement, and 2) we know the cost of one counselor for one year, then 3) since we know the technical relationship between teacher input and placement $\left(\frac{\delta x_i}{\delta z}\right)$ we can easily determine D_i, or the gain (or loss) to society resulting from one student being moved from high school to unsheltered full employment by the program. The total gain (or loss) to society from the program depends on how large the program is, or in terms of the above notation, how large is z^*, the input measured in terms of counselors employed.

Price Signals

There is nothing particularly arcane about the nature of benefit-cost judgments. They are contained at least implicitly in all decision processes. The effects of an intricate benefit-cost calculus, for example, are seen in the price signals generated by the market economy. Assume first an individual with given tastes, educational level, income and wealth. These in turn are aggregated over all consumers and, through interaction with market supply conditions, they determine the relative price structure, which is the private market's relative evaluation of all goods. Thus the consumer possessing his own peculiar material and psychic endowments performs at least implicitly a benefit-cost calculation whenever he chooses from the possibilities that confront him. These choices feed information back into the market system, which is in turn reflected in the relative prices of final products and factor inputs.

In the public sector, however, evaluative signals are generated only vaguely and intermittently through such devices as voting and the various modes of political action. The fact that no political mechanism attaches unequivocal dollar values to political actions does not mean that public services provide no benefits to individuals. Reality is more extensive, even when considering merely individual economic welfare, than can be recorded on the T-accounts of private enterprise. Benefit-cost analysis could at least partially overcome this informational lacuna by generating signals similar to those that are provided automatically in the private market by the "invisible hand."

There are thus three main tasks for benefit-cost analysis:
1. the identification and quantification of all the benefits attributable to a particular program,
2. the identification and quantification of all costs attributable to the program,
3. the translation of benefits and costs into a comparable common denominator, typically their present value.

Program Benefits

Public services provide both direct and indirect benefits to individuals. Direct benefits often cannot be essentially distinguished from the benefits individuals enjoy from the consumption of goods and services supplied by the private market. Water service, trash disposal, parking space, and medical treatment are sometimes provided privately, sometimes publicly. These services are often best financed through user fees which serve the same allocational function as do prices in the private market. Indirect benefits, however, which may be called external benefits, introduce us to the realm of collective goods, in which a service directly benefiting one individual also generates some value for others. In more formal terminology, a service generating indirect benefits may be said to enter as an argument in the utility functions of two or more individuals.

Since one person's enjoyment of a collective service does not preclude another's enjoyment and often is even necessary for it, services which generate indirect benefits are called nonrival in consumption. Public health, education, and welfare programs are examples of services which provide indirect benefits to groups other than the direct recipients of the program. Because the price mechanism usually cannot be used to ration services which are nonrival in consumption, it is often impossible to make a market-type evaluation of the indirect benefits of these programs, and thus program outcomes which would result simply from market interactions would not be welfare maxima. For example, to the extent that people in society other than mental retardates themselves receive some monetary or psychic gain from programs directly affecting mental retardates, there will be underprovision of these programs if only the mental retardates are called upon to pay for benefits received.

Program benefits can also be viewed as either consumption or investment benefits. A consumption benefit is any psychic satisfaction generated by a program. An investment benefit is any increased capitalized net economic worth attributable to a program. Investment benefits can be translated into consumption benefits in future periods. Consumption benefits generated by a mental retardation counseling program might, for example, be 1) the increased emotional adaptability of the retardate, 2) reduced anxiety and stress among his siblings, and 3) satisfaction that third parties in society derive from knowing that mental retardates are being given such assistance. Investment benefits from such a program might be 1) the present value of the increased income flow which the retardates would earn as a consequence of the counseling as well as 2) the economic value of the personal services and physical resources which are now freed for other uses due to the increased independence of the retardate. Despite computational complexities which may be encountered, it should usually be possible to make fairly accurate estimates of investment benefits. However, problems inherent in obtaining an accurate measure of such nonmarket values as individuals' attitudes toward programs make the measurement of total consumption benefits more problematic.

All program benefits, whether they are classified direct and indirect, or consumption and investment, should normatively be considered benefits only if they are actually judged to be such by some beneficiaries. The citizen alone must judge when a course of action benefits any other citizen.[4] Benefit-cost analysis therefore is a computational device for discovering this citizen evaluation when automatic evaluations from the private market are either deficient or totally wanting. Its ultimate grounding, however, is conceptually the evaluation of individuals.

Program Costs

Program costs should be measured in reference to the opportunity cost of a program, that is, what must be foregone in order to provide the service. The motto for decision-makers living in a world with limited resources should be: "There is no such thing as a free lunch." Program benefits are purchased only in return for certain costs. Hence it must be asked: How would these resources have been employed if they were not used here? If they would all have been totally unemployed, then the opportunity cost of this particular program is zero.[5] If they could have been used in some other program, however, then the value of the foregone benefits in the supplanted program is the real cost of the program in question.[6] In most instances, factor prices of program inputs are a reasonably good first approximation of the opportunity cost of resources utilized in any particular program.[7]

Discount Rate

An important final step must be taken before benefits and costs can be compared. Benefits and costs which are realized in the future must be discounted to a common present value basis by an appropriate discount rate. Discounting is especially important in the case of evaluations for human investment programs since the time horizon over which they generate benefits often varies notably across programs. The higher the discount rate, the more favorable will be the benefit-cost ratio for programs with a short payoff period relative to programs with a longer payoff period.[8] The effect of discounting can be seen by referring to the following generalized objective function characteristic of a benefit-cost analysis conducted with no budget constraint:

Equation 2.

$$\text{Max: Present Net Value of the Program} = \sum_{t=0}^{n} \frac{B_t - C_t}{(1 + r)^t}$$

Subject only to the constraint that the present value of the program ≥ 0

where B_t = program benefits in year t

C_t = program costs in year t

r = appropriate discount rate

n = time horizon for evaluation of the program

Assume that 1) the total cost of the project is 10, all incurred in period 0; and 2) benefits of 4, 4, and 4 are realized in periods 2, 3, and 4 with none realized after that. It is clear that there exists a discount rate which can reduce the present net value of the program below zero. For example, with a discount rate of six percent the present net value of the program is .09. However, if the discount rate is seven percent the present net value is a negative .19.[9] Under the simple decision rule that accepts any program whose benefit-cost ratio is greater than one, the program would be approved with a six percent discount rate but disallowed with a seven percent rate.

One of the most controversial aspects of benefit-cost analysis concerns precisely the choice of an appropriate discount rate. There are, in general, two contrary approaches to this problem based, respectively, on the contentions that the discount rate should reflect social time preference and private opportunity cost.[10] Those espousing social time preference contend that the choice of a rate for discounting benefits and costs of public projects is reductively a political determination of the relative value of present and future consumption. The private opportunity cost school, on the other hand, argues that since the real cost of public investment is the marginal rate of return on investment foregone in the private sector, this private rate of return should be used to discount future values. In practice, the social time preference school generally advocates the use of a lower discount rate than does that favoring a private opportunity rate. Consequently they implicitly favor more public investment than does the latter group. But even though a consensus does not exist concerning the rationale for choosing a rate of discount, there is absolutely no controverting the judgment that some nonzero discount rate must be used in benefit-cost analysis.[11]

Criteria for Choice

Once a program's benefits and costs have been estimated and discounted to a present value, a criterion must then be applied to determine which programs should be adopted.[12] Under the strong assumption that there is no budget constraint, two decision rules are applicable: 1) a program should be adopted on efficiency grounds if the present value of its total benefits is greater than the present value of its total costs; and 2) the scale of the program should be increased to the point where marginal benefits from the program equal marginal costs. However, if there is a budgetary constraint, which is the more typical situation, then the applicable decision rule is that the difference between the present value of benefits and costs should be maximized.

Constraints and Suboptimization

In the discussion to this point two important assumptions have been accepted: 1) that programs are to be evaluated with no operative budgetary constraints and from the viewpoint of society at large; and 2) that benefits and costs are to be calculated with no attention given to their equitable distribution. Both these assumptions warrant further attention. Actually, all benefit-cost analyses concern programs that exist in a context of financial budgetary constraint and suboptimizing behavior. Financial constraints prevent agencies from automatically either adopting a program with a positive net benefit or expanding it to the margin where program benefits equal costs. Instead some choice must be made among programs, all or many of which presumably have a benefit-cost ratio greater than one. Furthermore, governmental agencies may be assumed to suboptimize their behavior, that is, they maximize goals which may well be in conflict with goals of higher levels of government or of society at large. Shoup has pointed out two important benefit-cost problem areas where local government suboptimizing behavior ("worm's-eye local view") may well conflict with grand optimization ("bird's-eye national picture").[13] First, local governments seeking to maximize the welfare of their own citizens will discount the future at a lower rate than the opportunity cost to society of foregone investment if, as is the case in the United States, local government borrowing is subsidized by the federal and state governments. Second, they will also consider merely the locally borne tax-costs of a program rather than the real resource cost to society. To the extent local taxes are exported to other jurisdictions, decisions based on a local benefit-cost calculus will differ from those based on a national perspective. A similar distortion can arise if exported benefits are disregarded.

Distributional Pattern

There has been increasing uneasiness recently with the emphasis placed by benefit-cost analysis on maximizing aggregate output to the neglect of distributional outcomes. Formal welfare economics traditionally has been concerned with the analysis of criteria which assure that the Pareto frontier is reached. Since the Pareto criterion accepts as normative any existing distribution of resources it is essentially a conservative force.[14] It is not necessary, however, that even a program whose benefit-cost ratio is considerably in excess of one meets the Pareto requirement that some citizens enjoy thereby a welfare gain with no citizen suffering a welfare decrement. Typically, some people suffer reduced welfare from programs that notably increase total output. Even more disturbing is that the most efficient programs in benefit-cost terms may well have distributional implications which are directly contrary to public policy.[15]

A health or education project directed to a high income target population may often generate greater marginal benefits than one directed to a lower income population. For example, a screening program among high income professionals may discover fewer cases of disease than among a low income population; but efficiency benefits, measured in terms of aggregate increased income attributable to the screening, may well be greater for the program directed to the high income group. Similarly, if benefits are measured in terms of market productivity, there is a built-in bias against programs directed toward women, who have lower labor force participation rates than men, and older people who have retired from the work force. Likewise programs designed to serve profoundly or severely retarded individuals, who usually never enter the labor force, will necessarily have little or no payoff if measured in terms of increased market productivity.

Some distributional consideration can be introduced into benefit-cost analysis by modifying efficiency benefits with equity weights designed to reflect the relative value attached to a dollar payoff to different groups. Thus a disease screening program among high income professional people may well have a high dollar efficiency return, but no one other than the direct participants may be willing to support these programs. Consequently the equity weights for these benefit dollars would be zero and the weighted benefit-cost ratio would be zero. On the other hand, a program to improve the social adjustment of mental retardates in low income families might well possess a high equity weighting and thus, even though the efficiency return may be negligible, the program would have a weighted benefit-cost ratio considerably greater than one.

How should such weights be determined? The introduction of equity-weighted efficiency benefits into benefit-cost analysis has hitherto foundered on this practical question. Various approaches have been suggested: use the weights that are implicit in previous political decisions, such as in the determination of income tax rates; derive them by analyzing voting data, or from attitudinal surveys.[16] Each of these procedures, however, leaves something to be desired.[17] Harberger and Wisecarver capture fairly well the current skeptical attitude of economists concerning the feasibility of incorporating distributional considerations in benefit-cost analysis. "That this concern is justified in most cases cannot be denied, but no one has as yet come up with a systematic measure of net redistributional benefit or cost that has even a remote chance of commanding widespread professional support. In this area we must confess to being pessimists in the sense that we doubt that the profession will approach consensus on any formal mechanism for dealing quantitatively with the welfare impacts of distributional changes."[18]

Human Investment and Program Evaluation

Although Adam Smith considered human endowments to be part of the capital wealth of a nation, economists have only recently used the concept of human investment extensively in the analysis of health and education programs. Some of the reluctance to incorporate the human capital concept into economic analysis has been based on the feeling that it is somehow demeaning to an understanding of people as morally independent beings.[19] Such reluctance, however, seems misplaced in view of the analytical development and practical applications of this concept in the past decade which have proved valuable in evaluating health and education expenditures. In the only significant attempt to calculate the benefits and costs of mental retardation programs, Conley relies implicitly on the human capital model.

In his analysis, Conley first discusses the nature of programs in five major mental retardation program areas:

1. residential care
2. educational efforts for those not institutionalized
3. clinical services, such as diagnosis, evaluation, counseling, and referral
4. employment programs
5. income maintenance benefits under Social Security, public assistance, and the Veterans Administration [20]

Flowing from program expenditures in these five areas, four major types of benefits may be inferred which are potentially includable in a benefit-cost calculation:

1. increased productivity of retardates
2. reduced cost of care for retardates

3.   psychic gains to retardates

4.   psychic gains to the families of retardates and to others[21]

The first two of these benefits, increased productivity and reduced cost of care, are investment benefits. The psychic gains to both retardates and others are consumption benefits. Thus programs designed to assist mentally retarded persons to function more adequately in society may conceivably generate both investment and consumption benefits. Although there have been numerous evaluations of programs directed at the mentally retarded,[22] little attempt has been made to evaluate programs in terms of the human capital concepts which are typically employed in the benefit-cost studies of other health and education programs. Often costs of the program to be evaluated are not carefully computed, control groups have not been carefully selected, and the outcomes of programs have been only qualitatively estimated. Thus, in terms of Equation 1, neither $D_i(z)$ nor $\frac{\delta x_i}{\delta z}$ have been calculated.

A Specific Program Evaluation

Any number of examples can be offered of program evaluations which do not meet the criteria of benefit-cost analysis. However, one such example may be a useful illustration. A Texas program to help educable mental retardates move from high school to unsheltered employment has recently been evaluated.[23] In this program special education instructors helped the clients locate job training programs and provided them with counseling and vocational guidance support as they moved from high school to full employment. When it was judged that a student had become reasonably independent, he was graduated from high school and passed from the program. This study concerns approximately 600 of the over 1600 students enrolled in the program during 1962-63. These 600 were interviewed during January and February in 1963 and were given three tests, the Gordon Personal Profile, the Peck Sentence Completion, and the Brown Self-Report Inventory. On the basis of these tests administered to the 600 students, it was found that those students who were further along in the program, in general "...made better scores on a significant number of the attitudes and personality characteristics measured,"[24] even when allowance was made for sex, life style, and ethnic considerations. On the basis of these results it is concluded that the "action taken in the Texas Program to improve the attitudes of the students has been effective..."[25]

This study may be useful for some purposes but it is not a benefit-cost study. No mention is made of the costs of the program, although presumably estimates of its cost could be rather easily determined. The program benefits are said to be positive, but no attempt is made to quantify them in dollar terms so they can be compared with the program costs. The program may actually be a very efficient program or very inefficient but from the analysis presented there is no basis for making any judgment concerning the program's efficiency. Even if we assume that the resources used in the program are to be devoted to the service of the mentally retarded, we are not given any norm for judging whether they are used as effectively as they could be.

To recapitulate, a benefit-cost analysis must: 1) clearly define the objectives of the program; 2) relate these objectives to certain indices of performance, which can be evaluated and quantified as program benefits; and 3) link these program benefits with specified inputs through a production function which permits the inputs to be quantified in relation to specified benefits. In order to be able to evaluate the indices of performance, it is most important that relevant longitudinal data are collected pertaining to the experience of the target population and a control group.

Conley's Analysis

Conley's work represents the only existing comprehensive economic analysis of mental retardation.[26] It contains a useful institutional description of current programs relating to mental retardation and the manner in which they are funded. Particularly relevant to our discussion, however, is his chapter, "Benefit-Cost Analysis," in which the nature of his technique is described with particular focus on mental retardation programs. Even though Conley does not provide a strict benefit-cost study with marginal benefits and costs calculated for a specific program, he does estimate average benefits and costs of two mental retardation program areas.

Vocational rehabilitation is the first program area evaluated by Conley. Expenditures for vocational rehabilitation include outlays for case service, counseling, referral, training, and income grants during periods of training. On the basis of 1970 U. S. program data, the average lifetime costs for these services discounted to the present by a seven percent rate of discount are $3,703 for mildly retarded cases (IQ between 50 and 69) and $5,044 for moderately retarded cases (IQ between 40 and 49). Although both investment and consumption benefits might well be generated by these expenditures, the problem of estimating the value, for example, of increased productivity from homemaking services or the psychic gains to retardates and others are so formidable that Conley limits his analysis to the estimation of the increased lifetime earnings attributable to the vocational rehabilitation services. For this purpose he assumes that: 1) the trainees will remain in the work force until 69 years of age, 2) unemployment among the trainees will average 20 percent beginning five years after the training and 3) their lifetime earnings should be ascribed totally to the rehabilitation services they have received. Estimated lifetime earnings are discounted to a present value by a seven percent rate.[27] On the basis of these assumptions the estimated rate of return to vocational rehabilitation services varies with the age, sex, and degree of retardation of the trainees. As can be seen in **Table 1**, the benefit-cost ratio for vocational rehabilitation outlays ranges from 14.8 for male, mildly retarded trainees twenty and twenty-five years old down to 0.9 for female, moderately retarded trainees forty-five years old. The principal reasons for this discrepancy are 1) males generally earn more and have a higher labor force participation rate than do females; 2) the work opportunities available to mildly retarded individuals are much broader than for those moderately retarded; and 3) an older person has fewer years in which to recoup the costs of any human investment outlay than does a younger person.

Table 1 Value of future earnings generated by each dollar spent on the vocational rehabilitation of the retarded at different ages, discounted at 7 percent, 1970

	Age of Retardates When Rehabilitated				
	18 yrs.	20 yrs.	25 yrs.	35 yrs.	45 yrs.
Mildly retarded					
male	$14.2	$14.8	$14.8	$13.5	$10.7
female	8.3	8.4	7.8	6.9	5.7
Moderately retarded					
male	2.2	2.3	2.3	2.1	1.7
female	1.3	1.3	1.2	1.1	0.9

Source: Conley, *The Economics of Mental Retardation*, Table 53.

These results suggest that, on an efficiency basis, the outlays for vocational rehabilitation in the United States are justified. Only in one category of the program is the benefit-cost ratio less than one. Undoubtedly if benefits other than increased earnings had been evaluated, the benefit-cost ratio would have exceeded one even for the category "moderately-retarded-females-45-years-old." A completely unequivocal policy recommendation for altering the vocational rehabilitation program at the margin, however, cannot be inferred from these estimates of average benefits and costs. But, on the basis of these results and appealing strictly to the efficiency criterion, it does seem likely that total benefits would be increased by a shift of funds in favor of young males who are mildly retarded. Such a recommendation must be qualified once other considerations are introduced. There is, for example, necessarily a built-in bias against females when benefits are measured in terms of market wages. For the same reason programs directed toward older people fare poorly in comparison with those for younger people. The *reductio ad absurdum* of simple-minded emphasis on investment benefits is that it justifies the death of all retired persons on the grounds that per capita output for the population would thereby be increased.[28]

Conley has also estimated the relationship between lifetime earnings[29] of retardates and the cost of the education services provided them. He estimates that the ratio of the present value of lifetime earnings to these costs, both discounted by a rate of 7 percent, ranges between five and ten for mildly retarded males, between one and 2.5 for mildly retarded females, and ranges downward from 1.0 for all moderately retarded individuals. These are admittedly crude estimates based on the strong assumption that the entire earnings of retarded individuals are attributable to education. In defense of this assumption Conley argues that, in the absence of education, a retarded person is considerably more disadvantaged than the nonretarded person who can fall back on greater natural endowments. Totally bereft of training, a retarded individual may be simply unable to hold a remunerative job. Such is not as likely to be true of nonretarded individuals lacking formal education. But even if we accept this line of reasoning, these results give us little guidance as to how to adjust educational services at the margin since, as in the vocational rehabilitation analysis, the benefit-cost ratios are expressed in terms of average rather than marginal values. From an average benefit-cost ratio ranging between five and ten we cannot validly conclude that an additional dollar in educational expenditure, say for mildly retarded males, will generate investment benefits of between five and ten dollars. We merely know that this relationship exists for total program outlays in the past. The other caveats made above concerning the results of the vocational rehabilitation expenditures apply with equal force here.

Concluding Critique of Benefit-Cost Analysis

Over the past decade benefit-cost analysis has moved from the fairly restricted confines of water resource evaluation into general budgetary analysis touching all major governmental programs. Consequently its strengths and weaknesses are no longer matters for merely speculative discussion by a small group of specialists. The resolution of controverted questions can have considerable practical impact. In the light of its track record benefit-cost analysis may now itself be judged by a benefit-cost criterion. Has it proved to be a better mouse trap? Predictably the early sanguine hopes of some enthusiasts have not been fulfilled. The terrain of policy analysis seems as tangled and pock-marked by uncertainty, ignorance, and controversy as ever. Consequently, the naive euphoria concerning program evaluation in some quarters a few years back is clearly untenable today. Indeed, a policy cynicism is evident which contends that as we have muddled through in the past so we shall muddle through in the future.

Wildavsky's counsel, for example, is waxing. From the beginning he and other political scientists have been insistent and articulate critics of benefit-cost analysis, charging that policy analysis is radically changed rather than being aided by PPBS.[30] The consistent, central thrust of this complaint has been that the focus of benefit-cost analysis is unrealistically restrictive. Successful legislators and bureaucrats, so the brief reads, have developed a nuanced appreciation for all the factors contributing to successful policy decisions, with economic efficiency only one aspect of this whole pattern. Consequently any evaluation technique which fails to give overriding weight to larger political considerations must be rejected. Otherwise the careful balance between the legislative bodies and the line agencies will be upset.[31]

These contentions merit serious consideration. An inference sometimes drawn from them, however, seems more questionable. To establish that economic efficiency should not dominate policy considerations is one thing. To assert that economic costs are irrelevant is quite another. Efficiency presumably is an important aspect of all policy questions. It would seem especially to be a central consideration for humanitarians striving in the face of resource constraints to assist individuals that society has labeled "mentally retarded." In the field of health and welfare programs, "efficiency" and "effectiveness" are the synonyms, "efficiency" and "miserliness" the contraries. Considerable misunderstanding still shrouds these matters. As Williams has observed,

> ...it needs to be clearly understood that attempting to place a money value on non-traded 'goods' does not imply *either* that one is advocating the establishment of 'markets' in such goods *or* that one is restricting one's attention to their 'economic' attributes. Thus if I try to place a 'value' on the reduction of road accidents, I am not advocating that the victims should be required to pay for medical treatment or that they should be compensated, nor am I solely concerned with the effects on GNP. Thus use of money as a common measuring rod in making diverse values commensurable is not to be confused with an obsession with the more sordid aspects of profit-maximization.[32]

However, even if economic efficiency is accepted as bearing directly on the overall success of any program, this does not necessarily establish the usefulness of benefit-cost analysis. Precisely because it is used to evaluate programs for which commensurable values are not readily available, benefit-cost analysis is often beset with intractable technical problems. A major difficulty with any such evaluation pertains to the interpretation of a program's effects. Theoretically the effects of a program are the difference between the situation "with program" and "without program." Attributes of an experimental group are contrasted with attributes of a control group with the difference being the effect of the program. In practice, it may well be erroneous to assume that the "before program" values are a good proxy for the "without program" values. Phenomena may be invalidly attributed to the program in question when, in fact, other events occurring simultaneously with the program are at least partially responsible for the outcome.

Two further problems are potentially troublesome in the evaluation of mental retardation programs.[33] The first is the policy of "creaming." Typically the most likely subjects are the ones initially accepted into a program. To the extent that this practice occurs, the evaluation of any ongoing program provides an overly sanguine picture of what can be expected from a program extension with its likely lower benefits and higher costs. A second problem concerns program inter-dependency. A certain minimum level of education, for example, may be a necessary but not a sufficient condition for the realization of such diverse benefits as satisfactory adult adjustment and increased earnings. Unfortunately there is no entirely successful way of unequivocally allocating these benefits to the various programs responsible for them.

Indeed, in the final analysis, the major payoff from a benefit-cost analysis may well not be a specific number which represents the "commensurable net benefit" of a program. Of more importance may be the discipline imposed by the benefit-cost procedure which has focused attention on questions which might have gone unasked.[34] For example, a benefit-cost exercise may be the occasion for comparing the benefits from outlays for research and prevention programs with the return to treatment programs. Or the focus of attention may be broadened to extend beyond the spectrum of mental retardation programs to income maintenance programs. The strategy offering the most promise for reducing mental retardation in the future might well be the adoption of a generous income maintenance policy coupled with efforts to generate higher income for low-income families, such as a vigorous pursuit of full employment policies even in the face of considerable price inflation. The possibility of such a strategic approach to the problem of mental retardation is suggested by the often observed inverse correlation between family income and mental retardation. "Contrary to the mode of thinking illustrated by medical research, no spectacular breakthrough can be made until the whole structure of the culture of poverty is destroyed, a structure which includes sub-standard housing, under-employment, inferior education, inadequate health services, poor nutrition and discrimination. Each facet of poverty overlies the other in the etiology of pseudo-mental retardation."[35] In other words, the principal benefit from benefit-cost analysis may be that pertinent questions are formulated rather than definitive answers supplied.[36]

Footnotes

1.   I am grateful to Ronald W. Conley for his comments.

2.   For a survey article that discusses all the major problems associ-ated with benefit-cost analysis and reviews the literature to that date, see A. Prest and R. Turvey, "Cost-benefit analysis: A survey," *Economic Journal,* 75 (1965), pp. 683-735.

3.   Arnold C. Harberger, "Three basic postulates for applied welfare economics," *Journal of Economic Literature,* IX (1971), pp. 796-797. This article is reprinted in a volume that promises to be the first in an annual series of collected articles dealing with topics related to benefit-cost analysis. [A. C. Harberger, R. Haveman, J. Margolis, W. A. Niskanen, R. Turvey, and R. Zeckhauser (eds.) *Benefit-Cost Analysis 1971* (Chicago: Aldine-Atherton, 1972), 485 pp. There are several articles appearing in this first volume that are relevant to mental retardation program evaluation.]

4.   That the consumer's evaluation is the ultimate criterion of the economic benefits of a program was first sketched out nearly a century and a half ago by a French mathematician Jules Dupuit: "To sum up, political economy has to take as the measure of utility of an object the maximum sacrifice which each consumer would be willing to make in order to acquire the object... Thus when a bridge is built and the state establishes a tariff, the latter is not related to cost of production: the heavy cart is charged less than the sprung carriage even though it causes more wear to the timber of the carriageway. Why are there two different prices for the same service? Because the poor man does not attach the same value to crossing the bridge as the rich man does, and raising the charge would only prevent him from crossing. Canal and railway tariffs differentiate between the various classes of goods and passengers, and lay down markedly different rates for them although the costs are more or less the same... The purchaser never pays more for the product than the value he places on its utility." [Jules Depuit, "On the Measurement of the Utility of Public Works," in Kenneth J. Arrow and Tibor Scitovsky (eds.) *Readings in Welfare Economics* (Homewood: Richard D. Irwin, 1969), pp. 261-262.]

5.   Haveman and Krutilla contend that the existence of unemployment and excess capacity should be allowed for in calculating the costs of public works. They construct a social opportunity cost adjustment factor for the U. S. economy which allows for the possibility that resources used in public works may be drawn from otherwise unemployed resources. Consequently the real cost to society is less than would be estimated if actual factor prices were used in the estimation. Since benefit-cost ratios will thus necessarily be higher, more projects will be approved than when costs are based on factor prices. See Robert H. Haveman and John V. Krutilla, *Unemployment, idle capacity and the evaluation of public expenditures* (Baltimore: The Johns Hopkins Press, 1968), 159 pp.

Harberger, however, argues that in some instances the presence of chronic unemployment may mean that the opportunity cost of labor may be higher than a market wage. This could occur if there were individuals who were voluntarily unemployed vis-a-vis certain low-paying positions but involuntarily so vis-a-vis higher paying positions. Thus the supply price for these individuals would lie between the going wage in the low-paying and high-paying positions. When job opportunities develop in the latter category some of the positions would be filled by those whose supply price was between the two going rates. On the basis of this analysis Harberger contends that the social opportunity cost of such workers is definitely nonzero, even though they were previously unemployed, and indeed may well be greater than the current wage level for the low-paying positions. See Arnold C. Harberger, "On measuring the social opportunity cost of labour," *International Labour Review*, 103 (1971), pp. 559-579.

6.   For a rigorous discussion of the place of opportunity costs in economic evaluation, see James M. Buchanan, *Cost and Choice* (Chicago: Markham, 1969), 104 pp.

7.   Conley suggests that the negative effects of a mental retardation program should be considered as an offset to benefits rather than as an element of cost. Thus the "cost" concept would be reserved to measure resources consumed directly in the provision of a service. The hardship imposed on his family when an institutionalized retardate, for example, is returned to the community would in this scheme be considered a deduction from benefits rather than an addition to costs. See Ronald W. Conley, *The economics of mental retardation* (Baltimore: The Johns Hopkins University Press, 1973), Chapter VI. That this decision to treat adverse effects as negative benefits rather than positive costs has substantive significance for a benefit-cost calculation can be seen from this example. Assume that positive benefits from a program are 100, direct program costs 50, and adverse effects 10. If the adverse effects are deducted from benefits the benefit-cost ratio is 1.8. However, if the adverse effects are added to the direct costs then the benefit-cost ratio is only 1.7.

8.   DeAlessi has pointed out that an empire-building bureaucrat should prefer a low to a high discount rate. A low discount rate will generate the most favorable benefit-cost ratios for that subset of projects with the same total benefits and total costs which have 1) higher costs in the present and 2) larger benefits in the future. The

practical outcome is that large investment outlays will be approved for the present time with returns in the distant future. This in turn means greater authority for the bureaucrat. See Louis De~lessi, "Implications of property rights for government investments," *American Economic Review*, LIX (1969), pp. 13-24.

9. With a discount rate of .06 the present net value of the program is calculated as follows:

$$\frac{4.00}{(1.06)^2} + \frac{4.00}{(1.06)^3} + \frac{4.00}{(1.06)^4} - \frac{10.00}{1} = 10.09 - 10.00 = .09$$

With a discount rate of .07 the present net value of the program is:

$$\frac{4.00}{(1.07)^2} + \frac{4.00}{(1.07)^3} + \frac{4.00}{(1.07)^4} - \frac{10.00}{1} = 9.81 - 10.00 = -.19.$$

10. For a good, brief discussion of the issues involved in this controversy by an advocate of the social time preference approach, see Peter O. Steiner, *Public expenditure budgeting* (Washington: The Brookings Institution, 1969), pp. 42-57.

11. Even though there may be no controverting it in theory, there has been considerable disregard of discounting in practice. In a survey of twenty-three federal agencies a few years back only ten reported that they currently discounted benefits and costs. Another eight reported that they "planned to do so in the future" and five apparently did not even have plans to do so. See Elmer B. Staats, "Survey of use by federal agencies of the discounting technique in evaluating future programs,"in Harley H. Hinrichs and Graeme M. Taylor (eds.) *Program budgeting and benefit-cost analysis* (Pacific Palisades: Goodyear, 1969), pp. 212-228.

12. Three criteria have been proposed for evaluating programs: 1) the benefit-minus-cost, 2) the benefit-cost-ratio, and 3) the internal-rate-of-return criterion. The benefit-minus-cost criterion is the one adopted here. For a good discussion of these criteria and their particular strengths and weaknesses, see Jesse Burkhead and Jerry Miner, *Public expenditure* (Chicago: Aldine-Atherton, 1971), pp. 215-224.

13. Donald C. Shoup, "Effects of Suboptimization on Urban Government Decision-Making," *Journal of Finance*, XXVI (1971), pp. 547-564.

14.　However, some income redistribution may well be compatible with the Pareto criterion. See Harold M. Hochman and James D. Rodgers, "Pareto Optimal Redistributions," *American Economic Review,* LIX (1969), pp. 542-557.

15.　Kenneth Boulding expressed in verse his concern over precisely such a possible outcome of a California water development plan.

"It would be well to be quite sure
Just who are the deserving poor,
Or else the state-supported ditch
May serve the undeserving rich."

16.　For a critical discussion of these points, see Burton A. Weisbrod, "Income redistribution effects and benefit-cost analysis," in Samuel B. Chase, Jr. (ed.) *Problems in public expenditure analysis* (Washington: Brookings Institution, 1968), pp. 177-209; and Richard A. Musgrave, "Cost-benefit analysis and the theory of public finance," *Journal of Economic Literature,* VII (1969), pp. 797-806.

17.　For an attempt to measure the *de facto* distributional effects of a program by deducing the weights that are implicit in the outcomes of a tuberculosis screening program, see William B. Neenan, "Distribution and efficiency in benefit-cost analysis," *Canadian Journal of Economics,* IV (1971), pp. 216-224.

18.　Arnold C. Harberger and Daniel Wisecarver, "Preface," in A. C. Harberger, R. Haveman, J. Margolis, W. A. Niskanen, R. Turvey, and R. Zechkauser (eds.) *Benefit-cost analysis 1971* (Chicago: Aldine-Atherton 1972), p. xxi.

19.　For a history of the use of the "human capital" concept by economists, see B. F. Kiker, "The historical roots of the concept of human capital," *Journal of Political Economy,* 74 (1966), pp. 481-499. A landmark paper in this connection is Theodore Schultz' presidential address to the American Economic Association in 1960 on "Human Investment." An important seminal work is Gary Becker, *Human capital* (New York: Columbia University Press, 1964), 187 pp. Numerous monographs as well as articles in the major economic journals have appeared in recent years utilizing the human capital model. *The Journal of Human Resources* has, since its founding in 1966, specialized in human investment evaluations.

20. Ronald W. Conley, *The economics of mental retardation* (Baltimore: The Johns Hopkins University Press, 1973), Chapter IV.

21. Dodson and Cole provide this list of potential benefits to be included in a benefit-cost evaluation of vocational rehabilitation programs:

1. increase in earnings
2. increase in homemaking services and care of children
3. other nonpaid work, for example, farming
4. unpaid work beyond normal occupation, that is, work after hours
5. savings in medical and custodial costs incurred by the client
6. savings in medical, custodial, and institutional costs incurred by the state
7. changes in the output of other family members; for example, if a rehabilitant gets a job, another family member may leave the labor force
8. psychic benefits, such as
   a. improvements in functional capability for non-earnings-related activities, for example, recreation
   b. improvements in the family situation
   c. insurance for the effects of disability for society in general

Additional taxpayer benefits include:

1. increased taxes on the increased earnings
2. savings in transfer payments, such as Social Security, public assistance, and Workman's Compensation

Richard Dodson and Charles B. Cole, "An introduction to cost benefit analysis of the vocational rehabilitation program: A model for use by state agencies," Institute of Urban and Regional Development, University of California, Berkeley, October, 1972, p. 18.

The "additional taxpayer benefits" cannot properly be included in a benefit-cost calculation without double-counting. If gross earnings are counted as a benefit then the tax contribution out of these earnings pertains to the question of distribution which, as we have noted above, is not handled in a benefit-cost study *per se.*

22.   For a bibliography of "Follow-up studies" through 1964, see Joel R. Davitz, Lois J. Davitz, and Irving Lorge, *Terminology and concepts in mental retardation* (New York: Bureau of Publications, Teachers College, Columbia University, 1964), pp. 123-127.

For a list of research concerning mental retardation sponsored by the United States Department of Health, Education and Welfare, Social and Rehabilitation Service between 1955 and 1971, see Dorothy G. Jackson (ed.) *Research 1971* (Washington: U. S. Department of Health, Education and Welfare, 1972), pp. 24-32. Of the more than 100 studies listed here none is a *bona fide* benefit-cost study in the sense that the benefits and costs of a particular program have been identified and estimated in monetary terms.

Since 1964, *Mental Retardation Abstracts* has been published quarterly by the U. S. Public Health Service. This periodical abstracts journal articles on mental retardation. Although there are many program evaluations abstracted in these pages one looks in vain for a benefit-cost study.

A team at the Department of Social Work of Florida State University has recently issued an initial report on establishing evaluation procedures for Developmental Disabilities Services. The data gathering and evaluation suggested here would make possible cost-effectiveness studies. National Developmental Disabilities Evaluation Project, Department of Social Work, Florida State University, *Initial report.* Tallahassee, Florida, December, 1972, 189 pp.

23.   Wallace Bloom, "Effectiveness of a cooperative special education vocational rehabilitation program," *American Journal of Mental Deficiency,* 72 (November, 1967), pp. 393-403.

24.   *Ibid.,* p. 402.

25.   *Ibid.*

26.   A project concerning the economic evaluation of mental retardation programs was conducted at the Institute for the Study of Mental Retardation and Related Disabilities at the University of Michigan during 1970-71. A staff summary of the project's efforts and the papers and comments presented at a conference concluding the

year's work are included in J. S. Cohen, I. Butter, S. E. Deline, and R. E. Nutter (eds.) *Benefit-cost analysis for mental retardation programs: Theoretical considerations and a model for application* (Ann Arbor: University of Michigan Publications Distribution Service, 1972), 184 pp.

27.   With a seven percent rate of discount the present value of increased earnings in the distant future, for example, between 65 and 69 years of age, is negligible.

28.   Mishan, however, points out that even on an efficiency basis alone such a conclusion must be rejected because efficiency benefits include consumer as well as investment benefits and the feelings of potential decedents are consumer benefits. See E. J. Mishan, "Evaluation of life and limb: A theoretical approach," *Journal of Political Economy,* 79 (1971), p. 690. But such niggling serves only to point up the inherent limitation of all economic analysis.

29.   Estimates of lifetime earnings incorporate the effect of unemployment rates, which are derived from a number of studies.

30.   See, for example, Aaron Wildavsky, "Rescuing policy analysis from PPBS," *Public Administration Review,* 29 (1969), pp. 189-192; see also his "The political economy of efficiency: Cost benefit analysis, systems analysis and program budgeting," *Public Administration Review,* 26 (1966), pp. 292-310.

31.   However, rather than the whole political structure having been shaken by the narrow considerations of economic evaluation, it seems that sometimes administrators have used program evaluations themselves as political instruments: producing them when they are expected to give the "correct" political answer; failing to generate them, or suppressing them, when they might prove politically embarrassing. Perhaps "political" considerations mayaccount at least partially for the great variance across federal programs in the funds spent for program evaluation. In a study of fifteen federal programs in four federal agencies in 1969 it was found that the cost of evaluation ranged from zero to 6.3 percent of total program outlays. The average for all fifteen programs was 0.4 percent. See Joseph S. Wholey   *et al.   Federal evaluation policy*. (Washington: The Urban Institute, 1971), p. 79.

32.   Alan Williams, "Cost-benefit analysis: Bastard science? And/or

insidious poison in the body politick," *Journal of Public Economics,* 1 (1972), p. 209.

33.   For a discussion of such problems, see Ronald W. Conley, *The economics of mental retardations,* (Johns Hopkins University Press, 1973), Chapter VI.

34.   Another benefit is suggested by Millikan: "The purpose of social science research should be to deepen, broaden, and extend the policy maker's capacity for judgment—not to provide him with answers. Thus, the test of effectiveness will be not in whether the research leads to a new and unfamiliar conclusion but in whether it clarifies and makes explicit the logical bases for a conclusion already perceived or suspected." Max F. Millikan, "Inquiry and policy: The relation of knowledge to action," in *The human meaning of the social sciences* (New York: Meridian Books, 1959), p. 167.

35.   Rodger Hurley, *Poverty and mental retardation* (New York: Vintage Books, 1969), pp. 72-73.

36.   The focus of discussion in this paper has been on benefit-cost analysis, narrowly construed. However, it should not be inferred from this emphasis on one type of analysis that other forms of evaluation are not useful. For a brief discussion of types of evaluation undertaken by the federal government, see Joseph S. Wholey *et al., Federal evaluation policy* (Washington: The Urban Institute, 1971), pp. 24-27.

Evaluation of Living Environments: The MANIFEST Description of Ward Activities[1]

M. F. Cataldo and T. R. Risley

From early childhood, the institutionalized retarded eat, sleep, work and play within the confines of the living environment defined by the institution. Various measurable and manipulable factors of that environment determine whether retardates merely exist or experience life to the full extent of which they are capable. Therefore, an important aspect of the overall quality of an institution is the quality of the retardate's daily experience in his living environment.

There has been a current proliferation of special programs in institutions—programs for education, recreation, behavior modification, occupational and physical therapy, community readiness and even religion. In some institutions these programs are well conducted and organized so as to provide an adequate if not exceptional quality living environment. Too often, however, institutions have been studied simply as administrative conduits for specific training programs. While such programs are no doubt valuable, they often make up only a small part of the institutionalized retardate's day, and for the remainder of the day leave him to his own resources in an environment impoverished of materials and activities, and understaffed by personnel who are underpaid.

Further, regardless of the success of work training programs, community programs, and half-way houses; regardless of the current trend to reduce the size of institutions and incorporate them into community life; regardless of our expressed commitment to return institutionalized persons to the community, it is still a fact that many of the retarded do and will spend much if not all their lives in institutions. For many retarded the institution will be their home, their place of work, and their recreation center. In sum, for many retarded persons, the institution is their only living environment.

It is essential, therefore, that we ask questions about the institution as a living environment, taking note of the materials and activities that make up a resident's day.

It is necessary to identify, if you will, "good" as opposed to "poor" environments. It is essential that we identify poor and intolerable situations and demonstrate that good alternatives are possible. Conditions in many institutions are so inadequate as to seriously retard the development of a normal child let alone the development of a mentally handicapped child.

The Need for an Assessment of Living Environment Quality

The issue of the quality of institution environments has been the subject of comments by the President's Committee on Mental Retardation. The Committee has likened the living environments in many public residential facilities for the retarded to that experienced by prisoners of war in the past three decades (1968). And in addition, this committee has commented that:

> Many residential services and programs as they exist within the 50 states comprise a tragic paradox for the wealthiest nation in the world. On the one hand, our knowledge of environmental design and care for the retarded has never been greater and increases daily. On the other hand, the gap between what we know how to do and what we actually are doing seems to increase at an even more rapid rate. (1970)

Conditions at a number of institutions have been reported in exposes such as *Christmas in Purgatory* (Blatt and Kaplan, 1966) and *Exodus From Pandemonia* (Blatt, 1970). The news media have brought to the public's attention particular incidents in institutions such as Partlow and Willowbrook, as well as reports of grand jury investigations and law suits against institutions and their personnel.

However, while attention is drawn to the more unfavorable conditions in some institutions, the process for such identification of conditions and identification of particular institutions is unsystematic, often initiated by rumor and innuendo, resolved after the "damage" has been done and often resolved in contexts which make objectivity difficult.

What is needed are empirical measures for the objective and reliable assessment of conditions in institutions for the retarded. These measures should be able to be applied systematically so as to establish norms for care and to identify those facilities below these norms.

A review of available standardized tests such as the Stanford-Binet, Vineland Social Maturity Scale, AAMD Adaptive Behavior Scales, etc., shows that the majority of these tests are specific to the performance of individuals in the testing situation and are in no way descriptive of the conditions residents are confronted with daily.

The development of an evaluation descriptive of living environments is, in its initial stages, primarily a research function. Yet an interesting dichotemy exists between issues in residential care and empirical research.

This is aptly depicted by review of the last five volumes of two journals in the field of mental retardation, the *American Journal of Mental Deficiency* (AJMD) and *Mental Retardation* (MR). In *AJMD* some 86 percent of the articles reported data but most were either normative studies on such issues as sex ratio, incidence of various syndromes, retardates' reaction time, memory span, perception, etc. On the other hand, in *MR,* while many articles dealt with institution issues, all of the articles appearing in this journal only 2 percent reported data. Thus, while we tend to talk about the issues in institutions we conduct our research on other variables.

However, procedures for evaluation of institutions are currently being developed by the Joint Commission on Accreditation of Hospitals. The Commission has had an important twofold impact: first, it has provided information on institution quality, and, second, as more institutions seek accreditation, it has acted as an impetus for the improvement of institution quality. Review of the Joint Commission's standards shows a consideration of many aspects of many institutions' operations. As outlined in the Joint Commission's "Standards for Residential Facilities for the Mentally Retarded" (1971), 65 percent of these standards deal with professional and special programs, and 13 percent with administrative policies and practices; however, only about 1 percent deal with resident living staff, another 1 percent with design and equipment of living units and .5 percent with group and organized living units.

By and large, then, the Joint Commission has sought to ask questions primarily about the institution's role in providing professional and special programs for its residents, and to a much lesser degree about the institution's role as a living environment. The Commission itself has identified this area as a most pressing topic for empirical efforts.

Prior Research of Living Environments

For the past several years, we have empirically investigated procedures for evaluating living environments for the retarded. The tactics for this work have been similar to those in our previous research for developing evaluations and procedural technologies for a number of areas including: language assessment (Hart, 1969; Hursh and Risley, 1971); language development and remediation (Reynolds and Risley, 1968; Risley, Reynolds and Hart, 1970; Risley, Hart and Doke, 1971; Risley, 1972); classroom activity planning and implementation (LeLaurin and Risley, 1972; Doke and Risley, 1972); recreation management (Pierce, 1972); toy evaluation (Quilitch, Christophersen and Risley, 1972); day care for infants, toddlers and preschoolers (Jacobson, Bushell and Risley, 1969; Cataldo and Risley, 1972; Krantz and Risley, 1972; Valdivieso, 1972; LeLaurin, 1973); day programs for children on pediatric wards (Benefiel, 1973); and activity programs in nursing homes for the elderly (McClannahan and Risley, 1972). Each of these considerations has proceeded from empirical evaluations of the environment and identification of variables which appear to affect environmental quality.

In developing measures for evaluating living environments for the retarded, we have noted that such environments can vary considerably from institution to institution, or even within an institution. Therefore, measures for such environments must provide the maximum amount of flexibility possible. That is, measures must be able to assess any situation encountered. Many observation procedures code behavior to facilitate recording. If measures for evaluation of environments for the retarded are to employ such code procedures, then an extensive enough code must be employed to be applicable to any situation encountered. Often construction of such a code or behavior classification system becomes a 'cart-and-horse' problem: one cannot construct an inclusive measure until one has knowledge of the observable events which will be encountered, yet observable events are best identified only when objectively and reliably measured.

What, then, is a broad and comprehensive enough categorization scheme for such a problem? Probably the *most* flexible method would be the English language, since we have no broader written method for describing a particular event. English description recording procedures have been used to provide daily ecological records (Barker and Wright, 1951; Barker, Schoggen and Barker, 1955; Barker, Wright, Barker and Schoggen, 1961) and to assess a variety of variables in such diverse environments as psychiatric wards (Gump and Jones, 1970; Ittelson,

Rivlin and Proshansky, 1970) to classrooms (Barker, Dembo and Lewin, 1943; Gump, 1969). Therefore, we have considered the use of exact English descriptions as the most viable means for recording, in as flexible a manner as possible, the conditions of the various living environments for the retarded.

However, the issues involved in descriptive recording procedures are quite different from those employing observation codes (cf. Bijou, Peterson and Ault, 1968). We have found that the particular problem with descriptive data collection lies not in the method of collecting observational data but in procedures for determining observer reliability and for analyzing and quantifying the massive amounts of data collected by this type of recording procedure.

The Resident Activity MANIFEST

From our research and observation of institutions and programs for the retarded we have noted children in various types of environments and thus have considered comparative measures of these environments accordingly. The result has been the development of procedures for providing a MANIFEST Description of Resident Activity. These procedures consist of three measures:

1. A *Stimulation* measure which provides information on what the residents are experiencing.

2. An *Interaction* measure which provides information on what the residents are doing.

3. An *Activity* measure which provides information on the participation of the residents in organized activities.

Each measure is designed to be particularly sensitive in assessing a different quality of environment. The activity measure is applicable to the highest quality environment, and the stimulation measure to the lowest quality living environment. This Resident Activity MANIFEST can then be used to assess the range of environments encountered by employing the measure most sensitive to the situation.

Stimulation Measure

A situation which we have observed in many institutions is one in which children are in extremely poor, barren environments. In many such environments are non-ambulatory residents, who are often incapable of but the most limited movement and are often found to have concomitant physical anomalies. However, such environments also exist for ambulatory residents. These environments can be characterized by the fact that children receive little, if any, stimulation. Even though these represent the worst of environments, some can be found to be better than others. Therefore, the first approach we have considered for evaluating environments is observational procedures which are sensitive to differences in the stimulation provided by the environment. For situations in which children are most often observed to be doing nothing, we have asked the question, "What is the child experiencing?" This measure is particularly sensitive to changes in children moving or touching things or attending to things.

Figure 1 presents an example of the recording forms used for this measure. An observer notes whether each child is vocalizing (including unintelligible utterances), what he is attending to (i.e., what he is looking at), what his hands are touching, his position and motion and his location. This information is noted in exact English words or a brief phrase and is written on the data sheet for each child before the next child is observed.

Reliability of this measure can be determined from comparison of two observers' records when both observers have noted the same child at the same time. What is compared is the exact English word used to describe the various aspects of the child's behavior. An observation can be said to be reliable when observers agree on what they have observed, that is, if they employ the same words to describe the behavior.

In the example shown in Figure 1, both observers agree that the first resident was looking at the "WALL," the second resident was looking at an "AIDE," and so forth. Agreement was also considered to occur when similar words with almost the same meaning were used, as in the case of what the second resident was touching: One observer recorded "KNEE" and the other recorded "LEG." Disagreement occurred when words clearly differed. For example, for the third resident, observers disagreed on attention: one observer recorded "AIDE"; the other recorded "BOY."

The percentage of agreement between observers (reliability) is computed by: No. of agreements ÷ No. of agreements + No. of dis-

Figure 1 Recording forms used in the stimulation measure to determine what children are experiencing. Observers record whether children are vocalizing, what they are looking at, what they are touching and their position, motion and location. Reliability of observations is assessed by determining whether two observers write the same words describing what they have observed.

Place_____ Name_____ Date_____ Time _____ Over-all Reliability $\frac{A}{A+D}$ = ____%

CHILD'S NAME	VOCAL %= $\frac{A}{A+D}$	ATTENTION %=	HANDS %=	POSITION/MOTION %=	LOCATION %=
E.B.	NO	WALL	KNEE / PAPER Towel	SIT	DAYROOM
J.B	NO	AIDE	KNEE / KNEE	SIT	DAYROOM
J.S	NO	AIDE	FREE / CHAIR	SIT	DAYROOM
K.C.	YES	AIDE	FREE / SHIRT	STAND	DAYROOM
E.C.	NO	OBSCURE	RADIATOR WINDOW	STAND	DAYROOM
P.D.	NO	THREAD	THREAD / THREAD	STAND	DAYROOM
R.F	NO	OBSERVER	CLASPED	STAND	DAYROOM
D.G.	NO	OBSCURE	HEAD / FREE	SIT	DAYROOM
D.H.	NO	LAP	OBSCURE LAP	SIT	DAYROOM
A.H.	YES	AIDE	CLOTHES / CLOTHES	SIT	DAYROOM
B.H.	YES	BOYS	FREE / TWIRLING FREE	SIT	DAYROOM
C.J.	NO	BOYS	OBSCURE / GATE	STAND	DAYROOM
P.K.	NO	OBSERVER	LAP / LAP	SIT/ROCKING	DAYROOM
J.M.	NO	OBSERVER	HEAD / HEAD	STAND	DAYROOM
M.M.	NO	OBSERVER	FREE / HEAD	SIT	DAYROOM
S.P.	NO	CEILING	CHEST / OBSCURE	WALK	DAYROOM
M.W.	NO	AIDE	TABLE / TABLE	SIT	DAYROOM

Place _____ Name _____ Date _____ Time_____ Over-all Reliability $\frac{A}{A+D}$ = ____%

CHILD'S NAME	VOCAL 100 %= $\frac{A}{A+D}$ 17/17	ATTENTION 76%= 13/17	HANDS 88%= 30/34	POSITION/MOTION 100 %= 17/17	LOCATION 100%= 17/17
E.B	No	A Wall	A Knee / Paper Towel	A Sit	A Dayroom A
J.B.	No	A Aide	A Leg / Leg	A Sit	A Dayroom A
J.S.	No	A Boy	D Free / Chair	A Sit	A Dayroom A
K.C.	Yes	A Aide	A Free / Shirt	A Stand	A Dayroom A
E.C.	No	A Obscure	A Radiator / Window	A Stand	A Dayroom A
P.D.	No	A Thread	A Thread / Thread	A Stand	A Dayroom A
R.F	No	A Observer	A Hand / Shirt	D Stand	A Dayroom A
D.G.	No	A Obscure	A Head / Free	A Sit	A Dayroom A
D.H.	No	A Floor	D Obscure Lap	A Sit	A Dayroom A
A.H.	Yes	A Boys	D Pants / Hand	D Sit	A Dayroom A
B.H.	Yes	A Boys	A Free / Twirling Free	A Sit	A Dayroom A
C.J.	No	A Boys	A Gate / Obscure	A Stand	A Dayroom A
P.K.	No	A Observer	A Lap / Lap	A Sit/Rocking	A Dayroom A
J.M.	No	A Observer	A Head / Head	A Stand	A Dayroom A
M.M	No	A Observer	A Head / Head	A Sit	A Dayroom A
S.P.	No	A Ceiling	A Chest / Free	D Walk	A Dayroom A
M.W.	No	A Boys	D Table / Table	A Sit	A Dayroom A

agreements x 100. Overall reliability for use of this measure has been 90 percent.

This level of reliability on plain English words allows us the flexibility to classify these words into larger categories, thus allowing us to evaluate the children's engagement into any number of different categories.

Figure 2 presents a simple and basic analysis: what children were observed to be touching. Observations on a residential unit for retarded children were made every fifteen minutes between 6 a.m. and 9 p.m. In this case four such "full-day" observations were made. The first observation is shown by the bars, and the second, third, and fourth are shown by the open circles, closed circles and open triangles respectively.

This provides an environmental profile showing two important comparisons: 1) the comparative levels of behavior under each of the six categories; and 2) the consistency of the data across successive observations. An example of the first point is that one can readily determine from the data that about as many children were observed to be touching movable objects as were described to be touching nothing or themselves. The second point is illustrated by the fact that the levels of behavior on the first observation, as indicated by the bars, are comparable to those indicated by the other symbols for the second, third, and fourth days, thus demonstrating the day-to-day consistency of the measure.

It is interesting to note that the fourth set of observations, those represented by the open triangles, were taken in a different environment. One of the recommendations made for improvements for the retarded is relocation to a different environment. Children on the residential unit for which data is presented in Figure 2 were relocated soon after the third set of observations were made. This provided us with the opportunity to investigate any differences after this relocation. The new environment had a larger day room. A picture window provided more daylight and the ward had been recently painted. Thus, a month after the move, observations were again made every 15 minutes from 6 a.m. to 9 p.m. As the data indicate by comparison of the open triangles with the rest of the data in this figure, little difference can be seen between environments in terms of what the children were touching.

The data presented in this paper are intended to consider the utility of measurement procedures for evaluating living environments for the retarded, not to draw conclusions about the relative merit of

Figure 2 What retarded children in a residential unit were observed to be touching using the stimulation measure. Observations were made every fifteen minutes from 6 a.m. to 9 p.m. on four different days. Day 1 observations are shown by the bars, day 2 by the open circles, day 3 by the closed circles, day 4 by the open triangles. The environmental profile thus obtained reveals that approximately the same number of children were touching movable objects as were touching nothing or themselves. The consistency of the measure is also clear, even though on the fourth day the children had been relocated to a different location.

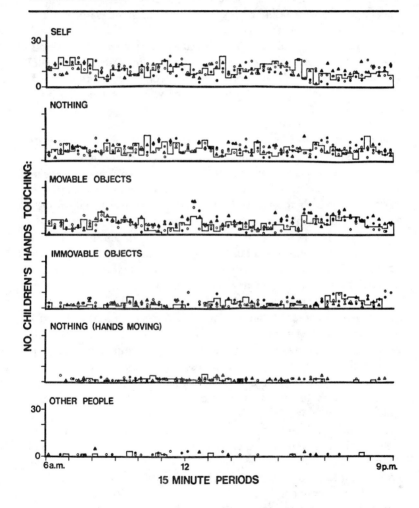

various environments nor identify "therapeutic" aspects of environments. That should be the result of effective comparative evaluation and the subject of future papers. Thus, these results should not be construed to mean that changes in environment do not result in changes in behavior; on the contrary, we would assert that they may, but perhaps they did not in this particular case. And the *perhaps* should be stressed—first, because this comparison between wards is the product of happenstance, making any conclusions at best correlational and not causal; and, second, because it is very likely that some aspects of behavior did change as a result of the move to a different ward, but the changes were not in these categories.

However, the necessity of a measure's being comparative across types of conditions is paramount if the measure is to be useful to evaluate and identify "good" vs. "poor" environments. Another analysis which is, therefore, most useful is one which compares environments.

Figure 3 shows such a comparison between environment *A* and *B*. (Throughout the paper each figure representing an across-environment comparison will identify environments by letters. This does not mean that the same letters on different graphs represent the same environment; in most cases they do not. It does, however, mean that we wish to avoid identifying particular institutions or particular aspects of the program which may or may not be the contributing factors in the level of behavior observed—this should be the scope of future research with this type of measure.) Nonetheless, the data show that in environment *A* as compared to environment *B* a higher percentage of time was spent by retarded children engaged with (touching) play materials, both were comparable on contact with non-play items, while environment *B* had a proportionately higher percentage of time spent by retarded children touching physical (non-movable) aspects of the environment, touching nothing and touching themselves. This serves to illustrate the comparative nature of the measure across environments. One environment can be identified as better or worse than another in terms of what the children are experiencing (in this case stimulation by being in contact with materials). Therefore, we consider this primarily a stimulation measure. The question can then be asked as to the cause of this difference—attractiveness of the materials, availability of materials, the program for selection and display of materials, etc.

We have presented the use of this stimulation measure in terms of providing information on children's contact with materials; other aspects of behavior noted in making these types of observations, i.e.,

Figure 3 A comparison using the stimulation measure of what retarded children were touching in two different environments. In Environment A, children spent a greater percentage of time in contact with play materials whereas in Environment B, children spent a greater percentage of time touching physical aspects of the environment, nothing, or themselves. This type of comparison enables an identification of "good" vs "poor" environments in terms of what the children are experiencing, or how they are being stimulated. Once the differences have been identified, the cause of the difference can be investigated.

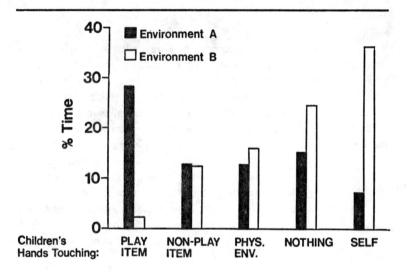

vocalization, attention, position, motion and location, can also provide useful analyses when considered individually or in combination; such as, what children attend to when seated, or locations in which high rates of vocalization occur, etc.

We have considered the stimulation measure to be particularly suitable for and sensitive to identifying differences between environments where little stimulation is provided and residents are largely inactive. We have found the measure to be reliable and useful in that it can provide within- and between-environment evaluation. In the case of between-environment evaluation, the measure is most useful in identifying environments which are quite poor, with little stimulation, as compared to environments in which more children are exposed to a variety of experiences and things. However, given that an environment provides things for children, the next level of question to be asked is what children are doing with these things. Thus, evaluation of two environments might show both to have comparable levels of children in contact with materials yet in one environment children may dismantle toy trucks, use blocks as missiles or clubs, or sit for hours holding a ball, compared to another environment in which children play with toys and games both individually or with other children and adults. The stimulation measure would not necessarily show these two environments to differ while in fact they do so considerably.

Interaction Measure

Thus, we have considered a second measure which is designed to be sensitive to describing children's interaction with their environment, and to the interrelation between objects and events and the children's actions. This requires a measure with a good deal of flexibility, not only in describing the objects or attention of the child, as in the previous measure, but also in describing the child's interaction with the things in his environment.

This second measurement procedure entails an observer noting in a plain English sentence what each child is *doing*, including information about the materials used and the interaction with the materials.

This type of data is analyzed by having someone "rate" the sentences as to whether particular aspects of behavior occurred. A "Rater" is asked to consider questions about the sentence recorded by an observer, such as:

> Was the child in contact with materials? Key words to look for were "touching," "holding," etc.

> Was the child interacting with the materials? Key words to look for included words such as "playing," "talking" and "looking."

Thus, "standing holding a toy truck" would be rated as contact with materials (i.e., a toy truck) but not as interacting, whereas "playing with a toy truck" would be rated as both contact with materials and interacting. We found that observers could reliably agree on this type of distinction. By comparing two observers' records on data taken simultaneously but independently, inter-observer reliability on all types of questions asked by each rater was 93 percent.

To determine the objectivity of raters, reliability between pairs of raters independently evaluating each observer's records was determined and also found to be high, averaging 95 percent.

As mentioned, the interaction measure was considered to be sensitive to environments in which children's contact with objects and events was comparable but their interaction with these differed. **Figure 4** demonstrates the utility of the interaction measure in making such a comparison. The figure shows the percentage of time children were in contact with materials and interacting with materials in four environments again identified only by letters. The results show these environments differ little in children's contact with materials, the highest percentage being 59 percent and the lowest, 46 percent. However, the interaction with the materials did vary considerably between environments, from 39 percent of the children interacting in environment A to 11 percent in environment D.

From the point of view of the interaction measure, this example demonstrates that reliable data can be obtained on differences between environments along dimensions of children's interaction with materials. This does not, of course, identify the reason for the differences. It could be because, in spite of our opinion, the children were really different, say intellectually; perhaps the environments were different, the materials better, the personnel and staff program more conducive to engaging children in play in one environment than the other. Hypotheses on what contributes to increased interaction should be investigated.

An example of what such an investigation might look like is provided in **Figure 5.** Here observations were made of retarded adults in a nursing home. The percentage of residents in contact with materials and interacting with materials were compared in a lounge area of the home when residents used the area as a lounge or when a music activity was presented. During both times residents were free to do as they pleased and a variety of recreation materials were always present. However, during music time some of the chairs were arranged in a semi-circle about a piano and two volunteers distributed hand instruments, played music and sang songs. The data show that music activity increased contact with things. The fourth observation during the music activity occurred as the activity ended. The prescription suggested here, instituting activities for people, is simple, certainly not profound and surely described extensively in many studies. But it does aptly demonstrate the utility which can be made of the interaction measure in describing variables affecting resident behavior.

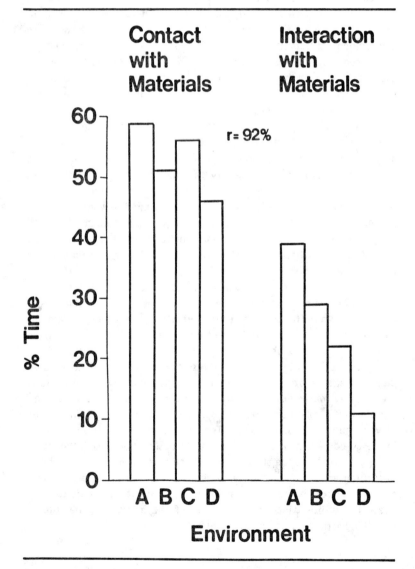

Figure 4 A comparison of four environments employing the interaction measure. While the four environments show little
difference in time spent in contact with materials time spent in interaction differed appreciably. In environments where children are brought
into contact with a variety of objects, this comparison enables an
identification of "good" vs "poor" environments in terms of what the
children are doing. The reasons for these differences can then be
investigated.

Contact with Materials

Interaction with Materials

r= 92%

% Time

Environment

Figure 5 Observations using the interaction measure to determine the cause of increased interaction with materials, carried out among retarded adults in a nursing home. When the lounge area was used simply as a lounge even with a variety of recreation materials available, very little interaction with the environment occurred. When a music activity was presented, however, the percent of time residents spent interacting increased considerably. The interaction measure is clearly useful in cases such as this in demonstrating variables which affect behavior.

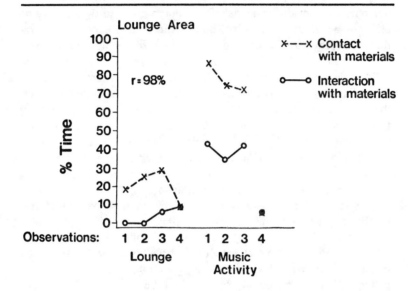

The interaction measure can be expanded to include any situation which can be observed and recorded by simply priming the observer and requiring the appropriate rater evaluation of observer's transcriptions. For example, suppose one were interested in the variables discussed above and in addition the types of furniture used most appropriately by retarded children. Observers could be instructed to write a brief description of what each child was doing, and, if the child were using a piece of furniture, to note especially what kind it was and how he was using it. The Rater could then be instructed to evaluate transcriptions in terms of the furniture used, as well as other aspects such as playing, contact with materials, interaction, etc.

However, we have noted cases in which children in two different environments are equally interacting with their environment, but the environments differ greatly in variety and type of organized activities available to the children. A measurement system of observers and raters employing English sentence description as the primary datum to distinguish between these would be cumbersome and expensive.

Activity Measure

Environments which provide a good activity program are characterized not only by providing materials for children but also by a variety of different activities, group play, opportunities to observe demonstrations, etc. The best indicator of the quality with which activities are implemented by staff and the attractiveness of the activities to the children is the degree to which children participate in activities. Thus, given that environments provide materials with which children interact, the next level of question is to what degree an effective activity structure is provided. The appropriate measure for answering this question must identify activity structure and determine the degree of children's participation or non-participation in the activities. The third measure we have considered, then, is an activity measure for identifying activities and children's participation in them.

The activity measure is employed by an observer noting at a specific point in time, say every 15 minutes, each activity going on at that time, and then counting the number of children present and the number participating in each activity. We have found that observers can readily identify activities and agree on the number of children participating. Reliability on identifying activities is 96 percent, and agreement on the number of children participating is 94 percent.[2]

Figure 6 demonstrates the utility of this measure in distinguishing among environments. Here the percentage of children's time participating and the number of activities is presented for 30-minute sample observations in six different environments. Data range from six activities with an average of 83 percent of the children participating in Environment A, to one activity and only 3 percent of the children participating in Environment F. Again, in this presentation we do not wish to draw conclusions nor speculate on reasons for these differences but rather demonstrate that they may be reliably observed.

216

Figure 6 Use of the activity measure in comparison of six environments as to the effectiveness of their planned activity
structures. The degree to which children participate is the best indication of the quality with which staff are implementing activities and the
attractiveness of the activities to the children.

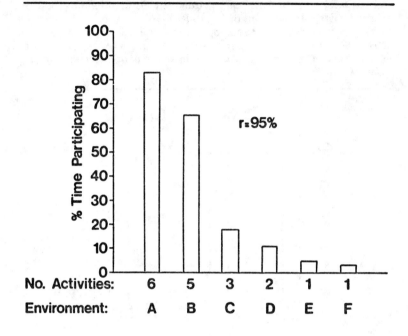

Figure 7 presents two examples of how this measure might be used to
identify variables affecting participation. In the first part of the figure
the percentage of time participating by one group of children in
Environment *A* is presented when that group was in two different
activity situations. In the first situation two activities were presented—
T.V. and FREE TIME. In FREE TIME children were free to use a
variety of materials usually found on the ward. In this situation 10
percent of the children were observed to be participating. In the second
situation two activities were also presented—LEARNING TO WASH
and COLORING. For these activities participation was 29 percent.
Thus, activity selection is one variable which should be considered.

Figure 7   The activity measure can be used both within and across
environments. In Environment A, a comparison was made
of the effect of different activities on children's participation. When the
activities presented were F R E E T I M E and T V, participation was 10%;
when L E A R N I N G T O W A S H and C O L O R I N G were presented, the
activity level rose to 29%. In Environment B, a different group of
children were observed in their residential unit when one activity,
F R E E T I M E, was being presented, and in a recreation hall where three
activities—E X E R C I S E T I M E, I N S T R U C T I O N I N G A M E S, and F R E E
P L A Y—were in progress. The change in participation level is notable,
from 1% to 22%

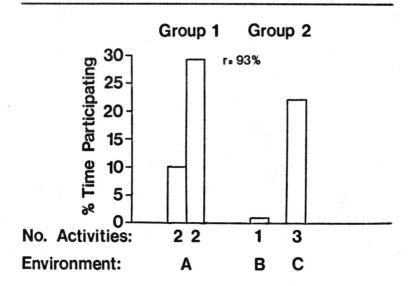

The second part of the figure shows the results of a second group
of children observed in two different environments, *B* and *C*. Environment *B* was the residential unit and one activity was presented, F R E E
T I M E, in which children were free to use any of the materials on the
unit; participation was 1 percent. Environment *C* was a recreation hall
designed to provide and promote activities. During one 15-minute
sample observation, three activities took place: E X E R C I S E T I M E,
I N S T R U C T I O N I N G A M E S, and F R E E P L A Y with a variety of
materials. Participation here was 22 percent. Thus, the activity measure
enables the comparison of environments according to their effective
activity structure.

Summary

Taken as a whole, all three measures comprise the Resident Activity MANIFEST which can be used as an assessment hierarchy. In assessments the *activity* measure is employed first. Those environments with extremely low scores are then assessed with the *interaction* measure. If scores are still low, the *stimulation* measure is used. Thus, the type of measure used, as well as the level of behavior, provides an index of the quality of the environment.

In developing the MANIFEST we have considered not only assessment of good environments for residents by employing the activity measure, but also use of the stimulation measure to compare and evaluate even the worst back wards, those wards with children at the lowest level of development. Differences do exist among these back ward situations, and we must identify these differences in our institutions. We must do so to be able to encompass in our evaluations the full range of situations which presently exist in institutions and to be able to determine progress as environments begin to more closely approximate our standards. Using the Resident Activity MANIFEST, even small improvements in barren back wards, as well as at every other level of institutional environment, can be detected and encouraged.

The Resident Activity MANIFEST has thus been designed to develop empirically based norms and in so doing to provide an evaluation procedure which will enable the beginnings of a set of standards for the quality of living environments in residential institutions for the retarded. The MANIFEST is explicitly designed in a format suitable for testing and inclusion in formal accreditation procedures.

Footnotes

1. This is one of a series of studies conducted by the Living Environments Group at the University of Kansas under the direction of Todd R. Risley. This project was supported in part by a grant HD-05-720-01 to the Bureau of Child Research and the Department of Human Development. The authors are indebted to Linda K. Haskins and Julie Sheppard for their assistance in conducting this research.

2. A training manual for use of the Planned Activity Check, a participation measure for classroom evaluation, has been prepared and is available upon request from the authors.

References

Barker, R. G., Dembo, T., and Lewin, K. Frustration and regression. In R. G. Barker, J. S. Kounin and H. F. Wright, *Child behavior and development*. New York: McGraw-Hill, 1943.

Barker, R. G. and Wright, H. F. *One boy's day: A specimen record of behavior*. New York: Harper and Brothers, 1951.

Barker, R. G., Schoggen, M., and Barker, L. S. Hemerography of Mary Ennis. In A. Burton and R. E. Harris (Eds.), *Clinical studies of personality*. New York: Harper and Brothers, 1955.

Barker, R. G., Wright, H. F., Barker, L. S., and Schoggen, M. *Specimen records of American and English children*. Lawrence, Kansas: University of Kansas Press, 1961.

Benefiel, D. Unpublished Master's Thesis under the direction of Todd R. Risley, University of Kansas, 1973.

Bijou, S. W., Peterson, R. F., and Ault, M. H. A method to integrate descriptive and experimental field studies at the level of data and empirical concepts. *Journal of Applied Behavior Analysis*, 1968, *1*, 175-191.

Blatt, B. *Exodus from pandemonium: Human abuse and a reformation of public policy*. Boston: Allyn and Bacon, Inc., 1970.

Blatt, B. and Kaplan, F. *Christmas in purgatory: A photographic essay on mental retardation*. Boston: Allyn and Bacon, 1966.

Cataldo, M. F. and Risley, T. R. The organization of group care environments: The infant daycare center. Paper presented at the American Psychological Association, Honolulu, Hawaii, 1972.

Doke, L. A. and Risley, T. R. The organization of daycare environments: Required versus optional activities. *Journal of Applied Behavior Analysis*, 1972, *5*, 405-420.

Gump, P. V. and James, E. V. *Patient behavior in wards of traditional and of modern design*. Topeka, Kansas: The Environmental Research Foundation, 1970.

Gump, P. V. Intra-setting analysis: The third grade classroom as a special but instructive case. In E. P. Willems and H. L. Raush (Eds.), *Naturalistic viewpoints in psychological research.* New York: Holt, Rinehart and Winston, 1969.

Hart, B. M. and Risley, T. R. Establishing use of descriptive adjectives in the spontaneous speech of disadvantaged preschool children. *Journal of Applied Behavior Analysis,* 1968, *1,* 109-120.

Hursh, D. E. and Risley, T. R. Normative data from and procedures for the recording of spontaneous speech in preschool children. Paper presented at the Kansas Psychological Association, Overland Park, Kansas, April, 1971.

Ittelson, W. H., Rivlin, L. G., and Proshansky, H. M. The use of behavioral maps in environmental psychology. In H. M. Proshansky, W. H. Ittelson, and L. G. Rivlin (Eds.), *Environmental psychology: Man and his physical setting.* New York: Holt, Rinehart and Winston, Inc., 1970.

Jacobson, J. M., Bushell, D. B., and Risley, T. R. Switching requirements in a Head Start classroom. *Journal of Applied Behavior Analysis,* 1969, *2,* 43-47.

Joint Commission on Accreditation of Hospitals. *Standards for residential facilities for the mentally retarded.* Chicago: Joint Commission, 1971.

Krantz, P. J. and Risley, T. R. The organization of group care environments: Behavioral ecology in the classroom. Paper presented at the American Psychological Association, Honolulu, Hawaii, 1972.

LeLaurin, K. Unpublished Doctoral Dissertation under the direction of Todd R. Risley, University of Kansas, 1973.

LeLaurin, K. and Risley, T. R. The organization of daycare environments: "Zone" versus "man-to-man" staff assignments. *Journal of Applied Behavior Analysis,* 1972, *5,* 25-232.

McClannahan, L. E. and Risley, T. R. The organization of group care environments: Recreation for the aged. Paper presented at the American Psychological Association, Honolulu, Hawaii, 1972.

Pierce, C. Unpublished Doctoral Dissertation under the direction of Todd R. Risley, University of Kansas, 1972.

President's Committee on Mental Retardation. *Residential services for the mentally retarded: An action policy proposal.* Washington, D. C.: U. S. Government Printing Office, 1968.

President's Committee on Mental Retardation. *The decisive decade.* Washington, D. C.: U. S. Government Printing Office, 1970.

Quilitch, H. R., Christophersen, E. R., and Risley, T. R. The organization of group care environments: Toy evaluation. Paper presented at the American Psychological Association, Honolulu, Hawaii, 1972.

Reynolds, N. J. and Risley, T. R. The role of social and material reinforcers in increasing talking of a disadvantaged preschool child. *Journal of Applied Behavior Analysis,* 1968, *1,* 253-262.

Risley, T. R. Spontaneous language and the preschool environment. In J. C. Stanley (Ed.), *Preschool programs for the disadvantaged: Five experimental approaches to early childhood education.* Baltimore: Johns Hopkins University Press, 1972.

Risley, T. R., Hart, B., and Doke, L. A. Operant language development: The outline of a therapeutic technology. In R. L. Schiefelbusch (Ed.), *The language of the mentally retarded.* Baltimore: University Park Press, 1971.

Risley, T. R., Reynolds, N. J., and Hart, B. The disadvantaged: Behavior modification with disadvantaged preschool children. In R. Bradfield (Ed.), *Behavior modification: The human effort.* Palo Alto: Science and Behavior Books, 1970.

Valdivieso, L. Unpublished Master's Thesis under the direction of Todd R. Risley, University of Kansas, 1972.

Evaluation of Mental Health Programs for the Aged 10

Robert L. Kahn and Steven H. Zarit

Some years ago, one of us was engaged in a research study of a number of institutions providing services for the aged, and one day came to a home for the aged whose residents my colleagues and I considered to be perhaps the worst institutional group that we had ever seen. Almost all of the residents were psychotic or deteriorated, sitting like zombies in their foul-smelling rooms or shrieking some delusion or hallucination in the halls, many of them in restraints. With our gallows humor reaction to the place, my colleagues and I threatened one another with being locked up for two hours on one of the floors, guaranteeing that the victim would come out raving. Yet, as we left one day, we ran into some members of the Board of Trustees, and, after introductions and the usual polite interchanges, the President of the Board, with a big smile on his face, enunciated, "Our people come here to live and not to die." One gets used to the clichés in the field, but the contrast between this man's evident pride and our own depression was startling, and we were overwhelmed with the necessity for evaluation studies. In the fifteen years since then there have been many developments in evaluation of programs for the aged, but the clichés, the poor programs and the differences of opinion continue.

The importance of evaluation in mental health programs has been increasingly established in recent years, supported by the need to screen the many psychopharmacologic agents that have appeared, and has been conceptually and operationally built into community mental health center programs. The rationale of evaluation is twofold: first, that it provides a scientifically rigorous method of determining the therapeutic efficacy of the treatment or program, and secondly, that these results can exercise a feedback into the system, modifying the clinical operations. Ideally, such a system should lead inevitably to constant improvement of levels of care, reinforcing good programs and discouraging those programs that are poorer. Regrettably, the ideal has not been the reality.

The purpose of this chapter is to highlight what, we believe, are the important issues and the directions of change that are indicated. We will consider some of the usual Who, How, What variables: the specifications of the population studied, the procedures and interventions that were carried out, and the evaluative criteria employed. From a broader perspective these aspects of research design are related to a system of values and expectations which are characteristically implicit. These goals and assumptions, which are hardly hinted at in the restricted statements of explicit goals, could be called the Why variables, and need to be taken into account to place the individual studies in a proper context.

Although all the evaluation dimensions are interrelated, we will first consider the major types of evaluation studies, including some of the important population or subject issues, and then examine the complicated questions of evaluation criteria.

Types of Studies

Intra-institutional Studies

The basic design of the intra-institutional study is the introduction of a program for the inmates that is expected to have some ameliorative effect. One basic objection to such studies is that it is not clear what is being affected, the mental disorder itself, the effects of the institution, or the interaction of the two. In any case, the results of intra-institutional improvement studies suggest two general conclusions: 1) that almost anything helps, and 2) that almost nothing helps—or, at least, that nothing helps very much. These programs range from extensive milieu or rehabilitation treatment plans in which a variety of techniques are offered (such as, physical therapy, individual therapy, occupational therapy, work programs and, most frequently, some sort of social group), to more limited studies which employ one or two of these basic mental health techniques. No matter what the treatment, the results are generally described as favorable in such terms as "improved self concept," "increased group interaction," "more adaptive behavior," "activity and conversations increased" (Donahue et al., 1960; Gottesman, 1965; Rechtschaffen et al., 1954; Pappas et al., 1958; Cosin et al., 1958).

But even granting that such loosely defined and measured criteria mean anything, in the context of the primitive conditions and prevailing custodial attitudes within the institutions, it is likely that any change introduced will make some sort of improvement. Lieberman

(1969) feels that the described changes may well be a manifestation of a "Hawthorne" effect, in which any alteration in a boring and repetitive situation leads to increased behavioral output. One of us was studying patients in a particularly bad nursing home when a breakdown in the heating system led the usually withdrawn patients to huddle together for warmth and to a general increase in social interaction. In this case, an additional negative stimulus led to the same kind of improvement as reported with more benevolent planned changes.

There are other reservations about the intra-institutional studies. Improvements in functioning may be transitory, with behavior declining following the cessation of the intensive therapy (Pappas *et al.,* 1958; Cosin *et al.,* 1958). This is apparently the case even when the institution's staff has been especially trained in methods to counteract the harmful effects of custodial treatment (Penchansky and Taubenhaus, 1965). Negative behavior may also result from the treatment. Jones (1972) was able to increase social interaction through recreation therapy in a nursing home, but also noted much conflict, hostility and mistrust among the patients during the program. Changes in patient behavior within an institution may have little bearing on subsequent behavior (Erickson, 1962). In working with an adult hospitalized population, Forsyth and Fairweather (1961) found that the criteria of improvement within the institution, such as ward behavior ratings and MMPI scales, showed no relation to criteria of adjustment six months after discharge. Increased discharge rate is frequently used as an evaluation measure of a program's success, but this is equivocal, as it may well be more of an administrative decision than a reflection of substantial differences in the patients.

Behavior modification techniques appear to have obtained results comparable to other methods, and are subject to the same criticisms, although the number of studies on institutionalized geriatric subject is limited (Cautela, 1966). Methodological discussions of behavior modification and aging have been contributed by Lindsley (1964) and Cohen (1967). Cautela (1969) has described the utilization of such techniques as relaxation, desensitization and thought stopping, necessarily restricting himself to the less impaired patients. Libb and Clements (1969) used a token reinforcement system with four severely impaired patients and found some increase in rate of performance on an exercise task. Filer and O'Connell (1964) worked in a large V.A. hospital and operated a system of consistent and discriminate rewards and feedback. Grossman and Kilian (1972) attempted to apply the principles of the token economy on a mixed ward containing both chronic schizophrenic and senile geriatric patients. They felt the program was a success for most patients in improving their grooming and social interaction, but that it was very fragile and was not maintained without the leaders' presence; it also had negative consequences such as increasing staff friction, inducing regression in at least one patient, and being unsuccessful with patients who were extremely depressed and withdrawn or who had severe organic impairment. Davison (1969), in an appraisal of behavior modification techniques with adults in institutional settings criticizes such studies as those of Ayllon and Azrin (1968) by indicating that some behaviors could not be modified, particularly self-care, and that undesirable mechanisms were also reinforced.

One of the most glaring difficulties of these institutional studies is in the peculiar definition of a geriatric population in state mental hospitals. These include chronic schizophrenics and persons with other mental disorders with long histories of illness, some having been hospitalized for as much as forty years or longer. Although it is useful to study changes in these patients with increasing age, it is absurd to mix them up in a heterogeneous hodge-podge with patients whose mental disorders occurred late in life and consider the whole thing a "geriatric" study. These chronic patients are so different in so many critical areas that they should be studied separately. A chronic schizophrenic at age 75 who has been institutionalized for thirty years undoubtedly has more resemblance to another schizophrenic fifty years old and hospitalized for thirty years than with another 75-year-old with a six-month history of impaired behavior following a stroke.

To combine such diverse patients in an undifferentiated study seems so patently in error that it would seem surprising that it is done so frequently. The explanation may be found, we believe, in the administrative practices of state mental hospitals, given the context of our historic tradition of negative stereotypes about the aged. In state hospitals services are typically organized by chronological age, and the geriatric service is usually for all patients 65 years of age and older. Accordingly, when a patient in one of the other wards reaches his 65th birthday he is automatically transferred to the geriatric unit. He may have been on one ward for many years with other chronic patients, but he is now transferred as though he were a different kind of problem and needed a different staff. When new aged patients are admitted to the hospital they also go into the geriatric unit, and the whole melange is treated as "geriatric." Because of our negative stereotypes about aging, those who establish intervention programs in these units go unquestioningly along with this characterization, accepting all the distortions introduced by the contamination of populations, whether it is the apathy and withdrawal of institutionalism confused with the effects of aging, or inaccurate perception of the true geriatric problems because of the schizophrenics' superior cognitive functioning.

Since the chronic patients had already shown difficulty in responding to the hospital treatment program it is unlikely that the shift to a geriatric ward will make much difference. While working with chronic schizophrenics has its own merits, these intractable institutionalized subjects give a negative therapeutic aura to all aged persons. In actual studies, the inclusion of schizophrenics distorts our understanding of the effect of a given mental health program on persons with the mental disorders of later life.

Very similar in its effect to the inclusion of schizophrenics is the preoccupation with other chronic institutionalized populations in many studies. With so many old persons institutionalized in homes for the aged and nursing homes, and with so many of them showing mental disorders (Goldfarb, 1962), they seem to represent both a convenient and appropriate population for study. But focusing on such patients limits to an extreme the kind of questions or interventions that can be studied. They suffer from institutionalism, which has been defined as a "syndrome which develops in an institutional setting that limits the individual's capacity for extra-institutional living" (Ochberg, Zarcone and Hamburg, 1972). As Macmillan (1958) and others (e.g., Wing and Brown, 1970) have pointed out, the deleterious effect of the institution may be greater than the mental disorder itself. Therapeutic interactions in such a setting may just be attempts at reversing the very difficulties we have brought on by institutionalization rather than by mental problems of aging. This leads to a circular process in which the poor results serve to confirm the notion that the aged are so disabled as to have required institutionalization in the first place.

Let us consider two of the most important, well-controlled studies of attempts to alter the behavior of chronic populations which exemplify the difficulties of intra-institutional programs.

Study I. One of the most elaborate reports (Kelman, 1962) was an ambitious experiment in the rehabilitation of nursing home patients, undertaken by a cooperative group of leaders in rehabilitation medicine and public health in New York City. Despite earlier reports of the negative effects of rehabilitation programs with nursing home populations (Reynolds *et al.,* 1959; Moskowitz *et al.,* 1960) they undertook an especially intensive effort to alter the level of self-care, including transfer to special rehabilitation institutions. The study was based on the observation that there was a discrepancy between the poor self-care clinically shown by the patients in the nursing home and the abilities they demonstrated when tested in the hospital. Their experimental design employed matched samples of randomly assigned treated and untreated patients, 89 percent of whom were over age 60, compared before and after one year of intervention. The change criteria were levels of function in ambulation, dressing, feeding, toileting and transfer skills. The subjects were all welfare recipients residing in a group of proprietary nursing homes in New York City, who had physical impairments limiting function in one or more self-care areas. Originally there were two treatment and two control groups, with about 100 patients in each. One treatment group remained in the nursing home and was evaluated by a mobile rehabilitation team consisting of a psychiatrist, a social worker, physical and occupational therapists, speech therapist, nurse, psychologist and group worker. The team devised and carried out an individually planned therapeutic program for each patient. The hospital treatment group was transferred to an established rehabilitation hospital where they received the regular program and then returned to the nursing home. One control group consisted of similar patients in nursing homes not part of the regular study to avoid any contamination of effects. A third, unintentional, control group was the somewhat more than half of those selected for transfer to the rehabilitation hospital who actually refused to go.

The results showed no difference between the experimental and control groups and no significant change within any group. All groups contained some patients who improved and somewhat more who got worse with most remaining the same. About one-fifth of all patients died at the end of the year.

In their attempt to explain their negative results, it was pointed out that the patients were chronically ill, had mostly been institutionalized for over a year, were financially dependent, tended to have no actively interested families, and were all drawn from low and marginal socioeconomic groups. Clinically the patients were apathetic and reluctant participants in the rehabilitation process. It required intense exhortation to get even a minority of the designated group to the hospital treatment centers. The rehabilitation goals of more independent self-care had little relevance to either the patients or the nursing home staff. The patients were either so depressed and pessimistic about their futures, or were ideologically opposed, feeling that they had a "right" to be cared for. The nursing home staff felt that improved, but incomplete, independence in functioning only led to greater demands on their time and energy.

Study II. There have also been elaborate studies of efforts to improve behavior in homes for the aged. Probably the most ambitious and sophisticated have been the studies undertaken at the Philadelphia Geriatric Center (Brody *et al.*, 1971; Kleban and Brody, 1972; Kleban *et al.*, 1971). They started out with the observation that functional incapacity is frequently greater than that warranted by the actual impairment. This observation was also the basis of the Kelman (1962) nursing home study and was reported by Kahn (1965) to be a widespread characteristic of aged persons in institutions, and which he termed "excess disability." In the Philadelphia Geriatric Center studies 32 matched pairs of women, mean ages in the early 80's, were evaluated for individual areas of excess disability such as mobility, personal self-care, social or family relationships, organized activities, individualized activities and emotional discomfort. Each person had a baseline determination and was elaborately evaluated by the usual extensive interdisciplinary team on the basis of history, observation, and meetings with the family. Each person was also evaluated on 109 different variables on ten different tests. During the one-year study the staff worked intensively as they saw fit with each experimental subject, while the controls received the customary institutional program. When the year was up, each person was reevaluated for his excess disabilities and his behavior on the 109 variables. In addition, outside observers were brought in to evaluate the change in excess disabilities on the basis of chart and other staff notes.

The results showed that both experimental and control groups improved with respect to their excess disabilities, but that for two areas, family relationships and individualized activities, the experimental group did significantly better. A significant degree of improvement for those medical disabilities diagnosed as excessive was found for both experimental and control subjects. On the 109 variables significant change occurred for both groups, and for only five was the difference between the groups significant. Combining these meagre results with the death toll, 31 percent in the experimental group and 18 percent of the controls, indicates a very minimal outcome.

The difficulties encountered by these well-designed, intensive studies such as those of Kelman and the Philadelphia Geriatric Center indicate that, although their attempt to provide humane, individualized care for the institutionalized aged is laudable, the results are hardly worth the effort. At this stage of our knowledge, however, we must assume that these poor outcomes reflect on the deteriorative effect of institutions rather than the intractibility of the aged.

Effect of Changes in Institutionalization: Relocation

A special type of study in recent years has been on the effect of relocation of aged persons from one institutional setting to another. Already suffering from chronic institutionalization, these persons have proved to be very vulnerable to transfer from state hospitals to nursing homes (Jasnau, 1967), or from an old home to a new one (Kral *et al.*, 1968; Markus *et al.*, 1972; Aldrich and Mendkoff, 1963), or transfer from one hospital ward to another because of fire (Aleksandrowicz, 1961), with significant increases in mortality frequently, but not always, occurring. Lieberman (1961) has noted a similar increase in mortality when persons on a waiting list for admission to a home for the aged finally enter. The various studies are not consistent in identification of predictive factors, although persons with brain syndromes are generally reported with the highest death rates (Blenkner, 1967).

Admission to Institutions: Alternative Treatment

What has been done in the way of effective programming at the point of admission to the institution before the chronic effects set in?

Sklar and O'Neill (1961) randomly assigned newly admitted patients to an "intensive treatment" geriatric ward and a control group to a regular hospital ward. Although their experimental group had a markedly higher return rate to the community, their results are contaminated by the fact that as part of their intensive care they had a social worker to make placement plans with the family, obviously facilitating discharge.

An unusually effective and important study influenced by the critical views of institutions of Goffman (1957) and Kleemeier (1963), has been conducted by Kahana and Kahana (1970) on the factor of age-segregation in a mental hospital. They took 55 consecutive male admissions 60 years of age and older and randomly assigned them to one of three wards: an age-segregated custodial ward with only aged patients, an age-integrated custodial ward which included the whole adult range, and a special therapy ward which, although having only aged patients, had small numbers, a mixture of men and women, a high staff ratio, and an intense activity program. Each patient was evaluated for interaction in the areas of affect, responsiveness to the environment and mental status, by means of interviews, naturalistic observations and staff ratings. Retesting was done after three weeks, which was the outer limit of the hospital system's tolerance of the random assignments.

They found that patients placed in the age-integrated custodial ward and in the therapy ward showed significantly greater improvement in responsiveness and mental status than those in the age-segregated custodial ward.

Several factors are considered to have contributed to the results differentiating the age-integrated and segregated wards. Even though both were custodial, the integrated ward provided different role models because it had younger patients. There was more general activity, more visiting, more hope and more planning to leave the hospital. Two social workers were assigned to this ward, while the age-segregated ward obtained social service aid only upon request. Contrary to the expectations of some that the older persons would suffer from the activity and demands of the younger patients, they, in fact, benefitted from special privileges. Younger patients offered their superior physical and intellectual resources in a non-reciprocating friendship pattern (walking the older men to meals, showers and the canteen, and allowing them to spend time outside the ward because a younger patient was watching). The older persons were given such privileges as being allowed to go to the front of the foodline and take afternoon naps, and aides were more tolerant of incontinence, even passing it off as an accident. The services of the half-time physician, less in demand by the younger patients, were more readily available to the aged patients. Finally, on the age-integrated ward the aged developed a group cohesion and would help some of their feeble contemporaries, while on the age-segregated ward they seemed to have lost "even the identity of an old person."

This finding is analogous to the celebrated Skeels (1966) study in which he followed institutionalized children for 30 years. He made the startling observation that young children of normal intelligence who were raised in an orphan asylum deteriorated in time to the level of retardation and had to be kept in institutions; while children who initially tested as mentally retarded and were transferred to an institution for the retarded, grew up to have normal intellectual functioning and to lead normal lives in the community. Skeels accounted for the dramatic increase in the functioning of the children originally placed in the institution for the retarded by their uniqueness by virtue of being much younger than the other inmates. They consequently received much fussing and stimulation and special privilege.

The Kahana study represents a rarity, a well-controlled evaluative study demonstrating the application of theory to a type of intervention which is significantly effective. It should also be emphasized that this study is a clear-cut demonstration of the effectiveness of a special therapy ward with a newly admitted population, although such a program is obviously much more expensive than the age-integrated custodial ward without achieving any better results.

But the significance of this study must be qualified, partly because of the inclusion of patients with chronic disorders, although that data is handled separately, and mainly, because non-testables are excluded. This was a response to the pragmatic realities of the situation, since non-testables very likely would not have been tolerated on the research wards. But, like errors of inclusion, such as, combining chronic schizophrenics and persons with mental disorders of old age, exclusion errors can also be a significant problem in evaluation of mental health studies in the aged. This is expressed through the classic exclusion criterion of "testability" which is so characteristic of psychological methodology. The very need for evaluation data with its emphasis on tests thus can have the effect of paradoxically transforming the process it is designed to measure. It is likely that the non-testables, including even those who have died, may be the most critical subjects for the particular program being studied. Testability is largely affected by such factors as degree of cerebral impairment, severe depression and paranoid behavior, obviously major mental health problems of the aged. Meanwhile, we can applaud those researchers who have recognized the importance of total sampling, such as Markus *et al.* (1972). In their study on relocation, all residents were interviewed, they said, "whether or not they were bedridden, 'out of touch,' too sick or senile to be seen in the opinion of the nursing staff."

Alternatives to Institutionalization

In his review of the effects of institutionalization on the aged, Lieberman (1969) has summarized the many studies showing increased mortality rates and noxious psychological characteristics as "poor adjustment, depression and unhappiness, intellectual ineffectiveness because of increased rigidity and low energy..., negative self-image, feelings of personal insignificance and impotency, and a view of self as old. Residents tend to be docile, submissive, show a low range of interests and activities, and to live in the past rather than the future. They are withdrawn and unresponsive in relationship to others."

With the overwhelming numbers of aged in state mental hospitals, much of the criticism of institutional effects was focused on them, and the question was raised of how "appropriate" were many of the patient commitments there. Accordingly programs were developed aimed at screening the aged and finding alternatives to the state mental hospital "by making greater use of other community resources that were believed to be more suitable to the needs of the patients" (Epstein and Simon, 1968). The screening programs have been very successful when measured by their stated goal of reducing hospital admissions. Stotsky (1967) was able to successfully place in nursing homes 81 percent of 141 state hospital aged patients. Epstein and Simon (1968) set up such a preadmission screening unit in San Francisco General Hospital in 1964 and achieved a striking reduction in state hospital admissions from San Francisco, going from a previous mean base of 450 a year to 40 in 1965, 12 in 1966, and none in 1967. These results presumably confirmed the belief that old people didn't really have to be committed to state hospitals, and could be handled in other facilities, mainly nursing homes.

Epstein and Simon (1968) then proceeded to do a one-year follow-up on a three-month sample of 99 screened patients who were sent to nursing homes, compared to 436 patients sent to state hospitals prior to the implementation of the screening program. Only patients with no psychiatric illness before age 60 were studied, but there were far more with simultaneous acute and chronic brain syndromes in the state hospital group, 41 compared to 13 percent. They found that of the nursing home population 25 percent had died and 54 percent were still in institutions, while 39 percent of the state hospital patients had died and 36 percent were still institutionalized. Orientation was somewhat better in the state hospital patients. The greatest difference was in the area of self-maintenance, with the state hospital patients far superior to those in nursing homes in such areas as toileting, bathing, grooming and dressing. For example, in the state hospital population 38 percent needed no help in bathing compared to only 7 percent in the nursing home group. For dressing without assistance, it was 52 percent in the state hospital and only 20 percent in the nursing home. The same direction of difference was even found between the two groups for those patients who were no longer institutionalized, with those who had been assigned to nursing homes doing poorer. No help in bathing was required by 83 percent of the ex-state hospital patients, compared to 68 percent of those who had been in nursing homes.

So powerful was the set that led to the study in the first place that, despite their own evidence that patients placed in other facilities did more poorly, Epstein and Simon (1968) concluded that their hospitalization study "confirms that for elderly mental patients there are alternatives to hospitalization in a state mental hospital." What they failed to state is whether or not they have shown a *better* alternative to hospitalization. Their study represents a classic problem in evaluation studies, the confusion of means and ends. If placement is regarded as the evaluation criterion, then placing the patients in other than state hospitals indicates a great success. If functioning of the patient after placement is the evaluation criterion, as it should be, then placement in a nursing home is seen as having a more *deleterious* outcome.

The mistake made by the program to keep the aged out of state hospitals which ends by sending them to an even more deleterious place, the nursing home, is the failure to understand why the hospital was so noxious in the first place. Certainly many of the criticisms made of the state mental hospital (such as Goffman, 1957 or Kleemeier, 1963) are even more applicable to nursing homes. The reason for the distortion may be linked to social and historical characteristics. Grob (1966), in his fine historical study of the decline and fall of the Worcester State Hospital in Massachusetts, has traced the development of negative attitudes and practices that occurred when the patients began to be drawn from the waves of new immigrants.

Another reason for the error in overvaluation of other than state hospitals may be in naive definition of "in the community," a phrase so popular in current terminology. If the state hospital is considered the ultimate in being away from the community, any other facility, especially if more proximal to geographic population centers, becomes automatically considered as in the community and therefore better.

Alternatives to Institutionalization: Community Programs

Traditionally many studies of mental health services for the aged have focused on operations within encapsulated or total institutions: the state hospital, the nursing home, the home for the aged. But the very use of these facilities has been challenged by some of the newer conceptions of community mental health. The two major criticisms of these institutions is 1) that they present too limited a treatment alternative and 2) that what is really needed is a comprehensive system of care which includes many alternatives and continuity of care in relating to the different components. Some of the newer ideas have been expressed by Daniels and Kahn (1968) and in the Guide to Program Development put out by the Group for the Advancement of Psychiatry (1971). Actual programs which have attempted to put these ideas into practice are those of Macmillan (1958), Perlin and Kahn (1968) and Whitehead (1970).

One type of alternative to hospitalization is a system of coordinated care. Hacker and Gaitz (1972) established a team approach for elderly admissions to the county psychiatric screening ward. They also found they could greatly reduce the proportion of state hospitalization, but that comprehensive care plans were difficult to achieve because of resistance to change and the lack of community resources. They introduced a new twist to evaluation research in that they also measured the evaluation of the team's actions by the patients, families and other caregivers. They found that most patients and families had little appreciation of the value of the team.

There have been few attempts to establish really comprehensive community mental health programs for the aged, and those that have existed have not used control group comparisons which are really critical for evaluation purposes. One of the earliest and clinically most impressive was the program set up by Duncan Macmillan (1958, 1962) at Mapperley Hospital in Nottingham. With a catchment area of 390,000 people, Macmillan's program emphasized the open hospital, brief, time-limited hospitalization and continuity of care with the same professional following the patient in the hospital and community, with coordination of after-care, and emphasis on pre-admission domiciliary visitation for the aged. A geriatric day center was also established. With this combination of activities he felt that progress was made in prevention. He found that the interaction between the old person and the responsible relative was more important than the degree of senile psychosis in committing a patient to the hospital. A person with a severe organic brain syndrome could function outside the hospital in a favorable family setting. Lowenthal and Berkman (1967) in the San Francisco geriatric survey reported similar findings—that many persons who were as severely impaired as their hospitalized sample were able to be maintained in the community if there was an involved caretaker. They found that a major cause of hospitalization was the breakdown of the caretaking services that were maintaining the old person in the community, rather than an increase in psychopathology. This situation could be prevented in many cases by the supportive services of a comprehensive program. Given the problem with discharge figures, and the lack of mortality data, Macmillan does report that, with more than 25 percent of aged patients of a total of 1,196 patients admitted in 1954, only eleven were still in the hospital three years later.

Evaluation Criteria: Further Issues

Community Mental Health Programs

Some evaluation criteria that may have had some validity in the past are now meaningless in these new programs. Discharge from an institution, duration of hospitalization and readmission are good examples of variables which should be regarded as criteria of treatment rather than outcome. In a flexible program it may be considered worthwhile to have many brief admissions rather than one protracted hospitalization. The many admissions would reflect the flexibility of the program rather than the pathology of the patient.

Of course, such a comprehensive program as Macmillan's presents evaluation problems because it also involves a community and a change in attitude at all levels, so that an experimental-control group design is not feasible. It would obviously require comparisons with an entirely different community that differs in basic components of the geriatric program (Grad and Sainsbury, 1968).

Another evaluation problem in a comprehensive program is the impact of "potential therapy," in which a commitment to service may be a significant part of the program, but is not as easy to measure as direct service. Macmillan (1958), for example, committed himself to a program of "holiday relief," in which he guaranteed a family that he would hospitalize an aged person when it was desired so the others could take a vacation. In the Montefiore program (Perlin and Kahn, 1968) guarantees were made for hospitalization or any other mental health services to the aged when needed. A similar approach was described by Brody and Cole (1971) in working with applicants to a home for the aged. In selected cases the application was not immediately admitted but put on deferred status, keeping his place on the waiting list but assured that, if necessary, there would be more rapid admission than for a new applicant. They reported that 70 percent of their deferred status applicants were still living at home 14 months later and only 22 percent had been admitted. Theoretically, by virtue of providing this commitment to potential service, the pressure on the patient and his family can be considerably eased. They may test the commitment to see how firm it is, but then seem to be able to have less need of the service because of the very promise of it.

Value Judgments: The Contented vs. the Angry Patient

Many studies assume that criteria such as subjective feelings of comfort or contentment are indicative of improvement. Although this may be relatively valid when dealing with severe depression, negative feelings may sometimes be more significant. Several studies have shown that the best outcome was shown by persons who were angry or aggressive (Aldrich and Mendkoff, 1963; Turner *et al.*, 1972; Kleban and Brody, 1972; Gottesman, 1965). Naive notions of hope, happiness or life satisfaction may be more related to denial (Scott, 1970; Haberland, 1972) which can be regarded in both positive and negative terms.

Deterioration

Although we tend to think of mental health intervention studies in terms of whether or not there are positive results in which some improvement in behavior is shown by the experimental group, there is substantial evidence that many programs have harmful consequences. In reviewing the literature on psychotherapy studies, Bergin (1971) has pointed out that, in a high proportion, as many clients deteriorate as improve. In a review of all evaluation studies of casework using control groups, Fisher (1973) found that about half showed deterioration in the experimental group. Similarly, there is much deterioration reported in the aging studies. In the Epstein and Simon (1968) study, the experimental group placed in nursing homes instead of state hospitals showed poorer self-maintenance. Cautela (1969) and Grossman and Kilian (1972) have shown that negative effects can be produced in behavior modification studies. But perhaps the most important demonstrations of harmful effects of intervention can be found in several studies by Margaret Blenkner.

In an early study (Blenkner *et al.*, 1964), she and her colleagues evaluated an experiment to test the effects of social work and public health nursing services for non-institutionalized aged. The participants had been randomly assigned at the point of application for service into a minimal program consisting of providing information and referral, or an intensive program of direct service in which both the social worker and nurse were more active, or a program that fell in between on amount of service. At a six-month follow-up it was found that the maximal service group had twice the death rate of the middle group, and four times the rate of the minimal program, the rates ranging from 6 percent to 24 percent. As an explanation of this striking result they noted that persons in the maximal service were much more likely to have been offered a service providing a more protected environment. From this result they formulated the hypothesis that: "There is a negative association between placement and survival among older persons which prevails even when their physical condition is held constant."

In a later study, Blenkner *et al.* (1970) followed a sample of 164 aged persons who were referred to various community agencies for protective services. A control group of 88 subjects received ordinary community services, while the experimental group of 76 randomly assigned subjects received a highly developed demonstration service with experienced caseworkers directed toward maintaining them in their own homes and involving a battery of ancillary project services such as a home aide service. The outcome was operationalized in terms of four major aspects: competence, environmental protection, affect and effect on others. The data was collected through structured interviews and ratings by observers. At a one-year follow-up there were no significant differences on most measures, but the experimental group did better on measures of the adequacy of the physical environment and relief of stress on collaterals, both because of a higher rate of institutionalization. At this time, however, it was thought that the experimental group was beginning to show an accelerated decline. By the time of the five-year follow-up the experimental group showed significantly higher rates of institutionalization and death.

These deteriorative results seem to run counter to what could have been reasonably expected. The program sounds as progressive a one as could be defined today, making use of trained workers and a variety of social agencies and aimed toward keeping the aged out of institutions. Why, for example, shouldn't the results be as good as in Macmillan's program? This may be a complex question which has many relevant answers, but we might suggest one. The caseworker in the Blenkner study had to deal with many different agencies in the community, the coordination of which is very difficult, as Gaitz and Hacker (1970) have shown. The administrative and other coordination difficulties can leave the caseworker with limited alternatives no choice but to turn to the institution when the problems appear to be too great. In Macmillan's program he had the law especially changed so that hospital and community care were not separated, with the staff having "double appointments" in the hospital and the Ministry of Health. In this way the hospital was a resource rather than the end point of frustration, and the patient was quickly discharged with the same personnel at all times maintaining the continuity of care.

To prevent deterioration we may not only require more effective integrated programs, but also those which are more informal and decentralized.

Covert Deterioration: Limited and Basic Goals

Death as an evaluative criterion is an obvious example of overt deterioration. This can also be shown by such criteria as decline in mental status and self-maintenance. But we would like to suggest that covert deterioration must also be considered. This is a critical factor in mental health studies but, unfortunately, one that is subtle and therefore conceptually controversial and operationally difficult to demonstrate. A good example of the phenomenon is cited by Alexander (1964) as a problem in psychoanalytic treatment. The analyst may induce a dependent relationship in order to establish transference which he feels is a necessary step for successful treatment. But he may then have no way of providing for the person to take over and make the therapist unnecessary. This subversion of the goal of independent functioning means that the very success of the treatment in a limited sense means the failure of the treatment in a more basic sense. It is, unfortunately, almost literally exact to cite the old medical gag that the treatment was a success but the patient died.

The distinction between overt and covert measures of deterioration is one aspect of an important problem in all mental health programs—the difference between limited and basic goals. This problem is particularly important for those who deal with the aged. It is this difference in perspective that accounted for the contrasting perceptions of the trustees and researchers cited at the beginning of this chapter. It is this disparity that accounts for many of the sharply different orientations among professionals toward the use of institutions. This issue has also been touched upon in the discussion of intra-institutional intervention studies, where it was pointed out that many ostensibly reasonable treatment goals, such as increased sociability or changed attitudes, are irrelevant when viewed in the light of institutional effects and their significance for longer-term changes in individual functioning. We will attempt to clarify the issue by consideration of a number of important alternative evaluation criteria in which there are issues of covert deterioration.

Dependency. Analogous to the dilemma posed by Alexander for psychoanalysts is a situation common in dealing with the aged. It is obvious that the older person has increasing dependency needs, but a treatment plan which caters excessively to the dependency needs may undermine the necessary requirements of independent functioning. The mere act of institutionalization intensifies dependency aspects, and ameliorative efforts within the institution may actually make it harder for the person to leave. Nursing homes, after all, are organized around the function of "caring" for their patients, and will conceptualize amelioration as providing better care. To cite a concrete example, dressing may be a slow, painful task for many older persons, but the well-meaning assistance of nursing staff can result in the person's losing the capacity to dress independently. An occupational therapy program to teach dressing skills is likely to be undermined by the ready availability of assistance, and by a staff, since its function is caring, that will want to assist. This kind of process probably accounts for Epstein and Simon's (1968) finding that state hospital patients were better in self-care activities than those in nursing homes. More independent behavior in a nursing home may actually, in some situations, be viewed as an administrative problem, and thereby discouraged (Goldfarb, 1964).

Amelioration vs. Prevention. Many programs have attempted ameliorative effects with chronically institutionalized populations with questionable results. If, in fact, so much of the behavior of the aged person is the effect of deterioration induced by the institutionalization rather than mere changes in the individual, then the best way to treat it would be to prevent it from happening in the first place. The expenditure of major effort at an ameliorative level may only obscure the most effective way to deal with the problem. Prevention rather than amelioration or restitution may be the most important approach to such populations. The trap is that, granted that prevention is a large part of the answer, what do we do with those patients who are in institutions right now? Although they should certainly be treated humanely, any substantial expenditure of time or money in such settings would only be reinforcing the wrong system, and lead to the continued use of those institutions by subsequent aged populations with the same deleterious consequences. Making the institution a more pleasant place is an extremely limited goal compared to the more harmful effects of its continued operation.

Custodialism. Many of the services available to the aged are based on the premise of custodialism. According to this premise, what is necessary is a benign setting which takes care of the patient's basic needs, provides minimal medical care, has no expectation of improvement and will continue until the patient's death. In such a context even therapy programs, as occupational or recreational therapy, serve a custodial role, making the adaptation to the setting more tolerable.

In contrast to this conception, an expectation of improvement would lead to much different treatment. Going into an institution would be specified as a temporary component of a total program in which the aim is the therapeutic goal of restoring or enhancing independence. In a custodial context an institution becomes a container; in a therapeutic setting it will be a revolving door. It is not that institutions are inherently bad, since they can serve a very important role dealing with certain brief critical periods. An old person should only be confined to a long-term custodial setting when all other measures have failed.

Institutional vs. Individual Criteria. An important practical problem in our current system concerns the definition of a good nursing home. We once visited a nursing home that had been described in the literature as outstanding. Among its exceptional qualities were a program for the aides who were paid extra salary for two hours a week to come in for in-service training, and an active volunteer program. The in-service time was spent on a discussion of the Menninger system of classification of mental disorders, and the volunteer was a weak-voiced woman reading out of a dull book to withdrawn and unresponsive patients. In a two-story structure with 47 beds there was a dining room which seated six, no elevator, and access to the second floor only by a steep flight of stairs. The patients were as deteriorated as could be found in any other nursing home with the same type of patients.

This experience exemplifies a fundamental problem in evaluation, whether the criteria should be based on the institutional characteristics or the patients' behavior, or both. With the vast proliferation of proprietary nursing homes, there has been much concern with quality and standards. Kosberg and Tobin (1972) surveyed 214 nursing homes in the Metropolitan Chicago area and found that the treatment resources, such as professional staff characteristics, facilities and equipment, were highly associated with organizational characteristics such as source of payment and referral. The authors seem quite confident that they can formulate standards for nursing home operations. Others such as Beattie and Bullock (1964) and Homburger and Bonner (1964) likewise formulate criteria for nursing home evaluations emphasizing such criteria as staff ratios and Tender Loving Care.

These criteria can best be described as "window dressing," satisfying the needs of relatives, staff, board members, and local government regulating agencies, to see the facility as a clean and pleasant place. None of the rating systems is based on evaluation studies of what actually happens to patients subject to these programs. There are institutions, for example, where high staff ratios facilitate custodialism. By avoiding dealing with the actual fate of their patients and with no control group studies they are able to perpetuate their own wishful thinking. The mental health and aging fields have plenty of this kind of uncritical thinking in which the instrumental technique assumes more importance than the end result. It is likely that as an encapsulated institution the nursing home can have only limited usefulness. The really critical factor may be the degree to which the institution is part of a comprehensive system of care. It may be that a poorly staffed nursing home that is integrated in a comprehensive system will have better results than a well-staffed encapsulated institution.

Social Class:Ambience vs. Substance. One of the sources of bias affecting judgment of institutions and programs is the social class characteristics of the patients. Social class is related to morbidity, type of pathology, amount and kind of treatment, and therapeutic outcome following treatment (Hollingshead and Redlich, 1958; Srole *et al.,* 1962; Leighton *et al.,* 1963; Kahn *et al.,* 1959). Institutions tend to select certain kinds of populations because of their auspices and status value. In a study of homes for the aged, Goldfarb (1962) found an enormous range in the quality of the residents of the different homes. These differences reflected the social class composition of the residents, who tended to be relatively homogeneous in each setting and ranged from poorly-educated foreign-born to those who were native-born and had a superior cultural background. Although it is true that the social character of the residents influences the character of the program, it is a common error to rate institutions by criteria which reflect some of the trappings of the social differences rather than any independent qualities of the program. The ambience that accompanies higher social class is mistaken for the substance of better mental health. This type of error is very common in evaluating nursing homes, in which those with private patients are seen as superior to those with welfare residents. The basis of the reputation of many homes for the aged seems to depend on the social background of their residents.

Family vs. Patient. The relationship of the needs of the patient and his family raises some critical questions in evaluation but which are generally not even considered. The nature of the program seems to determine whether there is complimentarity or conflict in meeting the needs of the patient and his family. Macmillan uses institutionalization as a way of responding to the family's need, while maintaining the interests of the patient. For example, as mentioned earlier, one service he provided was "holiday relief," according to which he would hospitalize the patient for a brief period, not because of any clinical need, but in order to enable the family to take a holiday. He thus uses brief hospitalization as a way of preventing long hospitalization which might be necessary without such flexible support. But the traditional, restrictive system of care with few alternatives creates a situation in which the needs of the patient and his family, or society, may be in conflict. Relief of stress on the collaterals has been reported by Blenkner *et al.* (1971) and by Grad and Sainsbury (1968), in which, while the family "improved," the patients were not doing well. It is clear that there is a different goal and evaluation criteria depending on whether one looks at institutionalization from the point of view of the patient or his family and society. A patient who has difficulties which are excessively taxing his family, or who has problems because he doesn't have family supports, will then have to be institutionalized. Solving the family or social need, however, often leads to the patient's decline and death. In one sense, because of present limitations of service, we cannot take a moral stand on this dilemma, as at times it may be more desirable to protect the family's or the patient's interest. A successful outcome for one may mean a disaster for the other, so that the evaluation depends on your perspective. In Macmillan's type of program there is much more opportunity for helping both.

Conclusions

1. Most mental health studies with the aged have been designed to improve functioning of institutionalized populations, partly because of their easy accessibility. Although outcomes are generally considered positive by the experimenters, the results are questionable by virtue of population selectivity, lack of control groups, vague or inappropriate criteria, transitory outcomes, and "Hawthorne" effect artifacts. The most elaborate and carefully designed studies show negative or minimal results.

2. We are committed to means rather than ends. Little attention is paid to negative results. The very studies which demonstrate the poor or inconclusive outcomes invariably contain a last paragraph recommending more of the same.

3. Prevention may be more effective than restitution or ameliora-tion in countering the effects of institutionalization. At the present time most of our energies are involved with overcoming the deteriora-tive effects of our predominant systems of care.

4. Some of the attempts at prevention of institutionalization are either providing alternative kinds of treatment on admission to the hospital, such as an age-integrated ward, or actual alternatives to hos-pitalization. Although these show some promising results, there has been confusion in the differentiation of critical variables, so that such factors as admission, discharge, duration of treatment, or readmissions are incorrectly seen as outcome instead of intervention variables.

5. Not only do many outcomes show doubtful improvement but the experimental group, in many studies, may be more deteriorated in function than the controls.

6. In addition to overt deterioration, covert deterioration is an important evaluation component, characterized by improvement in a limited function, while deteriorating with respect to a more basic goal. The very qualities, for example, that contribute to a person's adapt-ability in an institution interfere with his capacity to function independently outside the institution.

7. The confusion of limited and basic goals is widespread, with such absurdities as evaluating institutions by their resources and organi-zation, rather than by what happens to the patient.

8. Other conspicuous criteria problems are mistaking the social class characteristics of the patient for the quality of the program, or failing to differentiate the purpose of a program for the usually antagonistic goals of helping the family or the patient.

9. It is considered that the best hope for the future is a compre-hensive mental health system, with many flexible alternatives, integra-tion of community and institution, and continuity of care. All of these terms, however, can be clichés, receiving much lip service and little substance. An interagency cooperative operation may be so difficult to achieve that a program can result in more harm than good. When a crisis develops in such a situation, the staff may utilize traditional interven-tions, despite their community-treatment ideology.

10. Comprehensive mental health programs are hard to establish, and present complicated problems in evaluation. Some programs, how-ever, have been achieved which seem vastly superior to traditional practices, but good evaluation studies of these remain to be done.

References

Aldrich, C. K. and Mendkoff, E. Relocation of the aged and disabled: A mortality study. *Journal of the American Geriatric Society,* 1963, *11,* 185-194.

Aleksandrowicz, D. Fire and its aftermath on a geriatric ward. *Bulletin of the Menninger Clinic,* 1961, *25,* 23-32.

Alexander, F. Evaluation of psychotherapy. In P. Hoch and J. Zubin (Eds.), *The evaluation of psychiatric treatment.* New York: Grune and Stratton, 1964.

Ayllon, T. and Azrin, N. *The token economy.* New York, Appleton-Crofts, 1968.

Beattie, W. M. and Bullock, J. Evaluating services and personnel in facilities for the aged. In M. Leeds and H. Shore (Eds.), *Geriatric institutional management.* New York: G. P. Putnam and Sons, 1964. Pp. 389-397.

Bergin, A. E. The evaluation of therapeutic outcomes. In A. E. Bergin and S. Garfield (Eds.), *Handbook of psychotherapy and social change.* New York: John Wiley and Sons, 1971.

Blenkner, M., Jahn, J., and Wasser, E. *Serving the aging: An experiment in social work and public health nursing.* Community Service Society, New York, 1964.

Blenkner, M. Environmental change and the aging individual. *Gerontologist,* 1967, *7,* 101-105.

Blenkner, M., Bloom, M., and Nielsen, M. A research and demonstration project of protective services. *Social Casework,* 1971, *52,* 483-499.

Brody, E. M., Kleban, M. M., Lawton, M. P., and Silverman, H. A. Excess disabilities of mental impaired aged: Impact of individualized treatment. *Gerontologist,* 1971, *11,* 124-132.

Brody, E. M. and Cole, C. Deferred status: Applicants to a voluntary home for the aged. *Gerontologist,* 1971, *11,* 219-225.

Cautela, J. R. Behavior therapy and geriatrics. *Journal of Genetic Psychology,* 1966, *108,* 9-17.

Cautela, J. R. A classical conditioning approach to the development and modification of behavior in the aged. *Gerontologist,* 1969, *9,* 109-113.

Cohen, D. Research problems and concepts in the study of aging: Assessment and behavior modification. *Gerontologist,* 1967, *7,* 13-19.

Cosin, L. Z., Mort, M., Post, F., Westrupp, C., and Williams, M. Experimental treatment of persistent senile confusion. *International Journal of Social Psychiatry,* 1958, *4,* 24-42.

Daniels, R. S. and Kahn, R. L. Community mental health and programs for the aged. *Geriatrics,* 1968, *23,* 121-125.

Davison, G. C. Appraisal of behavior modification techniques with adults in institutional settings. In C. M. Franks (Ed.), *Behavior therapy.* New York: McGraw Hill, 1969. Pp. 220-278.

Donahue, W., Hunter, W. W., Coons, D., and Maurice, H. Rehabilitation of geriatric patients in county hospitals. *Geriatrics,* 1960, *15,* 263-274.

Epstein, L. J. and Simon, A. Alternatives to state hospitalization for the geriatric mentally ill. *American Journal of Psychiatry,* 1968, *124,* 955-961.

Erickson, R. C. Outcome studies in mental hospitals: A search for criteria. *Journal of Consulting and Clinical Psychology,* 1972, *39,* 75-77.

Filer, R. N. and O'Connell, D. D. Motivation of aging persons in an institutional setting. *Journal of Gerontology,* 1964, *19,* 15-22.

Fisher, J. Is casework effective? A review. *Social Work,* 1973, *18,* 5-20.

Forsyth, R. P. and Fairweather, G. W. Psychotherapeutic and other hospital treatment criteria. *Journal of Abnormal and Social Psychology,* 1961, *62,* 598-604.

Gaitz, C. M. and Hacker, S. Obstacles in coordinating services for the care of the psychiatrically ill aged. *Journal of the American Geriatrics Society,* 1970, *18,* 172-182.

Goffman, E. The characteristics of total institutions. In Walter Reed Institute of Research, Symposium on Preventive and Social Psychiatry. Wash. D. C., U. S. Government Printing Office, 1957. Pp. 43-84.

Goldfarb, A. I. Prevalence of psychiatric disorders in metropolitan old age and nursing homes. *Journal of the American Geriatric Society,* 1962, *10,* 77-84.

Goldfarb, A. I. The evaluation of geriatric patients following treatment. In P. Hoch and J. Zubin (Eds.), *The evaluation of psychiatric treatment.* New York: Grune and Stratton, 1964.

Gottesman, L. E. Resocialization of the geriatric mental patient. *American Journal of Public Health,* 1965, *55,* 1964-1970.

Grad, J. and Sainsbury, P. The effect that patients have on their families in a community care and a control psychiatric service: A two-year follow-up. *British Journal of Psychiatry,* 1968, *114,* 265-278.

Grob, G. N. *The state and the mentally ill.* University of North Carolina Press, 1966.

Group for the Advancement of Psychiatry. *The aged and community mental health: A guide to program development.* GAP Report, No. 81, New York, 1965.

Haberland, H. Psychological dimensions of hope in the aged: Relationship to adaptation, survival and institutionalization. Unpublished Doctoral Dissertation, University of Chicago, 1972.

Hacker, S. L. and Gaitz, C. M. Evaluating the actions of a mental health team. *Gerontologist,* 1972, *12,* 155-162.

Hollingshead, A. B. and Redlich, F. C. *Social class and mental illness: A community study.* New York: John Wiley and Sons, Inc., 1958.

Homburger, F. and Bonner, C. D. *Medical care and rehabilitation of the aged and chronically ill* (2nd edition). Boston: Little, Brown and Co., 1964.

Jasnau, K. Individualized versus mass transfer of nonpsychotic geriatric patients from mental hospitals to nursing homes with special reference to death rate. *Journal of the American Geriatrics Society,* 1967, *15,* 280-284.

Jones, D. C. Social isolation, interaction and conflict in two nursing homes. *Gerontologist,* 1972, *12,* 230-234.

Kahana, E. and Kahana, B. Therapeutic potential of age integration: Effects of age-integrated hospital environments on elderly psychiatric patients. *Archives of General Psychiatry,* 1970, *23,* 20-29.

Kahn, R. L., Pollock, M., and Fink, M. Sociopsychologic aspects of psychiatric treatment in a voluntary mental hospital: Duration of hospitalization, discharge rating and diagnosis. *A.M.A. Archives of General Psychiatry,* 1959, *1,* 565-574.

Kahn, R. L. Comments. In *Proceedings of the York House Institute on the Mentally Impaired Aged.* Philadelphia: Philadelphia Geriatric Center, 1965.

Kelman, H. R. An experiment in the rehabilitation of nursing home patients. *Public Health Reports.* Public Health Service, U. S. Department of Health, Education and Welfare, 1962, *77,* 356-366.

Kleban, M. M., Brody, E. M., and Lawton, M. P. Personality traits in the mentally-impaired aged and their relationship to improvements in current functioning. *Gerontologist,* 1971, *11,* 134-140.

Kleban, M. M. and Brody, E. M. Prediction of improvement in mentally impaired aged: Personality ratings by social workers. *Journal of Gerontology,* 1972, *27,* 69-76.

Kleemeier, R. W. Attitudes toward special settings for the aged. In R. H. Williams (Ed.), *Processes of aging,* Vol. 2. New York: Atherton Press, 1963. Pp. 101-123.

Kosberg, J. I. and Tobin, S. S. Variability among nursing homes.

Gerontologist, 1972, *12,* 214-219.

Kral, V., Grad, B., and Berenson, J. Stress reactions resulting from the relocation of an aged population. *Canadian Psychiatric Association Journal,* 1968, *13,* 201-209.

Leighton, D. C., Harding, J. S., Mecklin, D. B., Macmillan, A. M., and Leighton, A. H. *The character of danger: Psychiatric symptoms in selected communities.* New York: Basic Books, 1963.

Libb, J. W. and Clements, C. B. Token reinforcement in an exercise program for hospitalized geriatric patients. *Perception and Motor Skills,* 1969, *28,* 9-17.

Lieberman, M. A. Relation of mortality rates to entrance to a home for the aged. *Geriatrics,* 1961, *16,* 515-519.

Lieberman, M. A. Institutionalization of the aged: Effects on behavior. *Journal of Gerontology,* 1969, *24,* 330-340.

Lindsley, G. Geriatric behavioral prosthetics. In R. Kastenbaum (Ed.), *New thoughts on old age.* New York: Springer, 1964.

Lowenthal, M. F. and Berkman, P. L. *Aging and mental disorder in San Francisco.* San Francisco: Jossey-Bass, Inc., 1967.

Macmillan, D. Hospital-community relationships. In *An approach to the prevention of disability from chronic psychoses: The open mental hospital within the community.* Milbank Memorial Fund, New York, 1958, Pp. 29-39.

Macmillan, D. Mental health services for the aged: A British approach. Supplement No. 29: *Canada's Mental Health,* June, 1962.

Markus, E., Blenkner, M., Bloom, M., and Downs, T. Some factors and their association with post-relocation mortality among institutionalized aged persons. *Journal of Gerontology,* 1972, *27,* 376-382.

Moskowitz, E., *et al.* A controlled study of the rehabilitation potential of nursing home residents. *New York Journal of Medicine,* 1960, *60,* 1439-1444.

Ochberg, F. M., Zarcone, V., and Hamburg, D. A. Symposium on institutionalism. *Comprehensive Psychiatry,* 1972, *13,* 91-104.

Penchansky, R. and Taubenhaus, L. J. Institutional factors affecting the quality of care in nursing homes. *Geriatrics,* 1965, *20,* 591-598.

Perlin, S. and Kahn, R. L. A mental health center in a general hospital. In L. J. Duhl and R. L. Leopold (Eds.), *Mental health and urban social policy: A casebook of community actions.* San Francisco: Jossey-Bass, Inc., 1968. Pp. 185-212.

Reynolds, F. W., Abramson, M., and Young, A. The rehabilitation potential of patients in chronic-disease institutions. *Journal of Chronic Disease,* 1959, *10,* 152-159.

Scott, W. A. Research definitions of mental health and mental illness. In H. Wechsler, L. Solomon and B. M. Kramer (Eds.), *Social psychology and mental health.* New York: Holt, Rinehart and Winston, 1970. Pp. 13-27.

Skeels, H. M. Adult status of children with contrasting early life experiences. Monographs of the Society for Research in Child Development, 1966, *31,* No. 3

Sklar, J. and O'Neill, F. J. Experiments with intensive treatment in a geriatric ward. In P. H. Hoch and J. Zubin (Eds.), *Psychopathology of aging.* New York: Grune and Stratton, 1961.

Strole, L., Langner, T., *et al. Mental health in the metropolis: The Midtown Manhattan study.* New York: McGraw-Hill, 1962.

Stotsky, B. A. A controlled study of factors in the successful adjustment of mental patients in nursing homes. *American Journal of Psychiatry,* 1967, *123,* 1243-1251.

Turner, B. F., Tobin, S. S., and Lieberman, M. A. Personality traits as predictors of institutional adaptation among the aged. *Journal of Gerontology,* 1972, *27,* 61-68.

Whitehead, A. *In the service of old age: The welfare of psychogeriatric patients.* Baltimore: Penguin Books, 1970.

Wing, J. K. and Brown, G. W. *Institutionalism and schizophrenia.* Cambridge, U. K.: Cambridge University Press, 1970.

Evaluation Process and Outcome in Juvenile Corrections: Musings on a Grim Tale

11

Rosemary C. Sarri[1] and Elaine Selo

> Once upon a time, 1940 to be exact, a sociologist wrote of a strange community to which men were temporarily banished because they were possessed by evil spirits. Although high priests were sent to visit the banished men, their efforts to drive out the evil spirits proved in vain. The banished men resisted the efforts of the high priests and withdrew from them, speaking in a strange language and living by rules foreign to the high priests. Under these conditions, the evil spirits in many of the men, instead of withering away, increased and multiplied. Thus, when the men were finally allowed to return to the land from which they came, the people found them possessed by spirits more numerous and more evil than before, and they caused the men to be banished again and again.
>
> (Slosar, 1972)

More than thirty years ago, Clemmer (1940) presented his prisonization hypothesis about the effects on human beings of isolation in closed institutions. Although the prison epitomizes the extreme in corrections programs, it is probable that all correctional programs are afflicted with the "grim reality" of ineffectiveness in the rehabilitation of offenders. Certainly juvenile corrections is no exception! Evaluation of program processes and outcomes has been less extensive than in adult corrections, but it is still apparent that juvenile intervention seldom succeeds to anyone's satisfaction. The juvenile justice system is falling far short of its objectives: serving the best interests of individual youth and contributing to public safety by controlling and reducing youthful crime. Disappointment with juvenile justice is especially strong because of the humanitarian hopes generated by the founding of the juvenile court at the beginning of the century. One method for resolving at least part of the difficulty is to focus greater resources on thorough evaluation of correctional programs so that decisions can be made on the basis of greater knowledge about the probability of attaining a given outcome from a specified program of intervention. As in other human

253

service organizations today, evaluation is one of the "in" activities in juvenile corrections. Legislators and boards increasingly request that there be systematic evaluation of newly-funded programs. Unfortunately, very little of the activity that is subsumed under "evaluation" could be classified as research, but there is a consistent groping for more effective methods of intervention. Any review of the evaluative research literature in juvenile corrections would draw essentially the same conclusions as those drawn by Rossi in his assessment of the evaluation of poverty, education, and other social action programs (Rossi and Williams, 1972). He concluded that there were few sufficiently powerful research designs among those studied to permit unequivocal statements that could be used for policy formulation.

This chapter reviews some of the issues, dilemmas, and constraints in the evaluation of juvenile corrections. It examines the implications of organizational goals for the evaluation of processes and outcomes, and following that, a series of contrasting studies of juvenile corrections are analyzed with reference to their goals, characteristics of subjects, treatment technologies, organizational efforts and processes and outcomes. Societal values as a constraint on criteria for assessment and on means of intervention are considered along with particular problems of measurement in this category of human service organizations. Lastly, elements of the plan are proposed for the evaluation in which we are engaged at this time. When this plan is fully operationalized, we hope that it will enable us to assess significant aspects of the effectiveness of variant types of juvenile correctional programs in a large number of states.

Issues and Dilemmas in Evaluation

What should be evaluated in the assessment of juvenile corrections? At least three orders of phenomena are of importance in any evaluation that has explanatory, as well as policy, implications:

1.   the personal and social characteristics of the target population that the organization seeks to change;
2.   the structures and practices within the organization that must be implemented if an offender is to be changed from Condition A to Condition B;

3.   the inter-organizational exchange among
     units within or linked to the juvenile
     justice system that have consequences for
     the varying careers of juvenile offenders.

Most evaluative research to date has addressed the personal and social characteristics of the individual offender—personality, behavior, values, attitudes and capabilities (Schrag, 1971; Suchman, 1967). Insufficient attention has been directed to organizational goal implementation, stability and adaptability, technological feasibility, referral rates, and organizational structures required for quality performance (Mott, 1972). Programs typically are judged as effective or ineffective by reference only to individual level results (California Youth Authority, 1973). Moreover, even the latter type of evaluation often fails to consider sufficiently the selective input of offenders into different types of programs. When selective assignment occurs, as it does in most correctional classifications, methods must be devised for taking this factor into consideration before there can be comparative evaluation across programs or organizations. "Tracking" is an observable phenomenon in juvenile corrections, as it is in public schools and other human service organizations (Cicourel and Kitsuse, 1964; Schafer and Olexa, 1971; Burghardt et al., 1974; Sarri et al., 1970). Again, individual characteristics are used as the basis for assignment to a given program which has a greater or lesser probability for successful outcome, independent of those individual characteristics. For example, a juvenile assigned to probation has greater opportunities for education and employment than most youth assigned to institutions. Yet the criteria for assignment may be race, sex, family composition and so forth, characteristics unrelated to ability to take advantage of education or employment. Furthermore, "time of the year" is a factor that may affect the processing of a juvenile. The probability of commitment by a juvenile court to an institution is lower in the spring quartile than in other months of the year because the court is likely to have expended its resources toward the end of the fiscal year and cannot afford institutionalization. In addition to the above factor, there are many other organizational conditions which should be considered in evaluation, but too often they are ignored or an assumption about randomized effects is proposed as a general explanation.

Standards of performance at the organizational and inter-organizational levels have been almost non-existent in corrections; where they were found, they were based largely on the collective subjective opinions of administrators. Objective criteria and ongoing

program evaluation are only now being developed. At least five categories of criteria can be delineated for organizational evaluation to then
be linked with outcome evaluation. These include: (1) *effort* (e.g., cost,
time, and types of personnel expended to achieve goals); (2) *level of
performance* (e.g., the number of individuals who complete Program X
of those who enroll); (3) *adequacy of performance* (e.g., value of the
program to offenders); (4) *efficiency* (e.g., relative cost of Program X);
and (5) *organizational processes* (e.g., program attributes which relate
to success or failure, recipients who benefit, service delivery, and first
order effects produced during the period of intervention).

Recidivism: A Criterion for All Seasons

A second and equally important question is: Should recidivism be the
primary outcome criteria in the evaluation of juvenile corrections, and
if so, how is it to be defined? When one thinks of effectiveness and
outcomes in corrections, the concept "recidivism" inevitably is considered. Most often it is used to refer to some absolute measurement of
post-program law-violative or morally disapproved behavior. This is particularly problematic in the case of juvenile offenders because data
about recidivism reinforces the "criminal" label; yet, a large proportion
of juvenile offenders in many programs are guilty only of status
offenses—truancy, running away, promiscuity, incorrigibility, and so
forth. None of these behaviors are crimes for adults, but juvenile
"recidivists" are labeled as law-violators along with adults who commit
felonies. Even in states or communities where status offenses are not
sufficient basis for state intervention, their repeated commission may
be a basis for the label "recidivist" and for incarceration, often in jails
and for longer periods of time than for offenders who do violate the
law.
    Another problem associated with the use of recidivism in absolute
rather than in relative terms is that positive results may be obscured.
Thus, a single arrest or violation is enough to classify the person as a
"recidivist" and an outcome failure. If recidivism is conceived in relative terms, there is an expectation that the program will result in fewer
and less serious offenses by participants. The addition of other outcome
measures reduces reliance on recidivism as an absolute criterion. Thus,
positive changes in education, employment, family life, and so forth
may be linked to program experiences. The recently published results
of the Provo and Silverlake Experiments (Empey and Erickson, 1972;
Empey and Lubeck, 1971) indicate very clearly a relative reduction in

the seriousness and frequency of law-violative behavior when pre-program results are compared with post-program behavior. Further-more, they were also able to identify important differences in behavior in relation to age. Their findings are similar to those obtained by Miller (1962) in a study of a community delinquency prevention program. Both observed that the program results varied according to the age of the youth at the time of entrance and exit from the program. These patterns could be linked to general patterns of criminal behavior for all youth at different ages. Thus, youth who entered the program at younger ages would be expected to demonstrate a slower reduction of criminal behavior than those who entered and left at older ages because criminal behavior peaks in the late teens and then tapers off sharply. It is also possible that other general developmental patterns of youth will produce variable outcome patterns from similar program experiences. When known, these can be considered in the program design and in the development of "base expectancy" criteria for the categorization of populations according to the probability of success or failure in the community. Moberg and Ericson (1972) argue that if recidivism is to be used meaningfully as an outcome criterion, it must be conceptualized as a continuum with variable probabilities developed for programs and individuals. They also assert that it is wholly unrealistic to expect "total conversion," as we apparently do at the present time, in measuring change from criminal to non-criminal behavior. For purposes of pro-gram planning, knowledge about the length of time and phases of change are as important as ultimate outcomes.

Recidivism is also a problematic criterion for the measurement of effectiveness because it obscures differentiation between short-run and long-run consequences for the society. In the case of youth, that inter-vention which may protect society in the short-run (e.g., incarceration in a closed institution) may have long-run negative consequences and vice versa. The effectiveness of any intervention is to be assessed on the basis of its ability to rehabilitate and reintegrate juveniles into meaning-ful social roles, not merely to reduce immediate law-violative behavior. Furthermore, over-reliance on absolute measures of recidivism obscures negative or no impact from correctional experiences. Far too few studies ever measure negative impact other than recidivism, despite general awareness of the inevitability of this outcome in many programs. Were these data to be made as routinely available as is recidivist data, opportunities for change in custodial programs might be vastly increased (Kassebaum, Ward and Wilner, 1970). Only recently in the plethora of legal actions against correctional agencies has there been any substantial effort to measure negative impact.

Ward and Kassebaum (1972) contend that the lack of concern about the overwhelming evidence of negative results from correctional intervention occurs because departments of corrections are concerned more with surveillance and control than rehabilitation. Thus, it makes little sense to measure their present outcomes in terms of rehabilitated individuals, because that is not their primary goal. Obviously, much evaluation has failed to address this phenomenon.

The unreliability of crime statistics and the manipulation of data by administrative boards, police and other agencies is another reason for caution in the use of recidivist data in the evaluation of correctional programs. Police, courts, parole boards, and other agencies may seek to improve or depreciate the public status of a particular program and, in order to do so, may covertly manipulate the data about individual behavior. The unreliability of crime statistics was recently documented in an analysis by Seidman and Couzens (1972). They analyzed police reports in several metropolitan communities and observed reports of reductions in selected types of crime which corresponded with political pressures to reduce such crime. Thus, they conclude "crime statistics...are highly misleading indicators of what they are used to measure, at least in part, simply because they are used as measures" (p. 29). It has also been recognized for a long time that persons in programs or releasees may be surveilled and harrassed by law enforcement officials far more than the rest of the population.

Experimental Design Dilemmas

Thus far, we have been concerned with issues in evaluation that involve measurement of outcome. Another set of issues which has been discussed extensively in recent years in the evaluation literature concerns problems in the use of experimental designs (Weiss, 1972; Rossi and Williams, 1972; Caro, 1971). Seldom do researchers in juvenile corrections have the authority or resources to exert the necessary controls required by powerful experimental designs, nor are they able to measure objectively ultimate and process goals as these relate to behavioral outcome criteria. Many assume that correctional decision-makers can select variable types of programs for youthful offenders; thus, there should be few limits on application of experimental designs in evaluation. Seldom, however, do administrators have such discretion; in fact, in many communities, judges wholly control where juveniles will be placed, for how long, and when they may return to their home communities.

Campbell's (1966) proposals for quasi-experimental designs offer some solutions for sound evaluative research, as do those by Guttentag (1971) for decision-theoretic models. Assumptions about interchangeability of units and definitions of variables must be made with great caution. Guttentag (1971) points to some of the problems which occurred in the Westinghouse Study of Head Start programs where the assumption was made that these programs throughout the country could be viewed as unitary variables. Our field research in juvenile corrections in several states indicates clearly that regional, cultural, and socio-economic differences must be examined and controlled if comparisons are to be made among organizations and persons. Furthermore, statutory variations and judicial decisions may dramatically alter conditions in the middle of an evaluation experiment. It is inevitable that much research in corrections will continue to be done on a non-experimental basis, but knowledge about effectiveness in corrections can evolve as a consequence of multiple types of experimentation rather than from a few definitive classical experiments.

Humaneness and Justice vs. Effectiveness

Recent statements by organizations such as the American Friends Service Committee (1971), the American Association of University Women (1970), and by social researchers such as Lerman (1968), as well as judicial decisions have highlighted consideration of the relationship between effectiveness and conditions of fairness, humaneness, and justice in the operation of correctional programs. The National Conference on Criminal Justice (1973) has now articulated a set of standards which provides behavioral guidelines regarding humaneness and justice. Enforcement of these standards through the courts will undoubtedly have an impact on program operation and evaluation, for not only is the "right to treatment" at issue, but so are the general social and physical conditions under which the juvenile offender must exist. It is possible for a program to be effective (at least hypothetically) and yet not meet criteria of humaneness, fairness, and justice. The evidence, however, appears to be overwhelming that these three conditions are necessary to, but not sufficient for, effectiveness.

Behavior modification technologies and the conditions governing their use pose another issue to be addressed by those interested in evaluation of such programs. More and more juvenile correctional programs are instituting behavioral modification technologies, and recently, electronic devices for remote observation and control of behavior have been proposed for juveniles, as well as adults, by Ingraham and Smith (1972), and by Schwitzgebel (1967). There is considerable debate about the use of these latter technologies, but the position paper by the American Friends Service Committee (1971) and the legal critiques by Shapiro (1972) and his colleagues in Southern California (1972) raise broad philosophical questions about freedom and psychic autonomy. Ingraham and Smith (1972) argue that electronic and other behavioral control procedures are preferable because the offender who accepts these devices has far greater freedom in other sectors of his life than if he were incarcerated. In rebuttal, Shapiro (1972) asserts that there is considerable risk of abuse of these technologies and that, if behavioral control through electronics is instituted, we will have effected a fundamental change in values about personal privacy and freedom. Thus far, evaluators of behavior modification technologies in juvenile corrections have avoided dealing directly with these issues in their assessment of programs, but they will need to be addressed in the near future. Obviously the use of any interpersonal change technology raises ethical dilemmas regarding freedom of choice. The external manipulation of behavior should not be pursued without reference to the social values at issue. More than a decade ago, Krasner (1962) offered the following caution about the use of these technologies:

> Behavior control represents a relatively new, important and very useful development in psychological research. It also may be horribly misused unless the psychologist is constantly alert to what is taking place in society and unless he is active in investigating and controlling the social uses of behavioral control.

Our delineation of issues and dilemmas in evaluation in juvenile corrections would be incomplete if we did not refer to involvement of the offender population directly in the assessment of the program. Much evaluation is completed in corrections without any direct participation of offenders, and where they do participate, it is only to comment positively or negatively about the program as it is presented to them. They are not permitted to formulate expectations or suggest means for achieving objectives. This continues despite the suggestive data in the literature that one's expectations and assessments are critically linked to one's behavior. Certainly, this is the case when negative consequences occur. The youth who views his experience negatively, who is pessimistic about the future and his behavior, is not likely to succeed in post-program situations. Youth are committed to correctional programs for vastly different behaviors and attitudes—yet much evaluation starts from the assumption that there will be similar responses among offenders given a standardized program experience.

Program Goals—Can They Be Measured?

Mott (1972) and others have proposed that effectiveness is to be defined with reference to the extent to which organizational goals are attained. Difficulties arise because of the ambiguity of the goals of corrections agencies, because some goals may be covert, and because there may be actual or potential contradictions among multiple goals. For example, protection of society is a typical goal in a correctional agency, but if it is carried to an extreme state, it would mean that an agency would seldom release an offender who was a "risk." Not to do so, however, would jeopardize the goal of rehabilitation.

The researcher, in his effort to measure organizational goals, must distinguish between ultimate goals and process or intermediate goals. These objectives must then be linked to each other as we suggested earlier and they must also be measured in relation to the behavioral outcomes for juvenile offenders. Implicated in any effort at delineation and measurement of organizational goals is the definition of the *problem* that is or will be the *target* for change. The way in which the problem is defined influences the means of intervention for resolution of the problem. Thus, if delinquency is defined primarily in terms of the individual person rather than in relation to the peer group, neighborhood, or other social situation, then the goals, targets, and technologies should relate to individual level phenomena. On the other hand, if the problem is viewed as situational, then the physical, social or economic environments would be the targets for change.

The use of goals in evaluation is also complicated by lack of clarity both in definition and in measurement techniques. Objective procedures for measurement of organizational goal attainment are presently not available for human service organizations. The research, therefore, must examine official mandates, objectives and priorities of the executive cadre, and staff perceptions of what should be the desired ends for the organization. The latter approach was utilized by Ullman (1967) in his study of the relative effectiveness of mental hospitals. He developed two normative measures of outcome which were independent of organizational definitions of the phenomena. The normative approach was the basis for recommendations of the President's Commission on Crime and in the recently published Criminal Justice Standards of the National Advisory Commission on Correctional Goals and Standards (1973). The general assumption underlying these normative approaches is that the primary function of juvenile corrections is the rapid reintegration of the offender into his usual social roles with as little severing as possible of ties with the external environment throughout the period of intervention and/or incarceration. Given this assumption, goals of custody and protection are of secondary importance and should be so assessed in evaluation. In the case of juvenile corrections, there is wide-spread consensus that the primary mandate is rehabilitation, but when staff perceptions are measured, custodial ends often are asserted to be of equal importance. Thus, evaluative procedures have to include multiple measures and variable weighting of goal priorities if these are to be utilized appropriately. The analysis of five programs in the following section highlights some of the many problems involved in defining and measuring goals and in tracing out the consequences of goals for program performance.

A Critique of Five Studies in Juvenile Corrections

Five studies which deal with evaluation in juvenile corrections were selected to illustrate a variety of settings, programs, and populations, and to highlight various questions and modus operandi for this kind of scientific endeavor. These selected studies are not representative of the entire range of research in this area, nor do they necessarily represent the most fruitful work. Rather, they are examples whose strengths and weaknesses can serve as guidelines for further refinement and elaboration of evaluative methodologies.

These five studies encompass a selection of research in juvenile corrections over a 15-year period—research which looks at a variety of ways of trying to effect change in youth in a variety of settings in various regions of the United States.

First, *the subject population*. What personal and social background characteristics were measured, what attitudinal, behavioral and personality characteristics were assessed; and how were subjects selected? If there were both an experimental and control group, how were they compared and were they adequately matched? To what extent were these differences in the subject population related to later differences in outcome?

Second, *the setting in which the intervention took place.* What were the milieu and situational characteristics, the characteristics of staff both in terms of background and attitudes, the goals of the program, the inter-organizational network in which it functions and the constraints upon it in general in terms of realizing program goals? To what extent are these programs differentiated along organizational dimensions; and if they are, how are these differences considered in the overall evaluation of the program?

Third, *the treatment technology* being used on the subject population. Are the intervention strategies or technologies being used clearly and precisely specified and are there real differences for the control and experimental populations? Can we separate the effects of various segments of the intervention process? Is the technology consistent over different periods in the history of the project and, if not, are these differences taken into account?

The next step is to examine to what extent they sought to discover the *effort* expended to effect change. One cannot really compare technologies or programs with regard to their intrinsic value if they are not implemented with the same degree of intensity and if they are differentially embraced or resisted by their subject population. To what extent are the efforts of staff, the efforts of subjects, the efforts of the organization, and the efforts of the community analyzed in relation to a discussion of the technology and its effects? If there are differences between the experimental and control programs, are differences in effort variables looked at as possible explanatory factors?

Process variables are defined as the effects produced during the period of intervention. These include the effects on a short-run basis, i.e., prior to termination or at the point of termination from the program. For reasons asserted earlier with regard to recidivism, process effectiveness measures are assumed to be of crucial importance in evaluation and should not be viewed as inherently "softer" data than long-range effectiveness measures. Along with traditional types of process measures such as offenders' attitudes toward self, expectations for success on the outside, and views toward peers and staff, other behaviors engaged in during treatment are also considered including: objective measures of achievement while in the program and at point of termination, and preparation for future roles given by the program. The extent to which researchers examined humaneness, fairness, and justice for the subject population will also be considered. Also examined are length of stay, costs of program, and proportions of subjects completing the program, failing, or dropping out, as well as process effects on the staff and organization.

Finally, the *outcome or performance measures* are analyzed as is the extent to which these are related back to the other aspects of the analysis. For example, to what extent are differences in recidivism related to differences in subject characteristics and the effort expended by the subjects during treatment, as well as to differences in the treatment technology? In what different ways is recidivism measured and how adequately? To what extent are other measures utilized, such as stability and survival of the program itself, morale and quality of the staff, degree of community cooperation and concern with the program, as well as behavioral measures of the subject's long-range adjustment through vocation and education.

Social Structure, Identification, and Change in a Treatment-Oriented Institution.
Raymond J. Adamek and Edward Z. Dager, 1968.

Characteristics of subjects. The subject population consisted of the universe of girls resident in the institution and data are given about the variable percentages of these girls with respect to several background measures. No comparative information is provided about the distribution of these background characteristics for other institutionalized female delinquents. The institution had a selective admission policy with respect to age, educational level, and severity of emotional disturbance.

Subjects were also characterized by their entering scores on the ICL, the MMPI, and the IPAT Anxiety Scale, which were administered by the institutional staff at intake. These data were used without reference to the situational characteristics which might have affected responses.

Only five subject characteristics—intelligence quotient, social class, religion, age at entrance, and length of stay—were analyzed for relationships with degree of change. They found that length of stay and age at entrance were significantly related to change and degree of identification with staff, so these variables were controlled in the analysis.

Intervention setting. The intervention setting was described in terms of its location, auspices, authority structure, staffing, and structure and mechanisms of social control as they affect milieu. These data apparently were gathered through observation, analysis of institutional documents, and questionnaires to residents. Goals of the institution were not clearly identified nor was there any indication of how they were operationalized; thus effectiveness cannot be measured. With respect to the environmental context, only sketchy information was provided and there were no data about the opportunity for or frequency of contact with local community people. Information is needed about the extent and degree of available outside contact and the degree of congruence between the intervention setting and the usual social roles to which residents will return, for these are important in accounting for the success or failure of efforts to integrate offenders into conventional societal roles.

Treatment/technology. The most distinctive aspect of the treatment technology was that it was highly-structured, unambiguous, and consistent in the patterns of reward and punishment. It was described in terms of its mechanisms of social control, but no information was given about sanctions or rules. Also not presented was information about the relative emphasis of the individual or group in treatment, the problem focus of staff, the kinds of diagnostic categories or classification schemes used, and the variety of techniques employed.

Effort. Information about contact with group mothers was provided, but there were no data on frequency of contact with social workers, psychologists or psychiatrists, number of hours spent in school, emphasis placed on group or individual punishments and rewards, or even the kinds of contact and the quality of contact of staff with girls. Two effort measures of students—service as a group leader and conformity to institutional norms—were related to the degree of identification with the institution and staff—a process variable. It would have been helpful had the authors also analyzed the relationship between those effort measures and outcome variables but this was not done.

Process. Process measures of interest to the authors were: identification of students with the staff and institution, and degree of change in self-esteem, faith in people, psychological-behavioral adjustment, and anxiety. They were not interested in any behavioral measures.

In accounting for the development of identification with the institution and the staff, the researchers alluded to a number of other effects of treatment, or process effects, which were not measured but were described, such as: reduction of peer interaction, little or no peer support for "fighting the system," isolation from the outside, too much punishment for minor rule infractions, no legitimation of many of the rules by the girls, and so forth. Several of these potentially negative process effects required systematic study.

The measures of change were calculated for girls at various stages in the treatment process, i.e., they were not measured at point of termination, but rather all were obtained at the same time regardless of the phase of treatment. As indicated earlier there was almost total reliance on psychological assessment as a measure of change. Although the average length of stay was 18 to 24 months, information was not given about what types of data were considered in release decisions. No information was provided about changes in school performance, in peer relationships, in misbehavior, and so forth. Also unknown is the proportion of girls in this program who completed it, dropped out or were transferred. No information was given about program costs.

Outcome or performance. This study did not report any outcome or performance measures either at point of termination or after termination. All change considered was change within the institution during the process of treatment. But, there was no certainty that any of these indicators of process change were linked to any long-term changes for the subjects, either positive or negative.

A Follow-up Study of Boys Participating in the Positive Peer Culture Program at the Minnesota State Training School for Boys: An Analysis of 242 Boys Released During 1969.
Minnesota Department of Corrections, June 1972.

Characteristics of subjects. The subject population consisted of the boys released in 1969 from the Minnesota State Training School for Boys. All the boys were characterized on numerous dimensions of background, but for only three of these characteristics—area of residence at admission (urban/rural), racial/ethnic background, and intelligence estimate—were any comparisons made between this Training School population and the male population in that state between the ages of 10 and 19. And yet, comparison after comparison was made in these figures between boys who had their paroles revoked from those who did not. It seems likely that they collected information on every background characteristic that appeared in the file without any theoretical reason or conceptual framework for linking them to the dependent variable or measure of effect. This resulted in a number of comparisons between the background characteristics of boys whose paroles were revoked with those whose paroles were not revoked being made without any really sound reason. Therefore, it was not surprising that some significant relationships were observed. A number of the background characteristics which were analyzed were never operationalized clearly, e.g., "living situation" and "drug/alcohol and physical abuse."

Several intra-institutional program characteristics were also studied in relation to the subjects—that is, characteristics of the subjects that were related to their institutional experience. These included: the number of successful and unsuccessful truancies of boys from the institution, the differences in lengths of stay, the age at release from the institution, the school grade placement at release, the cottage lived in, and the living situation after release as related again to revocation or non-revocation of parole. As mentioned earlier, the reader was not informed as to how the data were collected, nor how variables were defined and operationalized.

This study relied almost completely on the characteristics of subjects for the explanation of effectiveness or ineffectiveness of the program technology. These characteristics of the subjects were related not only to the incidence of parole revocation or non-revocation, but also to comparisons between parolees and transfers from the institution.

Intervention setting. There was virtually no description or analysis of the intervention setting. It would have been helpful if the cottages which were analyzed in terms of the differences of the characteristics of the residents had been described in terms of any organizational or structural characteristics. It is critical to an adequate understanding of the process of treatment to determine the significant characteristics of the settings in which it occurs.

Treatment/technology. According to the report, the technology employed in treating these boys was Positive Peer Culture (PPC)—a type of group therapy, based on principles of guided group interaction, which utilizes peer pressure and staff guidance to treat delinquent youth. The description of PPC states that it was the basic treatment tool of the institution. Group meetings five nights a week were the focal point of the boys' daily activities. The group was also the focus for many other activities experienced by the youth in the institution.

This is fine as far as it goes, but it leaves a great many questions unanswered. What kinds of behaviors or attitudes did this technology really try to alter and what kinds of behaviors and attitudes did it accept or tolerate? To what extent were group meetings supplemented by other kinds of counseling such as individual counseling? To what extent did the group reward and/or punish its members at times other than in group meetings? To what extent did all staff really implement the PPC program—was it thwarted at all by custodial staff or other treatment programs? What particular parts of the PPC technology were crucial for effective treatment and what parts of it were adjuncts whose modification would leave the program relatively unchanged? Were all boys in the institution really subject to the same technology or were there differences in its application, intensity, or staffing patterns that might, in fact, have been related to the success or lack of success on parole? There was a difference in the parole success rate of different cottages in the institution—it is probable that some of this might have been explained by differences in the application of the technology in these different units. No effort was made to look at the actual implementation of the technology in the institution as a whole, in different sub-units of it, for different kinds of offenders, and by different kinds of staff. This is a crucial deficiency in a study which seeks to assess the effect of one kind of technology in a single institution. At the very least, it is necessary to examine the operation of that technology in depth in order to ascertain why it was or was not effective.

Effort. Ideally, the effort expended by staff and boys in implementing PPC should be considerable—after all, "they have the responsibility to help and care for each other 24 hours a day." They met as groups five nights a week for 90 minutes, but no information was provided on the total hours of contact with staff or with each other in discussing and working on individual or group problems, how much in-service training was given to institutional personnel in PPC, or how much of a commitment the institution itself gave to the program.

No data were provided about the relative priority of the PPC technology in the regular operation of the institution, nor about supports provided by the institution for re-entry under a PPC technology, and also none about the effort and commitment by boys to the PPC program. Such differences in such commitment and effort might well be related to differences in the success of parole outcome and probably were related to the selection of boys for transfer as opposed to those who completed the program.

Process. The process measures included the number of truancies from the institution, the success or failure of these truancies, academic school grade placement at release, and the placement or living situation at release. These measures were not only insufficiently defined but were also not easily comparable with other kinds of programs. Further, they were always analyzed for their relationship to the outcome characteristics of the subjects—whether or not they had successful parole outcomes—but they were not analyzed for possible relationship with personal and social characteristics of the subjects or to differences in treatment.

Although information could have been obtained about attitudes and behaviors assumed to be influenced by the PPC technology, none of these were, in fact, obtained. For example, they could have had pre- and post-program evaluation of school attendance and performance, employment expectations and behavior, attitudes toward delinquency, peers and self, or relationships with parents and relevant others. The only intra-organizational variable which was evaluated was transfer status. Transfers were compared with non-transfers with several important differences noted. Twenty-three boys were transferred to other juvenile correctional facilities because of repeated truancy and behavior which required closer supervision and control. But, these transfers had fewer incidents of all types of truancy prior to admission than did the parolees. Why then did these boys run more than other boys at Red Wing? What possible interactions might there have been between the program and the characteristics of the boys that produced a propensity to run? These questions remained unanswered.

Transfers were, on the average, younger and had a higher estimated intelligence level than parolees. A higher percentage of the transfers were from the Metropolitan area and were minority group members. Moreover, there were fewer known cases of alcohol, drug, and physical abuse among the transfers than among the parolees. Why these particular boys were not able to complete the program was not answered despite the differential effect of this program on boys. Rather than simply stating, as the researchers did, that "certain strengths and characteristics may be necessary for a boy's gainful participation in confrontive peer group treatment programs," it would certainly seem necessary to try and relate process measures to characteristics of the organization and treatment program, as well as to individual characteristics of participants.

Outcome or performance. The outcome measures used in this study were all variations on the general theme of recidivism. Of the 219 parolees, 51 percent had their paroles revoked while 49 percent did not, and the comparisons between these two groups and the transfers were made in terms of the previously-mentioned background characteristics and intra-institutional characteristics. Revocations of parole were more frequent for members of racial minority groups, especially American

Indians and Spanish Americans; for boys with more disruptive living situations; for younger boys; and for boys with more frequent truancies. In addition there were more revocations of parole of boys released from certain cottages and for boys with shortest lengths of stay in the institution. Along with this analysis, they collected data on the average number of months on parole before violation (6.8 months), the offenses resulting in revocation of parole, and the institution to which the revocations were returned. No other measures of outcome were attempted.

Girls at Vocational High: An Experiment in Social Work Intervention. Henry J. Meyer, Edgar F. Borgatta, and Wyatt C. Jones, 1965.

Characteristics of subjects. The subject population consisted of 400 girls who entered Vocational High between 1955 and 1958, and who had been identified as potential problem cases by the research staff in their examination of the school records. From this pool of four entering groups of students in four different years, a random procedure was used to select the girls for the experimental and control groups. Comparisons were made not only between the experimental and control groups on a variety of background and social characteristics, but also between the whole group of identified potential problems and the remainder of the high school population of the school.

Differences were observed among those girls identified as potential problem students and others on a number of dimensions, most of which were in the expected direction. The data indicate that the random procedure for selecting experimental and control cases among the potential problem population resulted in generally similar groups, at least on those variables for which comparisons were made.

Despite elaborate procedures devised for tapping background and social characteristics, these characteristics were, for the most part, not used in the later analysis of effectiveness and content of service. The reason for this we do not know because many of these characteristics might well be related to outcome and would present a more detailed and informative picture of the actual process of intervention and its effects. For example, individual therapy might be more effective for certain types of girls and group therapy more effective for other types, perhaps depending on racial background, sibling structure, or personality type.

Intervention setting. All subjects attended a vocational high school in New York City which had an enrollment of about 1,800 students admitted from all over the city. Subjects who had been randomly assigned to the experimental group were referred to Youth Consultation Service, a private non-sectarian social agency for individual casework and group therapy.

During the evaluation, a decision was made to switch from individual to group treatment because of evidence that it would prove to be more satisfactory. The approaches differed in their settings—casework in the traditional agency setting and group work in a more relaxed community setting. Although this was not ever explicitly stated, the differences in the setting alone could have been important in accounting for the differential impact of the two treatment modalities.

The goals specified for intervention were vague and not well-defined. They essentially revolved around trying to interrupt potential deviant careers and assumed that the agency was successful in diagnosing potential problems. Treatment objectives appeared to be multiple and individualized, so there were very real problems in defining effectiveness criteria. There was no information as to how many regular staff members were involved in this experimental program, the actual ratio of staff to girls in various phases of the project, the background characteristics of the staff that might be related to their differential effectiveness in working with these girls, or the relative priority of this project in the ongoing functioning of the agency.

Treatment/technology. Originally, the project sought to use casework services on an individualized treatment basis as the primary technology, but in the second year, they shifted to a process of group referral and treatment. These two technologies were compared and evaluated along with the comparison between the control and experimental groups. Unfortunately, there was a wholly inadequate presentation of the differences in the two technologies and how they were actually implemented. There was a much better description of the ways in which the group treatment processes operated than of the ways in which the individual treatment processes worked, probably because group treatment was seen as more novel and interesting in this setting.

The researchers remarked that one of the social workers asked them at the beginning of the study, "How can you possibly evaluate what we are trying to do when we do not know ourselves?" Unfortunately, we are faced with the same question and are forced to the same conclusion.

Effort. Fairly complete information was provided about the efforts made by the school, the agency, and the girls to implement and maintain this program. Effort variables on the part of the school and agency included: provision of physical facilities; scheduling changes; orientation of staff and shifting of resources, staffing patterns, and treatment strategies. For staff, there were measures of contact with parents, number of interviews, and content and depth of group sessions. In addition, the data indicated that, for the whole experimental group, 95 percent received some treatment services and half of these had 17 or more treatment contacts with social workers. Therefore, the experimental group was clearly well-exposed to the therapeutic program. In addition, girls in the experimental group reported more help from social workers and researchers than did those in the control group. The researchers were sensitive to their impact on the situation. Other effort measures collected for the experimental girls included judgments by the caseworkers and group therapists about their clients. The caseworkers felt that not many of their clients became seriously involved in a treatment relationship on an individual basis, but this was not the case for girls involved in group treatment. Unfortunately, the girls themselves were not asked to rate their own effort, and we have no information on the number of missed appointments or instances of late appointments.

Process. Because of the lack of precision in defining goals and technologies of this program, the researchers were confronted with a real problem in assessing effectiveness. They tried to resolve this dilemma by presenting an array of variables designed to measure the impact of service, all of which were variants of process measures. These process measures included:

> 1. Judgment by the caseworker as to the progress made by the girl in using the agency's services constructively. Background variables of the girls (race, religion, intelligence, and clinical diagnosis) were examined to determine whether they related to the degree to which the girls were involved in using such service. Unfortunately, there was no examination of the background characteristics of staff, as related to their ability to motivate or help their clients.

2. Judgment made by the caseworker as to the effects of treatment. The Hunt-Kogan Movement Scale showed more positive results for group treatment. For the experimental sample, only one-fifth of all the girls were judged to have changed or moved positively during treatment.

3. School status at the end of the project. Twenty-nine percent of both the experimental and control cases had graduated high school at the termination of the project. Equal proportions had dropped out. There was no discernible impact of the intervention on this measure.

4. Highest school grade completed. Extremely small differences in staying in school favor the experimental cases.

5. Academic performance. There was a positive selective effect of the treatment program in reducing failing grades in academic subjects.

6. School-related behavior. There were no significant differences in attendance records. There was slightly less truancy among experimental than among control subjects. There was no difference in conduct marks between the experimental and control subjects. There were no real differences in teacher ratings on character and work traits. There were no real differences in ratings by guidance and counseling staff between the experimental and control subjects.

7. Out of school behavior. There were no real differences in entries on health records, or in instances of out-of-wedlock pregnancy.

8. Client self-reports of effects. There are very scant differences, if any at all, on measures of well-being, perception of quality of interaction with others, psychological insight and reactions to help, or assessment by seniors of their present and future situations.

9. Personality tests. There were no real significant differences in responses on the Junior Personality Quiz or the Make a Sentence Test.

10. Sociometric measures. There is no evidence of effect.

Although there is an impressive array of these process measures which are analyzed, many were not systematically collected and were not really meaningful for purposes of analysis. Rather, they were interesting observations about adolescent girls and agency staff. Unfortunately, there were no process measures designed to look at the effect of this experimental program on the agency staff or the school. Such would seem to be almost as important as discerning the impact on the client if the program were to be generalized to other settings.

Outcome or performance. There were no long-range outcome or performance measures used in this study. It was apparently sufficient to show that even process or intermediate objectives were not fulfilled by the intervention strategy. But a study which sought to evaluate a delinquency prevention program would seem bound to at least try to assess a few long-term effects.

The Silverlake Experiment.
LaMar T. Empey and Steven G. Lubeck, 1971.

Characteristics of subjects. The subject population consisted of 261 boys who were assigned by the courts from a common population of delinquent offenders in Los Angeles County.

Once boys were selected for the project, they were randomly assigned to either the experimental or control program and the background characteristics of the subjects in these two programs were compared on a host of background variables. Few differences were observed, but the experimental program may have inadvertently been assigned more serious or more experienced offenders.

Many of these measures of background characteristics were combined into scales and were subsequently used in analysis of predictor variables for both process and outcome differences. Thus, the scales of peer influence, background, offense, and personality were consistently used throughout the report in explaining instances of critical incidents, runaways, program failures, and program successes.

Intervention setting. There were very clear distinctions in the setting for intervention for the control and experimental population and these differences were considered among the most crucial elements of the intervention strategy. The control program was housed in a large physical plant of the traditional institutional variety while the experimental program was located in a ranch-style house in a residential neighborhood. The two programs also differed in size; no more than 20 boys at a time in the experimental program but up to 125 boys in the control program. Boys in the experimental program returned to their own homes on weekends and attended high schools in the community while boys in the control program lived there all the time and attended high school on the grounds.

Actual differences in the staff-inmate ratio in the two programs were not given, but the quality and quantity of the interaction between staff and offenders differed between the two programs. A special questionnaire was constructed and administered to both the staff and boys in both the experimental and control programs. The instrument dealt with the perceptions of the setting, among other things, and it verified that there were indeed differences in the expected direction between the experimental and control programs.

The two programs differed considerably, not only in the flow and content of communication between staff and offenders, but also in the degree of community linkage with other agencies concerned with youth. The rule structure and sanctioning mechanisms also varied in accord with traditional differences between custodial and treatment-oriented programs.

Treatment/technology. The authors reported that the control program was highly structured and traditional with much emphasis on training and individual counseling. Custodial factors were of moderate importance. Far more detailed information is provided about the experimental program, about theories of causation, treatment modalities, and so forth. The basic technology was a variant of "Guided Group Interaction." The peer group was utilized as both the target and the medium of change. The second important component of the technology was community linkage, providing a way in which offenders could be reintegrated into normal community roles. The experimental unit was located within the community; youth attended neighborhood schools, and had weekend home visits.

During this research, both programs underwent a series of major organizational changes which were reflected in changes in treatment methods. The experimental program imposed a strong negative sanction against runaways 16 months after it began. The control program shifted from a concentration on one-to-one treatment to more group-oriented modes and to more participatory forms of decision-making by both staff and boys. Both sets of changes were analyzed in terms of their relation to changes in process and outcome efforts.

Effort. The amount of effort put forth by the staff in implementing the program cannot be determined accurately, because sufficient information was not given, but one got the impression of fairly high levels of effort in both the experimental and control programs. More attention was paid to the efforts of boys to embrace or resist the different programs by asking them through interviews, questionnaires, and informal conversations about their own and others' involvement in the treatment process. Information was not provided, however, on the amount of effort put forth by boys in the school (there was no comparison of attendance records) or at work (there were no records of work attendance or performance).

Process. Some interesting behavioral measures of the effects of treatment on participants were utilized, including runaway rates, participation in critical incidents, and program failures. The terminal runaway rates for both programs, covering a two-and-one-half year period, were relatively high and very similar—37 percent at the experimental program and 40 percent at the control program, but these rates were associated with different predictor variables in the two kinds of program.

Critical incidents were studied only in the experimental program, so cross-program comparisons of participation were impossible. This type of analysis is important in correctional program evaluations because it is an enlightening process measure, not only in delineating the types of concerns that are defined as crisis-provoking for the program, but also in terms of organizational handling of crisis and the participants' responses to it.

The program failure rates (those transferred or drop-outs) of both programs were much lower than the runaway rates. In both programs, failures were boys with the most persistent and serious offense backgrounds and personality problems.

The summary measure of the process effect of treatment in the two programs was that no more than 46 percent of the experimental subjects, as contrasted to 50 percent of the control subjects, successfully completed the program. The remainder were runaways or in-program terminees. Surprisingly, there was no information collected from the participants in either program at the point of termination or before with regard to their own evaluation of the experience or their assessment of the impact of it on their futures.

This study dealt rather thoroughly with some of the negative effects of treatment on participants. Two particular aspects stand out: (1) There was evidence that the experimental program may have been overly concerned with custody and control; (2) both programs were far more inclined to punish boys for undesirable behavior than to reward them for desirable behavior.

This study was one of the few which compared the costs of the two programs and the average lengths of stay. The average monthly cost for the experimental program was $302.86 per boy, while it was $362.18 per boy for the control program. But the average length of stay for experimentals was 5.73 months as compared to 12.65 months for controls; thus, the difference in cost was considerable. The human costs for the boys were also less, for they had much more contact with home and their usual environment with shorter periods of confinement in the experimental program. Costs were not examined with respect to relative differences in humaneness, fairness, or justice between the two programs, but this might have been part of this type of process evaluation.

Outcome. Outcome was analyzed only in terms of recidivism in this study, but the ways in which it was measured far surpassed the usual recidivism reports. All experimental and control subjects—runaways and failures, as well as successful graduates—were followed for at least a year after their termination from either program. Recidivism was analyzed in three different ways: (1) in terms of number of offenses committed by individuals; (2) in collective terms by comparing the total volume of delinquency committed by subjects a year before entering the program with their total volume committed a year after termination from the program; (3) in terms of the seriousness of the recidivistic offenses. This relative estimate of recidivism certainly has advantages over the more traditional absolute approach. Recidivism rates were compared in each of these three ways for graduates, in-program failures, and runaways in both types of programs.

Most subjects in both programs seemed to have been relatively free of post-program delinquency and there was relative similarity in the amount of individual recidivism from both experimental and control programs. Subjects who did not complete either program were much more likely to recidivate than those who did. There was a 73 percent reduction in the volume of delinquency committed by the experimental subjects and 71 percent for control subjects during the twelve-month period after release, as compared to the twelve-month period before assignments to the program, but these findings are possibly due to regression effects. Both programs brought about a significant reduction in the volume of serious offenses, suggesting that they were important sources of delinquency control. Although there was no assessment of long-term outcomes, these data do suggest that the experimental program, which was much shorter and thereby less costly, was at least as effective as the control program.

The Youth Center Research Project.
Carl F. Jesness, William J. DeRisi, Paul M. McCormick, and
Robert F. Wedge, 1972.

Characteristics of subjects. The subject population consisted of 904 wards of the California Youth Authority, who were randomly assigned to the two programs—O. H. Close School, which used transactional analysis, or Karl Holton School, which used behavior modification. These boys were compared on several dimensions of individual and background differences, but few differences were observed between the study populations at the two schools. Despite the impressive array of data that were collected, none of these measures were later analyzed for their relationship to measures of process our outcome effectiveness, with the exception of the personality classification measures.

Intervention setting. A primary objective of this research was to examine the differential impact of two technologies in two institutions, apparently alike in their organizational structure, staffing patterns, and physical layout. Throughout the period of the study, the organizational structure and the number and the types of personnel were almost identical. The existing treatment programs at the two schools were also almost identical, at baseline. The internal climate of the two schools was described in detail, but little information was provided about the environmental setting in which they existed. They were situated adjacent to each other in Stockton, California, but there was no specification of how isolated they were from the rest of the city, how much communication existed between the two schools, how much interaction there was between staff and boys from the two schools, or what network of community resources was linked to the schools.

Treatment/technology. The heart of this research was its differentiation and comparison of two treatment technologies—Transactional Analysis and Behavior Modification. The two technologies were presented as somewhat idealized conceptions of what should actually occur in their implementation, but differences were apparent in the goals for the two technologies, the content of in-service training sessions for the two sets of staff, the composition of treatment groups, the ways in which participants were rewarded and punished, the expected actions and routines of staff and boys under the two systems, and the expected changes in behavior and/or attitudes. The two strategies were supposed to be particularly effective for a broad range of behavior and personality.

Although the written conception of the operation of the two technologies varied, there was no indication that these differences pervaded all areas of institutional life. The boys in both programs went to school with their own hall group, and were taught in an individualized, non-competitive manner. Both technologies involved heavy use of group methods, contracts between staff and boys, emphasis on improved social adjustment, and a decrease in the probability of delinquency. Readers would be aided by having descriptions of instances of differences in handling of the same behaviors, or differences in the kinds of rewards given for the same behaviors. More clear-cut differentiations in the actual operation of the program components were necessary to really understand that the differences in the two technologies were more than a matter of differences in jargon.

Effort. The extent to which either or both of the treatment technologies were actually effectively implemented is debatable. There were apparently quite serious problems in conveying to line staff that these technologies were more important than the issues of security, paperwork, or housekeeping. The priority for the treatment program within each institution might have been different for there were data to suggest that Transactional Analysis was actually implemented more successfully than Behavior Modification. There was no continuing in-service training for the staff in Behavior Modification, but there was continuing training for Transactional Analysis.

The researchers also took considerable pains in measuring the effort of the subjects to embrace or resist the treatment technologies. These measures of effort of participants were then related to their maturity and ego levels. For all these measures of effort, it was determined that staff and boys of both schools approximated the original expectations of the project, but fell short of the ideal.

Process. One of the principal process effects examined was change in management problems within the institutions. Both programs had an eventual drop in the number of incidents of misconduct reported, although initially the number rose. They also discovered that there was a continuing reduction in the number of residents sent to detention for misconduct, and when it was used, it was used for briefer periods and "for promoting change in behavior rather than for retribution." However, since these data were based on special incident reports written by staff in both institutions, they may not be comparable. This indicator was more useful for examining trends within a single unit than in comparing two units.

Also examined were several psychological indices of process effects. Results from the Jesness Inventory and the Post Opinion Poll showed positive psychological change in both units, but again Transactional Analysis subjects evaluated the program more positively. Observer ratings of behavior indicated greater behavioral change in the other unit as might be anticipated.

There were many hypotheses which sought to relate the characteristics of subjects to the process effects of the different kinds of treatment and they were as follows:

1. Transactional Analysis will be more effective with higher maturity subjects, and this will be evident in their verbal behavior and in their observable behavior.
2. Transactional Analysis will be most effective with higher maturity subjects who enter treatment expecting to change, and who receive high intensity and high quality treatment.
3. Behavior Modification will be more effective in changing the behavior of lower maturity subjects.

None of these hypotheses were clearly substantiated. Indeed, they found that the more mature subjects did better in both treatment programs.

Unfortunately, negative process effects were not examined for either program. There was a consistently longer average stay for subjects in the Behavior Modification program than for those in Transactional Analysis. No information was provided about cost differences of the two programs, although one would assume that Behavior Modification was more expensive since it had a longer average length of stay.

Outcome or performance. Parole revocation was the only long-run outcome measure used, as was true in many of the earlier studies. They compared the subjects' rates of parole revocation for a 12-month period following release with those of inmates from the same institutions who had been released prior to the introduction of the treatment technologies and with inmates from two other institutions. It is important to note here that they only looked at the rates for successful graduates, not for runaways or in-program failures, and they did not, compare these rates with the prior delinquency of the subjects as was done in the Silverlake Experiment.

In a 12-month parole exposure period, only 31 percent of the Transactional Analysis subjects and 32 percent of the Behavior Modification subjects of the same age had been removed from parole, and these figures were significantly lower than those of the control groups. No other outcome measures were used so recidivism again reigned as the supreme criteria of effectiveness.

A Summary Critique

The adequacy with which the researchers in these five studies evaluated programs will be summarized in a series of small tables for each dimension followed by a brief discussion of the overall strengths and weaknesses of the analysis of these dimensions. The reader is cautioned, however, that these judgments are crude and somewhat subjective, and do not reflect the differences in objectives, units of analysis, problems, and resources available.

For the most part, researchers handled the explication and measurement of subject variables adequately (**Table 1**), though there was a tendency to measure a large number of them without any apparent theoretical reason for so doing. In most cases they were used

Table 1   Subject Characteristics

Excellent	Good	Fair	Poor
Empey and Lubeck	Adamek and Dager	Minnesota Dept. of Corrections	
	Meyer, Borgatta and Jones		
	Jesness, DeRisi, McCormick and Wedge		

primarily to show the comparability of the experimental and control populations but were not systematically analyzed for their relationship to the effects of treatment. For example, every one of the studies looked at race in comparing the experimental and control groups but race was never further analyzed in terms of the extent to which there were differential rates of effectiveness in process and outcome based on race of the subjects. This would seem to be a rather important omission in the study of programs which handle disproportionate numbers of minority group members. Finally, because there weren't many efforts to compare the population characteristics of the subjects with those of other correctional populations, these studies are subject to the criticism of the inability to generalize from them to the correctional population in general.

Most of these studies suffered from lack of attention to the effects of the intervention setting (**Table 2**) on evaluation process and outcome, particularly in the areas of goal description and analysis and the environmental context of the program. In only two of the studies (Jesness *et al.,* 1972, and Meyer *et al.,* 1965) was any mention made of any changes in aspects of the intervention setting during the course of the research but we suspect that such change is fairly common in most settings and must be dealt with in designing such evaluative research designs.

Table 2   Intervention Setting

Excellent	Good	Fair	Poor
Empey and Lubeck		Adamek and Dager	Minnesota Dept. of Corrections
Jesness, DeRisi, McCormick and Wedge		Meyer, Borgatta and Jones	

Table 3 Treatment/Technology

Excellent	Good	Fair	Poor
	Jesness, DeRisi, McCormick and Wedge	Adamek and Dager	Minnesota Dept. of Corrections
		Empey and Lubeck	Meyer, Borgatta and Jones

The delineation and description of the methods of treatment (**Table 3**) was clearly a problematic area although all authors described some abstract conceptions of technology. In many of them, there wasn't even any comparable information given for the experimental and control groups with regard to the relative amounts of individual or group treatment; the premises underlying the choice of the technology with regard to problem causation, types of subjects most amenable to treatment, and priorities for problem focus; or clearly stated treatment objectives. Moreover, none of them adequately handled the actual implementation of the technology with regard to differences in methods of social control, rewards, restrictions, content of treatment sessions, locus of authority and decision-making and backgrounds of treatment personnel. In two of these studies, there were very clearly reported shifts in the technology during the course of the research (Meyer *et al.,* 1965, and Empey *et al.,* 1971) and in both of these the results were clearly related to differences in process effects. This is an important step and future research designs should be flexible enough to incorporate such changes into the total assessment of impact.

Table 4 Effort

Excellent	Good	Fair	Poor
Jesness, DeRisi, McCormick and Wedge	Meyer, Borgatta and Jones	Adamek and Dager	Minnesota Dept. of Corrections
	Empey and Lubeck		

Most of these studies related few measures of the effort of staff to the goals and technologies of the program (**Table 4**). Usually effort meant the frequency of contact with subjects and/or the number of interviews, group meetings, or counseling sessions held. With few exceptions, there was no effort to relate these measures of effort to the eventual process or outcome effects. The attempt to measure the effort of the subjects was even more truncated, though one would assume that such effort should affect the kinds of individual effects that occurred.

Table 5   Process

Excellent	Good	Fair	Poor
	Empey and Lubeck	Adamek and Dager	Minnesota Dept. of Corrections
		Meyer, Borgatta and Jones	
		Jesness, DeRisi, McCormick and Wedge	

There are huge gaps in the conceptualization and measurement of process effects in most of these studies (**Table 5**) although a few of the studies used a multitude of them. Some of the studies used a variety of behavioral measures of process effects to the exclusion of the subject's own attitudes and evaluation while others proceeded in the opposite way. Few of these studies used any measures of the effects of the program on the staff or the agency with regard to staff morale, turnover, agency innovation, agency interaction with each other, organizational and community networks, and so forth. More than half of them did not include any statement of the costs of the program though most of them did evaluate the length of stay involved. Although the positive effects of these programs were always emphasized, little attention was given to the negative effects.

Table 6   Outcome

Excellent	Good	Fair	Poor
	Empey and Lubeck	Minnesota Dept. of Corrections	Adamek and Dager
		Jesness, DeRisi, McCormick and Wedge	Meyer, Borgatta and Jones

In half of these studies, there were no measures of long-run impact of the program on the offenders or program at all and in the other half, the only measures used were related to recidivism or parole revocation (**Table 6**). The measures of recidivism which were used, with one exception, were absolute and did not take into account the past history of offenses committed by the subjects. In an earlier section of the chapter we discussed the importance of relative measures if recidivism is used as an outcome criterion.

Because recidivism was used so extensively, there was virtually no attention paid to other possible negative long-run effects of these programs such as stigmatization, decreased educational and occupational achievement, and feelings of injustice and anger. Furthermore, there were no efforts to look at any long-run positive effects of these programs—such as, educational achievement, vocational training, increased positive interaction with family and friends. In many of the programs, because there were no discernible positive features of process, outcome measures were not attempted.

A Plan for Comparative Assessment

Our present research involves assessment of a limited number of varying types of juvenile correctional programs in a number of states in all regions of the country (Sarri and Vinter, 1972). This is policy-related research which seeks to identify the range and variety of present policies in juvenile correctional programs throughout the country: their relative effectiveness and ineffectiveness; what new alternatives might or are being developed; and how specific change can be brought about. Efforts are being made to measure critical experiences and outcomes for offenders in each of these programs. However, organizations, rather than individuals, are the primary object of analysis, so rations, rates and probabilities will be calculated for groups of individuals. Furthermore, the assessment focuses more on the events within the temporal and social boundaries of the organization providing service, although some attention is given to cross-boundary relations, offenders' careers within organization-sets, and post-program behavior.

In developing a plan for identifying operational criteria, we considered the three targets identified earlier: *program outcomes* for individuals and organizations; *organizational processes and effort,* and *inter-organizational processes and effort.* Correctional units were classified according to a typology of the major functions performed by different agencies within juvenile justice systems: *prevention and social control* (e.g., youth service bureaus and community diversion units); *identifying and nominating youth as offenders* (e.g., police and school referral units); *processing and referring offenders* (e.g., court intake, diagnostic services); *adjudicating offenders* (e.g., juvenile courts); *containing and controlling offenders* (e.g., detention facilities, jails, custodial institutions, some probation and parole services); *treating offenders* (e.g., some probation services, community-based programs, some rehabilitative institutions); and, *re-entry for offenders* (e.g., some parole services, work release, job placement, some ex-offender organizations). This typology facilitates differentiation between units having the same general labels, but which may employ contrasting technologies or whose intended purposes are clearly different.

Our more elaborate classification of the functional categories of juvenile corrections was collapsed into four major groups for purposes of assessment: detention programs, processing, change and control, and exit management or re-integration programs. This classification recognizes that some corrections service units employ a combination of programs for part or all of their offender populations. It combines organizations that may pursue contrasting goals because their functions, programs, and results must ultimately be compared.

Questions had to be resolved about the relationship of fairness, humaneness, and justice to effectiveness before operational criteria could be formulated, as we mentioned earlier. The assumption was made that humaneness, fairness, and justice are essential preconditions for any effective program. Thus, the decision was made to measure them independent of other measures of effectiveness. A set of standards of the National Advisory Commission of Standards and Goals (1973) is being adapted for this measurement. The following are illustrative of the criteria for humaneness and justice in handling offenders:

1. Adequacy of sustenance conditions.
2. Nature and scope of interaction with peers and family members.
3. Access to and use of community resources.
4. Due process and other protections of individual rights.
5. Degree of restrictions imposed on offenders.
6. Extent of segregation of facilities.
7. Extent of discriminatory handling due to offenders' ascribed characteristics.
8. Provisions for insuring the right to treatment.

The criteria for evaluation which are presented in the following section involve both program outcomes and organizational processes. They are drawn from our review of the evaluation literature on correctional programs and from studies of other human service organizations. The availability of several comparative studies of juvenile corrections was a great asset in selecting criteria. Among these studies are the Pappenfort and Kilpatrick (1970) census of children's institutions; the Street, Vinter, and Perrow (1966) study of institutions for male delinquents; the Lerman (1968) and Bailey (1966) reviews of correctional outcomes; and several extensive reports about evaluation design, methodology, process, and outcome, including the work of Rossi and Williams (1972), Weiss (1972), and Caro (1971). Criteria used for selection included the following: (1) linkage to major policy questions mandated for the research; (2) relative ease of measurement; (3) potential for achieving operational comparability across units, communities, and states; (4) theoretical relevance and potency; and (5) observed empirical potency.

Program Outcomes

These refer to the degree to which organizations achieve their intended results at both the individual offender (target population) and organizational levels. Since both manifest and latent (positive as well as negative) results are being observed, the ratio between them provides one summary measure of relative effectiveness. Illustrative variables about which data are being collected for each major program category are presented below. These criteria are not meant to be comprehensive; in general, the research strategy calls for a parsimonious range and choice of data collection measures. In the case of each type of program the criteria are being operationally defined. This process will be illustrated here only for one type of program, "detention," but the process is similar for the other types. Detention as a type of program is contrasted from the others because effectiveness is measured with respect to restrictiveness of the custody, the length of stay, the number of youth detained, and the presence of screening procedures, more than with respect to the quality of the detention care per se. This is not to indicate that quality of service delivered is unimportant, but to specify other important criteria for a unit that is only to hold youth for processing prior to adjudication or disposition.

1. Type of detention and average length of stay.

     The less restrictive the detention and the shorter the length of stay, the more effective the unit.

2. Proportion of persons detained who have hearings within 24 hours.

     The higher the proportion of hearings held within 24 hours, the more effective the unit.

3. Percentage of juveniles detained for felonies.

     The higher the proportion of the detained who are charged with serious felonies, the more effective the unit.

4. Percentage of juveniles who are subsequently institutionalized.

     The higher the proportion of those detained who are subsequently institutionalized, the more effective the unit.

5. Offenders' perception of living conditions, experiences and help received.

     The more positive offenders' perceptions are, the more effective the unit.

6. Staff effort to curtail the domain of detention.

     The greater the staff effort to limit the use of physically restricting custody and to develop other alternatives for assuring court appearance, the more effective the program.

7. Independent observers' assessment of detention programming.

The more positive the ratings of education, diagnosis, medical care, and so forth, the more effective the program.

Processing Programs

For units primarily concerned with screening, adjudication, and referral, the extent to which dispositions vary and correlate with differences in offenders' social characteristics (including offenses) constitutes a general measure of outcome. Organizational effort and process variables have particular importance for these organizations because of their crucial role in decision-making regarding the status of youth.

1. Extensiveness of offender screening and diagnosis.
2. Congruencies between diagnoses and disposition outcomes.
3. Percentage of juveniles referred to non--isolating and non-stigmatizing service programs.
4. Nature and amount of service delivered per offender.
5. Proportions and characteristics of juveniles whose case-processing shows adherence to due process procedures.
6. Offenders' generalized evaluations of the processing and quality of services received.

Change and Control Programs

Although these programs are differentiated according to community location, goals, degree of institutionalization, etc., key variables are isolated for the assessment of each type of unit. Three facets for measuring outcomes are considered: (a) offenders' generalized appraisals of the program and organization; (b) nature and extent of preparation for offenders' reintegration into the conventional world; (c) relation between service received and subsequent recidivist behavior of offenders.

(a) Generalized offender evaluation of the program, its goals, policies, and technologies; functions, patterns, and structure of friendships and other informal systems; offender growth in self-esteem and self-knowledge; ability to handle stress and frustration; independence and individuality; and relative optimism regarding future.

(b) Degree and type of preparation of offenders for reintegration into the conventional world.

1. Levels of educational preparation and achievement.
2. Extent and content of vocational training and levels of achievement.
3. Extent and scope of occupational experiences provided by the programs, and levels of participation.
4. Nature of preparation for return to family, peers, and community situations.
5. Behavior of youth in relating to conventional social roles (work release, passes, etc.).

(c) Recidivist behavior of offenders in relation to service received.

1. Extent and type of post-unit offenses by self-report with controls for age and pre-program offense history.
2. Duration of avoidance of new offenses.
3. Extent of integration into non-criminal social roles.

Exit Management and Reintegration Programs

Concrete examples of such programs are parole, aftercare, pre-release centers, etc. We expect to find fewer units providing such services and proportionately far fewer than for adult corrections systems.

1. Percentage of offenders recommitted to correctional programs.
2. Offenders' perceptions of and judgments about re-entry services received.
3. Offenders' self-reports of legally prescribed behavior.

4. Percentage of offenders in vocational or academic training programs.
5. Percentage of offenders employed.
6. Extent and frequency of staff intervention in the community on behalf of offenders.
7. Average amounts of service received by types of offenders.
8. Extent of offender-staff planning of the reintegration process.

Organizational Processes and Efforts

Measures of phenomena or results at one level of assessment may be analyzed as measures of effort or process at another level. In studying organizational processes and efforts, we will attempt to identify efficiently those elements that contribute most to units' intended results or purposes. Again, it is assumed that organizational processes may have either positive or negative consequences, or both, for these ends.

Organizational goals

1. Content and specificity of goals.
2. Priorities among multiple goals (e.g., treatment, rehabilitation, staff morale, custody, etc.).
3. Staff commitments to goal priorities.
4. Offenders' commitments to the organization's goals and their priorities.

Executive leadership

1. Executives' goal priorities and commitments.
2. Nature of executives' relations with external units within the juvenile justice system, and with other agencies providing services to juveniles, etc.
3. Commitments to change and innovation.
4. Staff identification with members of executive cadre.
5. Degree of centralization of policy-making and decentralization of operational decision-making.

6. Relative power of rehabilitation-treatment cadre in organizational decision-making.

Organizational structure and program technology

1. Specificity of objectives for components within units' technological systems.
2. Staff division of labor based on differential task and skill requirements.
3. Levels of staff skills and amount of training required for technological tasks.
4. Articulation between technical system components, and between these and staff structures and roles.
5. Amount of resources allocated to rehabilitation-treatment technologies.
6. Ratio of staff performing rehabilitation-treatment roles to those performing maintenance and custodial roles.
7. Patterns of interaction and communication among sub-units within the organization—formal and informal.
8. Degree of adaptability of the technical systems to changes in both offender populations and environmental conditions.
9. Offender truancy or "AWOL" rates.

Staff-Offender relations

1. Ratio of staff to offenders—both total and for staff sub-groups.
2. Degree of support by staff for development of informal offender systems.
3. Extent of positive primary group relations between staff and offenders and staff-offender social distance.
4. Degree of staffs' non-stigmatizing perceptions of offenders.
5. Offenders' perceptions of staff as helping persons.
6. Types of rewards and punishments employed by staff and organizational controls over their use.
7. Ratio of gratification to deprivation for offenders.
8. Degree of offenders' participation in decision-making about major areas of organizational activity.
9. Extent to which due process procedures are adhered to in managing daily living and control of offenders.

Inter-organizational Processes and Efforts

Our concern at this level will be directed toward the effectiveness of service units in relation to their environments. It is recognized that the nature of units' environments, including those under private auspices, may be variously manifested or defined within and between the states. Effectiveness at this level is to be assessed in terms of organizational adaptability; organizational legitimacy; relations with regulatory groups; mobilization of resources; control over input and output (including offenders); relations with complementary organizations; and total level of exchanges with other units and organizations in the external environment.

1. Degree of resource control by the service unit.
2. Degree of autonomy in determining service unit policies and program content.
3. Routinization of linking mechanisms for inter-organizational exchange.
4. Degree of monitoring of exchanges.
5. Provision for feedback and adaptation.
6. Degree of congruency in expectations between unit and external agencies relevant to the unit.
7. Stability and rate of increment in resources for priority goals.

Many of the above criteria require greater specification before they can be measured reliably and validly. It is also expected that the total number of criteria can be reduced as more information is obtained about each type of program so as to be able to determine relative criticality for comparative assessment of effectiveness.

Conclusion

We have attempted to delineate some of the major issues and dilemmas in the evaluation of effectiveness in juvenile corrections. The analysis of several programs reported in the literature highlighted the serious problems in evaluation methodology, as well as the grim picture with respect to knowledge about technologies that will produce greater outcome success. To achieve this end, evaluation of process is as important as is measurement of outcome per se. Only when we can establish linkages between events within the program and subsequent outcomes can we have the knowledge that is needed for policy recommendations. Yet, most evaluative research continues to expend more resources on unrelated measurement of inputs rather than process and outputs.

Correctional organizations employ highly varied people-process and people-changing technologies to achieve both manifest and latent ends. Yet, criteria for choice among technologies remain unclear and often are non-existent. Instead, choices are based on fads and hunches without reference to input characteristics or output objectives.

Thus far, evaluation in human service organizations has focused primarily on program implementation phases rather than on assessment of program design, planning, and formulation. Weiss (1972) argues that greater priority should be given to the latter so that knowledge will be obtained about how to avoid or cope with organizational and environmental problems which often occur. The evaluation literature is filled with reports on major organizational changes which have occurred in the middle of the evaluation effort. In most cases these were unanticipated and researchers decried the problems created in adaptation, measurement, and so forth.Such change needs to be anticipated as a likely rather than an unusual event. Evaluative research will also be different and probably more difficult than other types of social science research because it deals directly with reality in settings where research is not the primary activity.

The politics of evaluation were dealt with only peripherally in this chapter, but they are of critical importance to the researcher today whether he or she likes it or not (Rossi and Williams, 1972; Weiss, 1972). The scientist must anticipate how his findings will be read, misunderstood, ignored and distorted. He must be prepared to explain at other than a superficial level why the results were obtained and what alternative meanings they may have. Over and over the findings from evaluative research report that the null hypothesis of no change was supported. The question then arises: Does that mean that the organization had no impact or that the proper dimensions of organizational behavior were not measured? Only infrequently are such questions considered.

Evaluation inevitably has political implications, for it is the means by which the character of a program or organization is described and analyzed. Social values are always involved and must be addressed as such. Many recent observers have referred to the increasing politicization of juvenile justice systems in several countries. This phenomenon will further add to problems in evaluation, for increasing pressures will be exerted on researchers. For example, we are in a period of rapidly escalating costs in all correctional programs, so legislators and others are looking for information which will be of use in resource allocation decisions. When the cost of institutionalization for a juvenile offender now exceeds $20,000 per year (as it does in several places), decision-makers will exert great pressure to obtain evaluative data about both process and outcome. Of even greater importance than costs are the social consequences of correctional experience for individual youth and for the society as a whole. Social scientists must be willing to deal with these and other value and policy questions. Such situations provide opportunities to enhance the development of better evaluation methodologies and the utilization of research findings.

Footnotes

1.   Although the authors are responsible for the content of this chapter, they are especially appreciative of the comments and criticisms of their colleagues in the National Assessment of Juvenile Corrections, especially to Y. Hasenfeld, A. McNeece, W. Grichting, and R. D. Vinter.

References

Adamek, R. J. and Dager, E. Z. Social structure, identification and change in a treatment-oriented institution. *American Sociological Review,* 1968, *33,* 931-944.

American Association of University Women. *Survey of prisons for women in the United States.* Washington, D. C.: American Association of University Women, 1970.

American Friends' Service Committee. *Struggle for justice: A report on crime and punishment in America.* New York: Hill and Wang, 1971.

Aronson, S. and Sherwood, C. Researcher vs. practitioner: Problems in social action research. *Social Work,* 1967, *12,* October, 89-96.

Bailey, W. C. Correctional outcome: An evaluation of 100 reports. *Journal of Criminal Law, Criminology and Police Science,* 1966, *57,* June, 153-160.

Baum, M. and Wheeler, S. Becoming an inmate. In S. Wheeler (Ed.), *Controlling delinquents.* New York: John Wiley and Sons, 1968. Pp. 153-185.

Brim, O. and Wheeler, S. *Socialization after childhood.* New York: John Wiley and Sons, 1966.

Burghardt, S., Sarri, R. C., and Gohlke, C. A comparative assessment of probation practices and perspectives. In *A comparative study of federal correctional program for young offenders.* University of Michigan, School of Social Work, 1974.

California Youth Authority. Follow-up of wards discharged from California Youth Authority during 1965. Sacramento: *California Youth Authority Research Report,* 1973, No. 64.

Campbell, D. T. and Stanley, J. *Experimental and quasi-experimental design for research.* Chicago: Rand, McNally, 1966.

Caro, F. G. (Ed.) *Readings in evaluation research.* New York: Russell Sage, 1971.

Christie, N. *Scandanavian studies in criminology.* London: Tavistock, Vol. 2, 1968, 73-107.

Cicourel, A. and Kitsuse, J. *The educational decision makers.* Indianapolis: Bobbs-Merrill, 1964.

Clemmer, D. *The prison community.* New York: Holt, Rinehart and Winston, 1940.

Cressey, D. R. Prison organizations. In James Marsh (Ed.), *Handbook of organizations.* Chicago: Rand, McNally, 1965. Pp. 1023-1067.

Cressey, D. R. *The prison: Studies in institutional organization and change.* New York: Holt, Rinehart and Winston, 1961.

Deniston, O. L., Rosenstock, I. M., and Getting, V. A. Evaluation of program effectiveness. *Public Health Reports,* 1968, *83,* No. 4, 323-335.

Emerson, R. *Judging delinquents: Context and process in juvenile court.* Chicago: Aldine, 1969.

Empey, L. and Erickson, M. T. *The Provo experiment: Evaluating community control of delinquency.* Lexington, Massachusetts: C. C. Heath and Co., 1972.

Empey, L. and Lubeck, S. *The Silverlake Experiment.* Chicago: Aldine, 1971.

Erickson, R. J., Crow, W. J., Zurcher, L. A., Connett, A. V. and Stillwell, W. D. *The offender looks at his own needs.* La Jolla, California: Western Behavioral Sciences Institute, 1971.

Fogel, D. The fate of the rehabilitative ideal in California Youth Authority decisions. *Crime and Delinquency,* 1969, *15,* October, 479-498.

Gafni, M. and Welsh, B. Post-conviction problems and the defective delinquent. *Villanova Law Review,* 1969, *12,* Spring, 546-602.

Glaser, D. *The effectiveness of a prison and parole system.* Indianapolis: Bobbs-Merrill, 1964.

Glaser, D. and O'Leary, V. *Personal characteristics and parole outcome.* Washington, D. C.: Office of Juvenile Delinquency and Youth Development, U. S. Department of Health, Education and Welfare, 1966.

Gottfredson, D. Current information bases from evaluating correctional programs. In *Research in correctional rehabilitation.* Washington, D. C.: Joint Commission on Correctional Manpower and Training, 1967. Pp. 28-33.

Guttentag, M. Models and methods in evaluation research. Unpublished paper, New York University, 1971.

Ingraham, B. L. and Smith, G. L. The use of electronics in the observation and control of human behavior and its possible use in rehabilitation and parole. *Issues in Criminology*, 1972, *7*, Fall, 35-54.

James, G. Evaluation in public health practice. *American Journal of Public Health*, 1962, July, 1145-1154.

Jesness, C. F., DeRisi, W. McCormick, P. M. and Wedge, R. F. *The Youth Center Research Project.* Sacramento: American Justice Institute in cooperation with California Youth Authority, 1972, July.

Jones, W. C. and Borgatta, E. F. Methodology of evaluation. In F. J. Mullin and J. R. Dumpson *et al.* (Eds.), *Evaluation of social intervention.* San Francisco: Jossey, Bass, 1972.

Kandel, D. H. and Williams, R. H. *Psychiatric rehabilitation: Some problems of research.* New York: Atherton Press, 1964.

Kassebaum, G., Ward, D., and Wilner, D. *Prison treatment and its outcome.* New York: John Wiley and Sons, 1970.

Kitano, H. H. L. The concept of "precipitant" in evaluative research. *Social Work*, 1963, *VIII*, October, 34-38.

Kittrie, N. *The right to be different: Deviance and enforced therapy.* Baltimore: Johns Hopkins University Press, 1971.

Krasner, L. Behavior control and social responsibility. *American Psychologist*, 1962, *17*, No. 4, 199-203.

Lerman, P. Evaluative studies of institutions for delinquents: Implications for research and social policy. *Social Work*, 1968, *13*, July, 55-64.

Lohman, J. D., Wahl, A., and Carter, R. M. *The San Francisco Project.* Berkeley, California: University of California School of Criminology, 1967.

Mandell, N. Recidivism studied and defined. *Journal of Criminal Law, Criminology and Police Science*, 1965, March, 59-66.

Meyer, H. J., Borgatta, E. F., and Jones, W. C. *Girls at Vocational High: An experiment in social work intervention.* New York: Russell Sage Foundation, 1965.

Miller, W. B. The impact of a total-community delinquency control project. *Social Problems,* 1962, *10,* Fall, 168-191.

Minnesota Department of Corrections, A Follow-up study of boys participating in the positive peer culture program at the Minnesota State Training School for Boys: An analysis of 242 boys released during 1969. St. Paul: Minnesota Department of Corrections, 1972.

Moberg, D. O. and Ericson, R. A new recidivism outcome index. *Federal Probation,* 1972, *XXXVI,* June, 50-56.

Moos, R. H. Assessment of social climates of correctional institutions. *Journal of Research in Crime and Delinquency,* 1968, *5,* 174-188.

Morris, A. *A correctional administrators' guide to the evaluation of correctional programs, Bulletin No. 21.* Boston, Massachusetts: Massachusetts Corrections Association, 3 Mt. Vernon Street, 1971.

Morris, N. and Hawkins, G. *The honest politician's guide to crime control.* Chicago: University of Chicago Press, 1969.

Mott, P. *The characteristics of effective organizations.* New York: Harper and Row, 1972.

National Advisory Commission on Criminal Justice Standards and Goals. A national strategy to reduce crime. Washington, D. C.: United States Government Printing Office, 1973.

National Conference on Criminal Justice. *Working papers for the National Conference on Criminal Justice.* Washington, D. C.: LEAA, 1973.

Pappenfort, D. and Kilpatrick, D. *A census of residential institutions in the United States, Puerto Rico and the Virgin Islands, 1966.* Chicago: University of Chicago School of Social Service Administration, 1970.

Riecken, H. W. Memorandum on program evaluation. In C. H. Weiss (Ed.), *Evaluating action programs: Readings in social action and education.* Boston: Allyn and Bacon, Inc., 1972. Pp. 85-105.

Robinson, J. and Smith, G. The effectiveness of correctional programs. *Crime and Delinquency,* 1971, *17,* 67-80.

Rossi, P. H. and Williams, W. *Evaluating social programs: Theory, practice and politics.* New York: Seminar Press, 1972.

Sarri, R. C., Tropman, J., Silberman, M., Pawlak, E. J., and Badal, K. *Client careers and public welfare structures.* A Progress Report, U. S. Department of Health, Education, and Welfare, Social and Rehabilitation Service, Grant No. CRD-425-C1-9. Ann Arbor, Michigan: School of Social Work, 1970.

Sarri, R. C. and Vinter, R. D. Organizational requisites for a socio-behavioral technology. In E. J. Thomas (Ed.), *The socio-behavioral approach and applications to social work.* New York: Council on Social Work Education, 1967. Pp. 87-100.

Sarri, R. C. and Vinter, R. D. *National assessment of juvenile corrections: Research design statement.* Ann Arbor: University of Michigan, 1972.

Schafer, W. and Olexa, C. *Tracking and opportunity.* San Francisco: Chandler Press, 1971.

Schrag, C. *Crime and justice: American style.* Rockville, Maryland: National Institute of Mental Health, Center for Studies of Crime and Delinquency, Publication No. HSM-72-9052, 1971.

Schwitzgebel, R. Issues in the use of an electronic rehabilitation system with chronic residents. Unpublished paper, 1967

Seidman, D. and Couzens, M. Crime, crime statistics and the great American anti-crime crusade: Police misreports of crime and political pressures. Paper presented at the 1972 Annual Meeting of the American Political Science Association, 1972. Copyright 1972 by American Political Science Association.

Shapiro, M. The use of behavior control techniques: A response. *Issues in Criminology,* 1972, *7,* Fall, 55-93.

Sherwood, C. C. The testability of correctional goals. In *Research in correctional rehabilitation.* Washington, D. C.: Joint Commission on Correctional Manpower and Training, 1967. Pp. 24-32.

Slosar, J. Prisonization: Social relationships and leadership patterns in two federal youth centers. Unpublished paper, 1972.

Southern California Law School. Conditioning and other technologies used to "Treat?" "Rehabilitate?" "Demolish?" prisoners and mental patients. *Notes: Southern California Law Review,* 1972, *45,* 616-685.

Street, D., Vinter, R. D., and Perrow, C. *Organization for treatment.* New York: Free Press of Macmillan, 1966.

Suchman, E. *Evaluation research.* New York: Russell Sage Foundation, 1967.

Terry, R. M. Discrimination in the handling of juvenile offenders by social control agencies. In P. G. Garabedian and D. C. Gibbons (Eds.), *Becoming delinquent: Youthful offenders and the correctional system.* Chicago: Aldine, 1970. Pp. 79-92.

Thomas, C. and Foster, S. C. Prisonization in the inmate contra-culture. *Social Problems,* 1972, *20,* Fall, 229-239.

Ullman, L. *Institution and outcome: A comparative study of psychiatric hospitals.* London: Pergamon Press, 1967.

U. S. Bureau of the Census. *General population characteristics: Final report.* PC(1)-B40, 1970.

Vinter, R. D. Analysis of treatment organizations. *Social Work,* 1963, *8,* July, 3-15.

Warren, M. *et al.* Community treatment project: An evaluation of community treatment for delinquents. Sacramento, California: California Youth Authority CTP Research Report No. VII, 1966.

Ward, D. and Kassebaum, G. On biting the hand that feeds: Some implications of sociological evaluations of correctional effectiveness. In C. Weiss (Ed.), *Evaluating action programs.* Boston: Allyn and Bacon, Inc., 1972.

Webb, G. E. Re-thinking macro-system intervention. In E. J. Mullen, J. R. Dumpson *et al.* (Eds.), *Evaluation of social intervention.* San Francisco: Jossey—Bass, 1972.

Weiner, N. L. and Willie, C. V. Decisions by juvenile officers. *American Journal of Sociology,* 1971, *77,* September, 199-210.

Weiss, C. H. *Evaluating action programs: Readings in social action and education.* Boston: Allyn and Bacon, Inc., 1972.

Wolfgang, M. Making the criminal justice system accountable. *Crime and Delinquency,* 1972, *18,* January, 15-22.

Wolins, M. Measuring the effect of social work intervention. In N. Polansky (Ed.), *Social work research.* Chicago: University of Chicago Press, 1960. Pp. 247-273.

Cost Efficiency and Effectiveness in the Early Detection and Improvement of Learning Abilities 12

H. S. Pennypacker, Carl H. Koenig, and W. H. Seaver

It is now becoming clear that, stripped to its essentials, the task of education is to bring about changes in human behavior in the direction of improvement. It follows that evaluation of any educational program or enterprise must necessarily involve some form of measurement of behavior and behavior change. In a very real sense, the difficulties which the educational community has experienced in coming to grips with the questions of cost efficiency, cost effectiveness, and problems of accountability in general are traceable to its difficulty in defining and agreeing upon suitable units and procedures of behavioral measurement.

Out of the tradition of behavior analysis, however, comes a system of behavioral measurement which is both sufficiently exact and sufficiently general to permit its effective utilization in meeting the problems of educational accountability. Our purpose in the present chapter will be two-fold: first, we will briefly examine the history and describe the major components of this measurement system as it presently exists. Second, we will illustrate the applicability of this system by considering its use in the evaluation of a program aimed at the early identification and remediation of the academic problems of children possessing insufficiently developed learning abilities.

Of the many contributions made by B. F. Skinner to the experimental analysis of behavior, perhaps none is more significant than his early (1938) and repeated (e.g., 1950, 1953, 1957) identification of *frequency* (number of responses/unit of time) as the basic datum of the science and any subsequent technologies. Thus, in 1953, Skinner wrote, "When we extend an experimental analysis to human affairs in general, it is a great advantage to have a conceptual system which refers to the single individual, preferably without comparison with a group. The study of frequency of response appears to lead directly to such a system." Skinner also emphasized the importance of frequency as a continuous measure of behavior when he wrote, "...frequency of response provides a continuous account of many basic processes. This is in marked contrast to methods and techniques which merely sample a learning process from time to time where the whole process must be inferred. The sample is often so widely spaced that the kinds of details we have seen here are completely overlooked." It is perhaps unnecessary to add that frequency is also a *universal* unit of behavioral measurement; all behavior, regardless of its topography, may be defined in terms of instances of its occurrence and these instances are countable. Since countable instances of a repeatable behavior must take place in time, this second parameter, time, is also common to all behavior. Consequently, the combination of count and time into one unit—frequency—renders that unit *universal,* with respect to its appropriateness as a unit of behavioral measurement. Skinner's choice of frequency as the basic datum for the science of behavior was obviously a wise one.

We have already indicated that behavioral technologies, particularly education, are concerned primarily with *behavior change.* In 1969, O. R. Lindsley called attention to the fact that the first derivative of frequency with respect to time yields a measure of change in frequency over time. Applying this notion to the measurement of changing behavior frequencies, Lindsley produced a measure known as *celeration,* the units of which are of the general form: Number of Movements/unit of time/unit of time. Thus, by describing changes in the universal behavior unit (frequency) over time, Lindsley has given us an equally universal measure of behavior change. It is perhaps not surprising that from the two most productive pioneers in the experimental analysis of behavior (Skinner and Lindsley) have come the two measures necessary to meet the needs of evaluation and accountability in education.

One need must be met, however, before we can apply these universal measures to the problems of describing behavior and behavior change within broad programmatic and educational contexts. We must incorporate these conceptual units—frequency and celeration—into a measuring tool or instrument which, like the metric ruler or cumulative recorder, may be applied to the broadest possible class of events for which its units of measurement are appropriate. If it is to be useful within the context of educational measurement and evaluation, this instrument must at once possess sufficient sensitivity to immediately reveal changes in the behavior of an individual child while at the same time being of sufficient generality to measure—with equal sensitivity—all the behaviors of which individuals or groups of individuals are capable. Finally, if such a tool is to be used across any number of situations, it should be *standard* in nature so as to permit direct comparison among the variables which differentiate these several situations. A measurement tool meeting these specifications exists and is known as the Standard Behavior Chart.

Figure 1 is a reproduction of the Standard Behavior Chart showing diagrammatically the major types of measurement afforded by its use. One notes immediately that the ordinate of the chart is frequency, the fundamental unit of behavioral measurement. One also notes that frequencies are scaled in ratio or logarithmic fashion on the Standard Behavior Chart. Such a scale, familiar to natural scientists and engineers, is strange to many psychologists and educators and therefore requires some justification.

It should immediately be apparent that the *range* of frequency values afforded by this scale (1,000 per minute to 1 per 1,000 minutes) is many times greater than would be afforded by an interval scale of equal length and sensitivity. Thus, the ratio scale chosen more easily meets the needs for universality we require of any standard measuring device used in education.

There are a number of other advantages to the ratio, or semilogarithmic, scale which are succinctly described by Schmid (1954):

> The semilogarithmic chart is unequaled for many purposes, especially in portraying proportional and percentage relationships. In comparison with the arithmetic line chart, it possesses most of the advantages without the disadvantages. This type of chart not only correctly represents relative changes but also indicates absolute amounts at the same time....For the uninitiated, the term "semilogarithmic," as well as the characteristic ruling of the vertical axis, may seem formidable; but actually the theoretical principles on which this chart is based, and also its construction and use are comparatively simple. Prejudice and general lack of understanding unfortunately have resulted in considerable resistance to the use of semilogarithmic charts. Generally, rates of change (celeration) are more significant than absolute amounts of change in statistical analysis and presentation. In using the ratio chart, one can have confidence that relative changes

Figure 1   Standard Behavior Chart

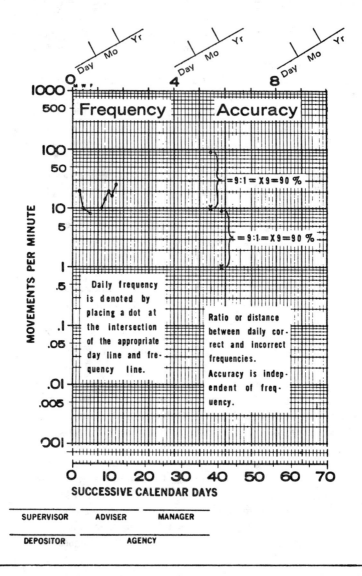

CALENDAR WEEKS

DAILY BEHAVIOR CHART (DC-8)
6 Cycle-140 days (20 wks.)
Behavior Research Co.
Box 3351 — Kansas City, Kans. 66103

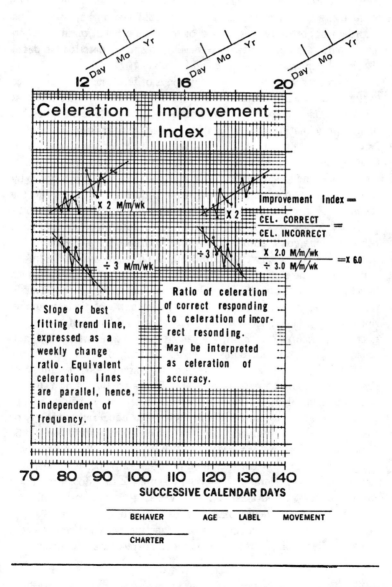

are portrayed without distortion and uncertainty. (P. 109)

As indicated in Panel A of Figure 1, daily frequencies are recorded on the Standard Behavior Chart by placing a dot at the intersection of the vertical line corresponding to the appropriate calendar day and the horizontal line representing the frequency of the behavior observed on that day. Conventions for displaying the length of the daily recording period, as well as for designating days where the recording opportunity was missed or where the behavior in question had no chance to occur have been developed and are described in detail elsewhere (Pennypacker, Koenig and Lindsley, 1972).

A property of the ratio scale which is of fundamental importance in the measurement of behavior and behavior change may be stated as follows: *equal distances represent equal ratios.* A valuable application of this principle in educational measurement may be seen in Panel B. Panel B shows that if, on a particular day, we chart the frequency of movements performed correctly in addition to the frequency of movements performed incorrectly on a given academic task, the distance by which these two points are separated provides a measure of the *accuracy* of the day's performance. This accuracy measure may be expressed either as a ratio, a multiple, or a percentage. In any case, because of the equal ratio nature of the frequency scale, it is clear that the distance on the chart corresponding to a given measure of accuracy will be the same regardless of the overall frequency of the performance being measured. Thus, it is possible to compare performances of vastly different frequencies with respect to this measure of their accuracy; since many educational objectives are stated in terms of either frequency, or accuracy, or both, the value of an instrument which simultaneously yields both measures would appear to be obvious.

In Panel C in Figure 1, graphic representation of Lindsley's *celeration* measure of behavior change is illustrated. By fitting a straight line to a series of daily behavior frequencies, celeration may be seen to be represented by the slope of such a line.[1] The equal ratio property of the frequency scale dictates that the slope of the celeration line will be a measure of the ratio or percentage of change taking place over a given period of time. A convenient time unit for assessing behavior change is one week; hence, celerations are usually expressed as ratios or multiples of frequency (x2 movements/minute/week, ÷ 5 movements/minute/week, etc.). These values may also be converted to percentages. A celeration of x2, for example, means that the behavior frequency is doubling each week, corresponding to a 100 percent weekly increase.

It is particularly important to note that the celeration measure, like the accuracy measure, is independent of frequency. Thus, equal proportions of change in the frequencies of two behaviors will be represented by parallel celeration lines possessing identical celeration values, regardless of the initial frequencies of either behavior. It is therefore possible to directly assess and compare rates of changes in behaviors that occur with vastly differing frequencies. As we shall see, this characteristic of the celeration measure obtained from the Standard Behavior Chart is extremely useful in the evaluation of the effectiveness of educational programs which are concerned with generating improvement in a wide variety of different behaviors.

Finally, the last panel of Figure 1 shows how accuracy and celeration may be combined to yield a composite measure known as the *improvement index.* The improvement index, defined as the ratio of the celeration of correct frequencies to the celeration of incorrect frequencies, may be regarded as a measure of the change in accuracy over time. One may calculate an improvement index either by forming a ratio of the two celerations as just described or by plotting the accuracy ratios on a daily basis and fitting a celeration line to the resulting display. The numerical result will be identical. The improvement index is, of course, independent of either celeration just as celeration and accuracy are independent of basic frequency.

These four measures—frequency, accuracy, celeration and improvement index—are easily obtained from the Standard Behavior Chart and provide us with direct measures of both the quantity and quality of behavior and behavior change. Thus, by using this one instrument, we have at our disposal a set of behavioral measures which are universal (may be applied to any behavior) and standard (the units remain the same regardless of the behavior being measured). Before illustrating the use of these measures in the evaluation of a particular educational program, let us briefly consider some of the general strategies for educational evaluation afforded by the availability of a measuring instrument with the characteristics of the Standard Behavior Chart.

Strategies for Educational Evaluation

It is widely held that effective teaching presupposes continuous evaluation. Since the Standard Behavior Chart utilizes both continuous and direct measures of behavior it is not surprising that its most effective application occurs when it is made an integral part of the teaching process. Both teachers and children must therefore become proficient in its use so that it may serve as an aid to individualized evaluation, decision-making, and planning. Experience has shown that training in classroom use of the Standard Behavior Chart can be both efficiently and economically accomplished on an inservice basis (e.g., Haughton, 1972; Pennypacker, 1973). Thus, our major strategy has been to introduce the evaluation process where and when it is needed most: at the level of individual teacher's daily interaction with individual children.

This strategy is at obvious variance with many traditional evaluation practices which require independent "pre-post measurement" with instruments presumed sensitive to the behavior changes assumed to be taking place. Evaluation practices of this sort are demonstrably *not* a part of the teaching process and are viewed by most, if not all, teachers as possessing scant validity, owing, as a rule, to the highly non-representative nature of the infrequent measurement occasions. Giving the evaluation tool directly to the teachers for daily use with children is, then, an effort to maximize the effectiveness of the evaluation process as an integral part of the teaching process, albeit at the expense of that form of "objectivity" which is thought to be a characteristic of infrequent, indirect measurement.

Instructing teachers and children in the use of the Standard Behavior Chart also insures that the data base for any evaluation will be orders of magnitude greater in quantity than that provided by virtually any other means. It is at this point that the universality and standard nature of the Standard Behavior Chart again prove their worth. This is because, as we have seen, the measures derived from the Standard Behavior Chart may be used to evaluate the quantity and quality of all human behavior and human behavior change. It is both possible and convenient to enlist the aid of the high speed computer in collating and analyzing the masses of data which inevitably result when teachers and children are encouraged to use the Chart.

The computer can easily digest and store these data to any desired level of sensitivity up to and including a single child's performance on a single page of a single arithmetic book on a specified day. In order, however, for the computer to analyze such data and render composite summaries with respect to meaningful parameters of an educational program, it is essential that an orderly and logically hierarchial relationship exist between the goals or objectives of a program and the behaviors emitted by the children in that program. It is therefore essential to involve program administrators at an early stage in the development of any evaluation format based on charts of daily behavior frequencies. The oft-mentioned requirement of stating program goals in behavioral terms now becomes an absolute necessity since the computer has no way of defining on its own which changing behavior frequencies are representative of which programmatic goals. Once a logical hierarchy relating charted behavior changes to program goals has been established, it is easy to have the computer provide composite statements, based on the daily records made in the classroom, of the degree to which the objectives have been attained.

Summarizing the data with respect to one or more of the measures of behavior change discussed above may be said to yield an overall measure of *effectiveness* derived from the program. This summarization can, of course, occur with respect to any independent parameter of the program or any sub-population of the participants in the program. Since all of the behavioral measures taken from the chart incorporate a time dimension, one can readily view any resultant behavior change in terms of the time taken to produce it and thus arrive at a measure of *efficiency*. Finally, one may add to such statements whatever cost figures are deemed appropriate and thereby provide a quantitative basis for statements of accountability in terms of cost effectiveness. We feel that a major virtue of this system lies in the fact that all such analyses are based entirely on the directly observed and recorded behavior of the individuals served by whatever program is being evaluated. The same information which guides the teacher in her daily planning and decision-making constitutes, when assembled across the appropriate units of a program, the data base for administrative planning and decision–making at any level of responsibility. Such a system virtually insures that educational decisions and policies are formulated in consultation with the ultimate experts—the children themselves (Lindsley, 1972).

Let us turn now to an illustration of this evaluative system as it was recently applied to an ESEA Title III Program designed to improve the learning abilities of first grade children of a county in North Carolina.

The Program

The Learning Abilities Development Program (LAD) of Albemarle and Stanly County, North Carolina, had two main objectives in its initial year of operation. First, it sought to screen all rising first graders in the district and identify those for whom subsequent success would depend upon marked enhancement of one or more of a variety of learning abilities.[2] Second, the program attempted to provide individualized service aimed at developing in each child sufficient proficiency in each of the isolated abilities to insure normal academic progress. This was attempted for each child selected by the screening process.

The program was situated in Stanly County, North Carolina, the county seat of which is the city of Ablemarle. Nearly all of the 42,000 residents of Ablemarle and Stanly County are native North Carolinians who enjoy a lower middle class way of life, supported predominantly by small farm agriculture and the textile industry. Although the median family income in the area is slightly above the median for the state, the average annual expenditure per child in the public school system ranks near the bottom of all districts in the state of North Carolina. Thus, the LAD Program was launched in a community whose cultural homogeneity might invite the label "provincial" and which is not given to displays of largesse on behalf of its educational institutions.

The staff of the LAD Program consisted of a director, three certified resource teachers, six teacher aides, and a secretary. The resource teachers, and frequently the teacher aides as well, spent a portion of each work day in the administrative center assembling materials, comparing procedures and progress, or participating in informal training sessions conducted by the director. The majority of their time, however, was spent in the 15 elementary schools scattered throughout the city and county. Although arrangements varied from school to school the teacher and her two aides typically removed target children from ongoing classroom activity and worked with them on an individual basis in storage closets, empty classrooms, empty offices or lounges.

The initial activity of the LAD staff involved assisting first grade teachers in the administration of a gross screening device to the approximately 720 first-graders in the district. The instrument used in the initial screening required the teacher to evaluate each child on a five point scale in each of nine areas: reasoning ability, speed of learning, ability to deal with abstract ideas, perceptual discrimination, psychomotor abilities, verbal comprehension, verbal expression, number and space relations, and creativity.

One hundred and eighty children were initially selected in the program on the basis of low evaluation in one or more of these nine areas. Each child selected was then further evaluated by a member of the LAD staff using the Remedial Diagnostic Form developed by Robert A. Farrald (1971). A total of 90 children were again selected as positive and were targeted for individualized assistance by the LAD staff. Of these, a total of 18 had only brief contact of a referral nature with the program, leaving 62 whose charted behavior formed the basis of our evaluation.

Early in the year, the director conducted extensive staff training in the area of remediation of learning abilities; the orientation of this training and the basic materials and techniques used may be found in the works of Farrold (1971) and Valett (1967). In addition, the first author and his staff conducted inservice training, marked by periodic follow-ups, in both the use of the Standard Behavior Chart and the tactics of precisely defining and recording appropriate target behaviors.

The professional staff then began, on an itinerant basis, the task of individually assisting each selected child in the enhancement of one or more of the learning abilities judged insufficient by the two screening devices. Specialized curricular materials were either developed or purchased for use with each child. The list of such materials is too extensive to be catalogued here; it ranged, however, from the Peabody Language Kit and Frostig materials to teacher-made card games, sandpaper letters, and macaroni stringing devices.

As soon as the child and the member of the LAD staff became acquainted, an effort was made to determine which behavior(s) was responsible for the judged insufficiency. For example, if the screening instruments indicated the presence of arrested gross motor development, the teacher might begin recording steps taken on a 10-foot balance beam. In the event this behavior showed a need for improvement, a variety of behavioral techniques such as shaping and fading were introduced, with the results recorded daily on the behavior chart. Similar tactics were used to enhance behaviors underlying academic abilities; for example, in order to enhance visual form discrimination, various symbol naming, letter naming, and matching-to-sample tasks would be tried and the results charted. Together, the teacher and child would view the progress displayed on the chart; in the event that improvement was not evident, new procedures would be tried until one was eventually found which produced success.

The Evaluation

A total of 337 charts resulted from the contact made by the LAD staff with the 62 children served directly during the first year. Each chart was a record of one child's performance of one particular behavior; e.g., "says alphabet letter correctly," "identifies missing object incorrectly," etc. In the appropriate blanks at the bottom of the chart (see Figure 1) were recorded the name and identifying numbers of the child, the resource teacher and/or teacher aide working with the child and the school attended. In the blank marked *Label* was put a number signifying which of the 53 possible learning abilities (Valett, 1967) the particular recorded behavior was judged to represent.

Vertical lines were drawn on each chart to identify points in time at which major curriculum or procedural changes were introduced, as well as at the beginning and end of each project. Thus, any adjacent pair of these so-called *phase lines* marks the temporal boundaries of the phases of a project, each phase corresponding to the period of application of a distinct set of materials or procedures. For each phase, the LAD teachers reported the number of contact minutes that had occurred during that phase. Celeration lines were fit, either freehand or by the method of least squares, to the frequencies plotted within each phase and the resulting numerical celeration value was entered on the chart. When all the charts had been prepared in this fashion, they were transferred to the Behavior Research Company for coding, computer storage, and analysis.

A macroscopic view of the temporal dimension of the service provided by the LAD Program is furnished by considering calendar weeks of involvement in the program on the part of the children served. A total of 2,058 child-project-weeks of service was provided during this first year; on the average, each child participated in 5.4 projects each of which lasted an average of 6.1 calendar weeks.

A total of 172 *different* behaviors were recorded in accumulating the total of 337 charts. This data testifies to the wide variety of observable behaviors which may be indicative of insufficient learning abilities and to the scope of the efforts on the part of the LAD staff to customize their tactics to meet the needs of the individual children. Another indicator of the extent of individualization of instruction is furnished by the fact that a total of 996 different phases were reported; a new phase was initiated whenever the charted data indicated that some procedural change would be required to generate further improvement.

For the entire program, a total of 85,230 teaching minutes were reported. The average number of teaching minutes per project, then, is 253; the average number of teaching minutes per child in the program is 1,373 while the average number of teaching minutes per phase was 86 (s.d. = 95.0).

A major conceptual parameter of the program was Valett's extensive list of learning abilities. Although Valett's list includes 53 such abilities, behaviors related to only 19 of these abilities were observed and recorded by the LAD staff. **Table 1** summarizes the amount of activity that occurred on behalf of remediation within each of these 19 ability areas. The total number of projects represented, 333, does not include four behavior modification projects, the targets of which are not readily classified under any of the listed learning abilities.

Table 1   Summary of Activity Within Each
Learning Ability Sampled

Learning Ability	Num. of Projects	Total Num. of Teaching Min.	Num. of Different Children
Throwing	4	400	2
Body Localization	2	180	1
Balance and Rhythm	18	3554	9
Directionality	6	1780	3
Laterality	6	1080	3
Auditory Acuity	26	7650	8
Auditory Decoding	14	3720	6
Auditory-Vocal Association	2	540	1
Auditory Memory	10	1140	4
Auditory Sequencing	8	2160	1
Visual Acuity	2	240	1
Visual-Form Discrimination	14	3988	6
Visual Memory	82	31165	30
Visual-Motor Fine Muscle Coordination	65	13360	21
Fluency and Encoding	18	3303	2
Word Attack Skills	2	600	1
Reading Comprehension	1	300	1
Number Concepts	49	9580	14
Social Maturity	4	190	2
	333	85230	116

Summing the number of children served within each ability area across the ability areas yields a total of 116, implying that most children received assistance with respect to more than one ability area. **Table 2** shows that, in fact, 60 percent of the target population were judged to require assistance in two or more ability areas. These data suggest that the listed learning abilities are not mutually exclusive at the functional level; if a child displays an insufficiency in one of the abilities, he is likely to display insufficiencies in others as well. It may be of interest to future researchers to attempt a functional redefinition of these ability areas in terms of non-overlapping behavior clusters.

Table 2   Frequencies of Children Served With Respect to Different Numbers of Abilities

Number of Abilities	Number of Children	% of Total
1	25	40
2	26	42
3	7	11
4	4	7
		100

The *effectiveness* of the services provided by the LAD Program within each of the ability areas is summarized in **Table 3**. The charts within each ability area were subdivided according to whether the aim of the project was to increase (accelerate) or decrease (decelerate) the behavior being recorded. The geometric means[3] of the within-phase celeration values within each ability area by target grouping were computed. These values, together with the total number of weeks for which each value is representative, are presented in Table 3.

Since the geometric mean represents the average weekly *ratio* of behavior change, raising the average value to the power given by the number of weeks yields a ratio value equivalent to the *average total* behavior change achieved in each ability area-target grouping. Consider, for example, the ability "auditory sequencing." The geometric mean weekly acceleration in those projects where the aim was to accelerate the behavior was x1.6. Since this rate of increase (which may also be read as 60 percent/week) occurred for a total of 7.1 weeks, the *average*

Table 3 Geometric Mean Weekly Celerations for Accelerate (A) Projects and Decelerate (D) Projects Grouped According to the Learning Ability Sampled

Learning Ability	Weekly Celeration^A	Total Projects Weeks	Weekly Celeration^D	Total Projects Weeks
Throwing	x1.9	4.3	÷1.7	4.30
Body Localization	÷10.0	.4	÷11.	.40
Balance and Rhythm	x1.3	62.0	÷1.2	58.70
Directionality	x1.2	8.6	÷1.8	8.60
Laterality	x1.2	28.0	÷1.5	28.00
Auditory Acuity	x1.3	55.2	÷1.7	55.50
Auditory Decoding	x1.4	27.2	÷1.3	27.20
Auditory-Vocal Association	x1.2	4.1	÷2.	4.10
Auditory Memory	x1.5	12.8	÷1.8	12.80
Auditory Sequencing	x1.6	7.1	÷4.3	7.10
Visual Acuity	x1.2	4.4	÷1.4	4.40
Visual-Form Discrimination	x1.6	25.9	÷1.8	25.90
Visual Memory	x1.2	322.4	÷1.2	317.20
Visual-Motor Fine Muscle Coordination	x1.1	207.8	÷1.8	167.10
Fluency and Encoding	x1.4	19.4	÷1.3	19.40
Word Attack Skills	x1.2	1.6	x1.	1.60
Reading Comprehension	x1.2	9.3	---	...
Number Concepts	x1.1	132.1	÷1.2	131.00
Social Maturity	x1.2	19.4	÷1.2	19.40
Grand Geometric Mean =	x1.2		Grand Geometric Mean =	÷1.3

total frequency change is x28.13; $(1.6^{7.1})$. Thus, we could say that if the aggregate of all the behaviors began at a frequency of 1 movement /minute, by the end of the intervention, that aggregate behavior was occurring at a frequency of 28.13 movements/minute. The reader may make similar interpretations concerning the other ability area-target combinations.

Perhaps the most interesting information to emerge from Table 3 is found on the bottom line. Across all children and all projects where the objective was to increase the frequency of the recorded behavior, the average weekly celeration was x1.2, meaning that, on the average, the program produced 20 percent per week improvement in all such charted behaviors. Similarly, where the objective was to decrease the frequency of the recorded behavior, the overall mean weekly celeration was $\div$1.3—the overall weekly reduction of these behaviors was, therefore, 23 percent. Assuming, for the sake of illustration, that in the absence of systematic intervention no change in these behavior frequencies would have been observed, we now have a useful approximation of the *composite effectiveness* resulting from the implementation of this program.

What of changes in accuracy of the academic performances charted? We recall that the measurement of accuracy requires the simultaneous charting of the frequencies with which a movement is performed both correctly and incorrectly on a given day. By forming the ratio of the celerations of these two sets of frequencies as they change over days, we produce, as the reader will recall, a measure known as the *improvement index* which, in essence, is the ratio describing the weekly rate of change in accuracy.

Of the 337 projects analyzed from the first year of the program, 324 were members of *accuracy pairs*—pairs of projects where correct and incorrect frequencies are charted simultaneously. In other words, a total of 162 different correct-incorrect pairs were recorded. The improvement index was computed for every phase within each of these pairs of projects. Collecting all of the improvement indices for each learning ability and computing their geometric mean yielded the results displayed in Table 4. Examination of Table 4 reveals that the greatest weekly improvement in accuracy was achieved in those projects falling in the ability category "auditory sequencing."

Reference to Table 3 shows that the major source of this improvement in accuracy is to be found in the extremely rapid deceleration of errors ($\div$4.3); the acceleration of correct frequencies being only x1.6. Further examination of Table 4 suggests that the abilities of "body localization" and "word attack skills" yielded the least improvement

Table 4   Geometric Means of Improvement Indices
           for Each Learning Ability

Learning Ability	Geometric Mean
Throwing	x3.2
Body Localization	x1.1
Balance and Rhythm	x1.6
Directionality	x2.2
Laterality	x1.8
Auditory Acuity	x2.2
Auditory Decoding	x1.8
Auditory-Vocal Association	x2.4
Auditory Memory	x2.7
Auditory Sequencing	x6.9
Visual Acuity	x1.7
Visual-Form Discrimination	x2.9
Visual Memory	x1.4
Visual-Motor Fine Muscle Coordination	x2.0
Fluency and Encoding	x1.8
Word Attack Skills	x1.2
Reading Comprehension	-------
Number Concepts	x1.3
Social Maturity	x1.4
Grand Geometric Mean	x1.6

in accuracy. For "word attack skills," for example, no general decrease in incorrect frequencies was observed so all the improvement is contained in the x1.2 geometric mean weekly acceleration of correct frequencies. The reader may make similar interpretations concerning the other ability areas for himself.

Overall, the geometric mean of all improvement indices (taken across children and abilities) is x1.6. In other words, in those cases where accuracy was recorded, the average weekly increase in accuracy was over 60 percent!

The foregoing analyses should be viewed not as exhaustive, but as illustrative of the class of evaluative analyses which result from the marriage of the Standard Behavior Chart and the high speed computer. For example, a complete analysis was performed using teachers as the major parameter so that the efficiency and productivity of each teacher working within each ability area was determined. These data are now guiding the director in deployment of his staff. Given summary data of this sort, it is a simple matter to take the final step of adding cost figures to arrive at cost effectiveness statements based on recorded changes in the behavior of the population served. For example, the reader will recall that a total of 2,058 child-project-weeks of data were accumulated during the first year. Dividing this number into the total cost of the program and multiplying the result by the average number of projects conducted on each child yields an estimate of the cost of bringing the services of this program to one child for one week. During that week, the average effect obtained was a 20 percent increase in the frequency of each acceleration target, and a 23 percent decrease in the frequency of each deceleration target, or, overall, a 60 percent increase in accuracy. One may regard the cost of these effects then, as being approximately equal to the cost of each child-project-week.

We must quickly add that these calculations do not take into account the cost to the children, and ultimately to society, of withholding such services. Only when accurate data become available relating drop-out rates, drug offenses and delinquent acts in general to the presence of undetected and/or unremediated early deficiencies in key learning abilities will the complete picture of the benefits provided by a program such as this become known. In the meantime, the potential contribution of continuous and direct measurement of behavior frequencies to an effective, humane and accountable educational technology has, we believe, finally been realized.

Footnotes

1.   Empirical validation of the practice of fitting straight lines to the logs of behavior frequencies has been established by Koenig, 1972.

2.   We eschew the term "learning disabilities" for its obvious negative connotations as well as the logical impossibility of its empirical definition. Observation of a child's behavior reveals only his abilities—inferring the presence of a disability provides nothing of additional value to those whose responsibility is improving the child's behavior.

3. Appropriate measure of central tendency for logarithmic values.

References

Farrald, R. A. Remedial diagnostic handbook for children with learning disabilities. Adopt Press, Inc., 104 E. 20 St., Sioux Falls, South Dakota 57105.

Haughton, E. Aims: Growing and sharing. In, *Let's try doing something else kind of thing.* Arlington, Virginia: Council for Exceptional Children, 1972.

Koenig, C. *Charting the future course of behavior.* Kansas City: Precision Media, 1972.

Lindsley, O. R. From Skinner to precision teaching: The child knows best. In, *Let's try doing something else kind of thing.* Arlington, Virginia: Council for Exceptional Children, 1972.

Lindsley, O. R. Personal communication. 1969.

Pennypacker, H. S., Koenig, C. and Lindsley, O. R. *Handbook of the Standard Behavior Chart.* Kansas City: Precision Media, 1972.

Pennypacker, H. S. How I spent my Christmas vacation. In R. Ulrich, T. Stachnik, and J. Mabry (Eds.), *Control of human behavior,* Vol. III. New York: Scott, Foresman. In press.

Schmid, C. F. *Handbook of graphic presentations.* New York: The Ronald Press Company, 1954.

Skinner, B. F. Are theories of learning necessary? *Psychological Review,* 1950, *57,* 193-216.

Skinner, B. F. *Behavior of organisms.* New York: Appleton-Century-Crofts, 1938.

Skinner, B. F. The experimental analysis of behavior. *American Scientist,* 1957, *45,* 343-371.

Skinner, B. F. Some contributions of an experimental analysis to behavior as a whole. *American Psychologist,* 1953, *8,* 69-79.

Valett, R. E. *The remediation of learning disabilities.* Fearon Publishers, 2165 Park Blvd., Palo Alto, California 94036.

Evaluating Individualized Education in the Elementary School

13

William W. Cooley and Gaea Leinhardt

The value which individuals will assign to a new product or procedure is a function of their perception of how well that new product or procedure will serve as a means to satisfy some need. Research designed to provide information for such value determinations is what we call evaluative research. If a program of evaluative research is to serve this function, then it must provide information related to the following:

1. How real is the need?

2. What priority does the need have relative to other needs?

3. Do the proposed means achieve the desired ends?

4. How competitive are the proposed means with those of available alternatives?

The purpose of this paper is to discuss and illustrate these different aspects of evaluative research. The context from which illustrations are drawn is a research and development center which must provide information regarding the value of a program of individualized instruction which it is developing. In that context, questions 1 and 3 are the more important concerns. Questions 2 and 4 are more appropriately dealt with by evaluators working directly with consumers, as opposed to developers.

This chapter also illustrates some convictions which we have about a particular kind of evaluation. What we are describing here is a continuous research process which is done as part of a general program of educational change. Evaluative research is not some final act of judgment which is made about some completed and installed innovation. One of the objectives of evaluative research is to provide information to developers and policy-makers about the shortcomings of current practices and about the kinds of changes which are likely to bring about desired improvements. In a sense, evaluation provides feedback to developers and feedforward to educational policy-makers and implementors. Thus, this chapter is not a report of a final evaluation of an individualized education program. Instead, it is a position paper on what a system of evaluative research should look like, one which parallels and compliments research and development efforts concerned with improving education. These efforts are directed toward an improved understanding of how children learn and the development of new products and procedures based upon these understandings.

How Real Is the Need?

Individuals differ greatly one from the other. Certain groups also differ greatly from certain others. Those differences are sometimes considered one of the greatest assets of the species. However, when the differences are extreme and in a certain direction, society generally ceases considering them virtues and attempts to modify the outlier. This is especially true in the case of academic aptitude and performance.

In the United States the one-standard-deviation school achievement difference between whites and blacks is an example of a difference that is of great concern to many. This concern focuses on the problem of what is to be done. Essentially, there are two basic solutions, which are espoused by four greatly antagonistic groups.

The solutions are either to do nothing or, as nearly as possible, to obliterate performance differences by rather dramatic methods. The two groups that conclude the problem should essentially be ignored appear to hold two very different philosophies. The first does not wish to have an intervention which would involve the sacrifice of anything they consider a source of freedom. It is the classical laissez-faire position. Differences are natural, the good can and should succeed, the bad can and should fail. This group does not really care why there are differences, but, in general, expresses no desire to alter them. The second group tends to move toward inaction from a rather convoluted sense of justice and equality—it might be considered the ostrich group. The observed differences are not real because: the tests are culturally biased, don't really test what they purport to test, or don't manage to reveal some basic equivalency between races or economic groups as they do between the sexes. (Girls are better than boys on verbal, but boys win in math so it's all even in the end!) The conclusion this group often comes to is to abandon all forms of standardized testing presumably hoping that if the evidence disappears, so will the problem—

symptomatic medicine in the extreme.

On the other hand, many recognize the differences in performance and acknowledge the necessity of doing something about the extreme failures. However, they also fall into basically two groups. Some suggest that complete environmental control will result in equality of performance. They trace the problem to the vast differences in wealth and in life style between groups in the United States. If culture, home environment, and schooling become equivalent, then certainly performance will too. Others, while recognizing the existence of differences, claim that nothing can be done through environment control because the cause is a genetic one. If pressed for a solution, they will offer genetic sterilization as the only logical alternative.

It is clear that educators, at least, must be concerned with extreme failures. One alternative which has emerged disregards the ultimate cause of the differences and assumes something can be done. It involves the development of instructional systems that are adaptive to differences among children. In such programs it is not necessary to teach all students in a given classroom the same things at the same time. Procedures and instructional materials are developed which allow each student to work on tasks from which he or she is prepared to learn. Such an instructional system requires: a structure for the basic skills to be learned; tests which assist the teacher in determining where each child is with respect to that structure; instructional materials which are largely self-instructional, so as to make it possible for different students to work on different skills at the same time without direct teacher tutoring; and management procedures which enable the teacher to operate a classroom in which all students can be working on different aspects and levels of the curriculum at the same time.

We suspect that if someone could devise an effective, adaptive system which costs no more than current programs cost, it would be highly competitive with those that are currently available for use in the schools. The problem is, such a system does not yet exist. Evaluative research becomes important because it is necessary to provide information to those who wish to weigh the increased benefits of adaptive systems against the increased costs. If adaptive systems are to be highly valued, it has to be shown that they can satisfy important societal needs.

But what are the real needs which such an adaptive system is likely to satisfy? One example is that the present conventional procedures currently allow over 10 percent of each age group to remain functionally illiterate. That is, they "complete" their education without the reading skills required for such functions as voting, finding a job, applying for a loan, or obtaining information on such basics as how to qualify for medical aid. This is probably an example of an undesirable situation. That is, a possible need of this society is to eliminate unnecessary and costly illiteracy. One function of evaluative research, then, is to document or demonstrate the validity of these illiteracy claims and show that this is a costly and unnecessary condition in our society. The value which people will assign to a remedy for this condition will be in part a function of how clearly the aversiveness of this condition is established.

We are not proposing that all children can be made to read equally well. We are proposing that functional illiteracy can and should be dramatically reduced. Providing empirical evidence for this proposition is one aspect of evaluative research. So is providing evidence for related propositions having to do with other minimum competencies people need to be effective individuals in society, competencies which adaptive educational systems could provide more effectively than do the present selective systems. (See, for example, Glaser (1972) for a more extensive discussion of this adaptive-selective distinction.)

There are, of course, other needs which individualized, adaptive education might help to satisfy. Many are related to the fact that present practices require classrooms full of children to "do" lessons together. This results in: fixed schedules, common starting and stopping times, instruction paced by a teacher's judgment of how the class as a whole is progressing, school facilities being used about one-sixth of the time, families converging upon our country's finite recreational resources at the same time, whether or not their work schedules are flexible, simply because they are afraid to take their children out of school for fear they might miss an important lesson, etc. Adaptive systems could free up the school and thus alleviate some of the problems associated with fixed systems.

Different people perceive different needs to be important. It may not be possible to have all of these various needs determine what a developer builds, but they will determine how others will value what gets built. For others to value a new system of individualized education highly, they have to see it as satisfying some need which they recognize as being important. Generating information which relates innovations to needs is one function of evaluative research.

What Priority Does the Need Have Relative to Others?

Perhaps the most difficult aspect of the valuing problem is this priority question. Certainly it is difficult from the standpoint of the evaluative researcher who is associated with a particular developmental effort. The decision to adopt an educational innovation is a local community/ school decision, and the evaluative researcher cannot anticipate the variety of local problems which will compete with the one the developer is helping to solve, especially problems outside of the educational sphere.

Although it is not possible to anticipate the total needs which will be competing for community resources, it is important for developers to recognize that if their innovation represents an increase in educational costs, they will have to be prepared to compete with other community programs for those finite resources. The best way of anticipating this problem is to be able to show how educational improvements can make a positive difference in extra-school affairs. For example, if a developer is building a new elementary school science program, and if it is going to mean an extra 20 dollars per child (say a 4 percent increase) then the developer is not going to have much impact on education if all he can tell the policy-makers (i.e., the resource allocators) is that the children taking this program score higher on the STEP Science test. Of course, if some communities happen to value high scores on that particular test, then the developer may get a few adoptions, but that is unlikely. What a program of evaluative research can do is provide information to the developers about the kinds of community needs a new science program might help to satisfy, such as improved citizen understanding of local ecological problems, and then provide information to the community about the effectiveness of the program in satisfying this need.

This aspect of evaluative research sounds like marketing research, but no one wants to spend five to eight years developing a new science program which does not get used because no one sees the need for it. Certainly few will support such a developmental effort. This is not to say that the evaluative researcher's job is to try to figure out how to unload a white elephant on the schools. But we are assuming that people engaged in educational research and development do have an interest in improving education. This implies activities directed toward designing and building innovations which will achieve important educational goals not now being achieved, or at least not as effectively as is desirable. Evaluative research can be viewed as the information network in this process. It provides information to developers about needs, and it provides information to consumers about the effectiveness of new methods for satisfying those needs.

The evaluator who is working as part of the development effort cannot deal with the priority question at the consumer end in any direct way. Information regarding the importance of the problem and the effectiveness of the developer's solution can be provided, but in the final analysis this gets weighed against other community/school problems and other solutions by the local decision-makers. (The role which the local evaluative researcher might play in this process is a different paper.) Of course the evaluative researcher can play an important role in determining the developer's priorities. This evaluator can also study possible displaceables. That is, although a given innovation might increase some operating costs, it could reduce others. Someone has to pull together this kind of information if an innovation is to have an impact. Once information is provided which establishes the reality and the priority of the need, the stage is set for what has classically been considered the sole function of evaluation: relating the new means to the desired end.

Do the Proposed Means Achieve the Desired End?

This is the evaluation question which requires the greatest effort as far as those evaluators associated with a research and development enterprise are concerned. Studies currently underway at the Learning Research and Development Center (LRDC) will be used here to illustrate this aspect of the evaluation problem.

LRDC has access to several settings in which evaluative research of this type can be carried out. First of all, in the laboratory itself, certain components of instructional programs can be validated prior to implementation in the schools. Secondly, evaluative research is conducted in two developmental schools in which the Center is directly responsible for the implementation of its new instructional programs. A third setting is a small network of schools participating in the national Follow—Through program, some of which have selected LRDC's instructional programs to be used in their classrooms. Although LRDC has the responsibility of implementing the programs in those schools, this is done only by training local administrators and supervisors. Also, our developers are not present on the site. It is in this network that we have a chance to see how well our programs can do outside of the "hothouse."

328

First, we shall illustrate what can be learned about a new program in one of our developmental schools. In this urban school, developmental efforts began in preschool and kindergarten in 1968-69, first grade was added in 1969-70, second grade in 1970-71, and third grade in 1971-72, with the fourth and fifth grades being added in 1972-73. In order to contrast LRDC's programs to the school practices they were replacing, control groups were established by taking advantage of the fact that the Center added one grade each year to its experimental program. As the program moved up from grade to grade, classrooms that were one and two grades ahead of the program were also tested. Table 1 illustrates the general design.

Table 1   Experimental (E) and Control (C) Groups
for Development School

Year	Pre-school	Kinder-garten	First	Second	Third	Fourth	Fifth
				GRADE			
1968-'69	E	E	C	C	----	----	----
1969-'70	E	E	E	C	C	----	----
1970-'71	E	E	E	E	C	C	----
1971-'72	E	E	E	E	E	C	C

No significant differences in achievement were observed between controls of a given grade from year to year. Also, no differences were found on variables, such as family socioeconomic status, known to be related to achievement but which could not have been affected by the program. Therefore, it seems safe to assume that from year to year children at a given grade level can be considered to be random samples from a common population, thus allowing us to compare the achievement level of children of a given grade prior to the implementation of our program with achievement following its implementation. It is also possible for us to compare down the columns of the chart, for example, children who were second-graders during the first year our program was implemented with second-graders of the second year to see whether changes made in the program from one year to the next resulted in improved performance. **Table 2** shows the average grade equivalents for the grades tested in reading achievement using the Wide Range Achievement Test (WRAT) (Jastak, Bijou, and Jastak, 1965).

Table 2   Reading Grade Equivalents on WRAT

	Pre	k	1st	2nd	3rd	4th	5th
'68-'69	.08	.69	1.8*	2.8*			
	(.40)	(.70)					
'69-'70	X	.99	1.81	2.3	3.40		
		(.41)	(.81)	(.85)	(1.30)		
'70-'71	1.0	.94	2.41	3.39	3.26	4.55	
	(.38)	(.50)	(1.2)	(1.89)	(1,3)	(1.64)	
'71-'72	.92	1.2	2.31	3.61	4.11	4.11	5.2
	(.31)	(.58)	(1.17)	(1.83)	(2.2)	(1.58)	(2.07)

*MAT medians
( ) = standard deviation

Examining Table 2 by column reveals the stability and change within a grade level over time. Starting with the second column (k), a reasonably steady improvement in grade equivalents from 1968 until 1971 can be seen. In the case of kindergarten all of the classrooms were under experimental treatment. However, reading as a separate subject was not introduced in kindergarten until 1969. Looking at the second-grade column, where there are two years of control scores (one of which is the median grade equivalent from the MAT) and two of experimental, we can see a difference of almost a year in grade equivalents between the two situations. Within the experimental situation, improvement continues.

Looking at the same table by row, the general trend of improvement across grades in any one year can be examined. The control group (the last two scores for each row) consistently shows an improvement of one year or more between first and second, third and fourth, etc. This is also true of the experimental group. However, on the average the experimental group is a year ahead of the controls. That is, second-graders at the end of the 1970-71 year were reading as well as third-graders in that school. The same was true for third- and fourth-graders the following year.

Of course, it is one thing to show that a new program can operate effectively in a laboratory or a developmental school setting in which the developers are available to facilitate proper implementation of the program, but quite another to show that the innovation will work in settings remote from the developer. Since the value which others will place on our programs is a function of the extent to which they perceive that people other than the developers can implement the program, as well as a function of their being able to understand how and why the program is effective, we have developed a set of implementation measures. Such measures are designed to reveal what a classroom looks like that has implemented LRDC programs.

Implementation measures have been missing in most previous efforts at evaluative research. We feel that it is essential to complete the evaluation picture because it establishes the extent to which an innovation can be implemented by teachers remote from the developer and because it contributes to an understanding of how the innovation achieves the desired ends through making its critical components more explicit.

Information regarding differences among classrooms and how they implement LRDC programs can be combined with information regarding students' entry-level abilities and end-of-year achievement to form an input-process-output analytical model for dealing with these data. That is, the measures of implementation become descriptors of the instructional process that has taken place in a classroom. Standardized ability measures given in the fall represent input measures, and standardized ability tests given at the end of the year represent output measures. We can then determine whether there is variation in output not explained by variation in input but which can be related to variation in process.

Before turning to empirical illustrations of the usefulness of implementation measures, the context in which the data were collected must be described. Included in the following illustrations are data from 30 second-grade classrooms, all of which were operating with LRDC's individualized instruction program in mathematics. Seven of the classrooms are from the two developmental schools with which LRDC works directly; the others are classrooms from the nationwide network of school systems participating in the national Follow–Through program. Seven school systems have selected the LRDC model for use in their Follow–Through schools, and the classrooms included here are from four of those systems.

Implementation measures serve several functions. First, they provide information which describes the implementation of the program in the field. Second, they permit a comparison of the implementation between the field and developmental schools. Third, the measures provide a mechanism for measuring how important specific components of the programs are to student achievement.

Table 3 shows averages by site on 16 variables. The variables fall into roughly two areas: context variables and process variables. The context variables consist of measures of: teacher experience with our program, class size, ratio of boys to girls, percentage of the children present,[1] and the amount of time spent in mathematics. The process variables consist of measures of: the percentage of unique assignments, the average number of days since the last test, the number of management and cognitive contacts, the number of adults traveling, the percentage of negative contacts, the distribution of total and cognitive contacts, whether or not play follows work, and if the children obtain their own work.

With one exception the context variables look similar between the laboratory and field sites. Class sizes when considered in light of the attendance seem to be smaller in the lab setting than in the field. That is, on the average, there are fewer children present in a laboratory classroom than in a field one. This is an important point to remember when one looks at the outcome measures and per pupil expenditures.

Some of the process variables also look similar (or equally different) across the field and laboratory sites. This is very encouraging as it indicates that the program is exportable on those dimensions. The process variables on which there are differences, however, are interesting to consider. In general, the laboratory schools test less frequently, make fewer cognitive contacts, more management contacts, and distribute teacher attention more evenly than the field sites do. It would appear that in some respects the field schools perform in a way which more closely resembles the expressed instructional model than do the laboratory schools. (A possible explanation of this is that developers are constantly changing the model in the schools to which they have access, placing other experimental demands on the teachers so that the classrooms do not strictly follow written guidelines.)

A more relevant question than the comparison of field and lab schools is how successful the schools have been in becoming adaptive. The answer cannot be given a precise value, but some general observations can be made. All of the classrooms are individualized to some extent. Some have modified the program in a specific way, such as having both the teacher and the aide travel, while others have extended

332

Table 3 Averages, by Site, of Context and Process Variables

Site	Experience $\bar{X}$	Experience SD	Class Size $\bar{X}$	Class Size SD	% Present $\bar{X}$	% Present SD	Ratio Boys to Girls $\bar{X}$	Ratio Boys to Girls SD	% Unique $\bar{X}$	% Unique SD	Average Number of Days since last test $\bar{X}$	SD
1	.2	.44	27.4	2.41	89	5	1.1	.13	57	8	9.06	9.4
2	1.83	.41	24	1.79	96.6	1	1.17	.25	51	4	6.85	2.61
3	1.3	1.03	21	1.90	92.5	5	1.18	.45	55	8	7.26	4.5
4	0	0	25	.63	87.8	7	1.04	.24	56	18	3.15	1.33
Lab 1	.4	.55	22.6	3.2	87.8	9	.78	.21	48	10	16.72	6.10
Lab 2	6	2.83	22.5	.7	84.5	14	1.15	.21	60	5	10.68	4.09

Site	No. of Cognitive Contacts $\bar{X}$	SD	No. of Management Contacts $\bar{X}$	SD	Percent Negative Contacts $\bar{X}$	SD	Distribution Total $\bar{X}$	SD	Distribution (Cognitive) $\bar{X}$	SD	Play Follows Work $\bar{X}$	SD
1	13.4	5.98	20.2	6.3	6	4	15.83	8.93	7.6	2.7	.4	.55
2	19.02	7.5	10.56	3.4	1	2	18.75	4.26	10.92	3.2	1	0
3	28	10.75	15.3	9.8	3	3	20.88	11.43	9.71	3.75	0	0
4	16.08	4.54	14.25	4.4	6	4	20.33	12.31	8.75	4.94	.33	.41
Lab 1	11.04	3.2	31-	19.33	2	2	11.87	10.65	8.74	6.6	.2	.45
Lab 2	16.5	10.6	19.5	9.19	5	7	4.45	.35	5.73	.03	.5	.07

Site	No. of Adults Traveling $\bar{X}$	SD	Child Obtains Own Work $\bar{X}$	SD	No. Minutes of Math Per Day $\bar{X}$	SD	No. Minutes of Reading Per Day $\bar{X}$	SD
1	1.8	.45	1	0	45	0	90	0
2	2.16	.41	.33	.52	60	0	120	0
3	1.5	.83	0	0	44.16	5.85	88.3	4.08
4	2.3	.82	0	0	60	0	120	0
Lab 1	1.4	.55	0	0	60	0	90	0
Lab 2	2	0	0	0	45	0	90	0

the management system from the specific program curriculum areas to all curriculum areas. Some classrooms test frequently, but tend to give children similar assignments rather than individual ones. No classroom assigns just those pages needed by the child as indicated by the test. Rather, most of them start at the first page a child needs, as indicated by a test, and assign a block of pages following that first needed page.

Turning now to the input-process-output model, this approach can be illustrated by using six of the best measures of classroom differences developed by Leinhardt (1972), together with input measures of students' entering ability as measured by the cognitive abilities test of Thorndike, Hagen, and Lorge (1968) and an output measure based on the arithmetic scores for the Wide Range Achievement Test (WRAT) given in the spring. The fall input measures are expressed as two statistics for each classroom, the mean and standard deviation. The output measure is simply the classroom mean for the arithmetic achievement test. As was indicated above, the 30 second-grade classrooms included here were all using some version of the LRDC individualized program during the academic year 1971-72.

Partial correlations were computed between output and process residuals after controlling for input abilities. The output and six process measures are listed in **Table 4** together with their partial correlations. The partial correlations of Column 7 in Table 4 show the relationship between the spring WRAT means and each of the six process measures, controlling for fall ability differences in classroom distributions. As can be seen there, class means tended to be lower for the

Table 4   Partial Correlations for Multiple Regression

	1	2	3	4	5	6	7
1. Class Size	1.00	-.27	-.34	.17	.09	.11	-.30
2. Boys/Girls	-.27	1.00	-.22	.22	-.21	-.36	-.30
3. Infrequent Testing	-.34	-.22	1.00	.00	-.08	.00	.32
4. Negative Contacts	.17	.22	.00	1.00	-.30	-.19	-.37
5. Dist. Cognitive Contacts	.09	-.21	-.08	-.30	1.00	.25	.20
6. Math Time	.11	-.36	.00	-.19	.25	1.00	.47
7. WRAT Math Means	-.30	-.30	.32	-.37	.20	.47	1.00

classrooms with large enrollments, a higher ratio of boys to girls, and with teachers making a large number of negative contacts in moving about the classroom. On the other hand, class means tended to be higher if teachers tested less frequently, distributed cognitive contacts evenly about the classroom, and allotted more time to mathematics each day.

A multiple correlational analysis of this matrix of partials revealed that the six context-process measures account for 46 percent of the variance in achievement residuals, that is, 46 percent of the achievement variation not explained by entering abilities. Of course, this large percentage is an exaggeration because of the small sample and the posterior selection of the best of Leinhardt's variables. However, if this general trend holds up in a replication of this study that includes more classrooms, then the results will have important implications for developers of the instructional model.

But what do these studies of input-process-output have to do with evaluation? They are related in two ways. First of all, they provide information about how well the new program can be replicated in the field, by considering both laboratory school and field-test school classrooms. For an instructional model to be of interest to others, there must be evidence that it works as well in the field as it does in the laboratory, or that the modifications made in the field are not dysfunctional to the program. Secondly, such analyses provide information regarding the validity of different components of the model, at least those components which show variation in implementation. For example, one surprising finding for the developers of the instructional program is that the "time since last testing" variable was positively correlated with student gain in abilities. Theoretically, the instructional model suggests that teachers should test frequently in order to make sure that students are working on appropriate units in the curriculum. However, the partial correlation of .32 suggests that about 10 percent of the variance in end-of-year class means not predicted from entering abilities is related positively to the average time since last testing (i.e., the more frequent the testing, the lower the achievement). This preliminary finding needs to be scrutinized very carefully by the developers in order to determine its validity. If it turns out that testing does not have to be as frequent as the current program prescribes, then costs can be reduced. It also will force the developers to re-examine the purpose of frequent testing and perhaps modify their instructional model.

A finding which is consistent with the instructional model is the negative relationship between percentage of negative teacher contacts and achievement. That is, the more the teacher bitched to students, the lower the achievement. The training program for the instructional model tells the teacher to ignore students who are exhibiting undesirable behaviors and attend to students who are "on-task," praising them for good work and avoiding negative statements.

Of course, the negative partial correlation between achievement and negative contacts does not prove the importance of this component of the instructional model. There are several alternatives to the hypothesis that negative contacts are dysfunctional. First of all, given the large number of relationships which were explored, this one may be a chance relationship that needs replication to be convincing. But even if it is a replicable relationship, it is possible that classrooms with trouble-makers force teachers to use more negative contacts, and at the same time, the trouble-makers disturb classrooms enough to reduce overall achievement. Laboratory results suggest, however, that teachers who make negative contacts actively generate disruptive behavior on the part of their students, by unintentionally reinforcing (through attention) the inappropriate behavior.

This last point illustrates the fact that evaluative research does indeed need to be concerned with how to support causal arguments from this type of panel data. One possibility is to go to path analysis and show how the observed relationships are consistent with some believable causal model. Another is to control the training program in a way which changes the behavior of randomly selected teachers with regard to aspects of their behavior such as distribution of contacts, then to determine if identified changes in teacher behavior result in changes in student performance.

How Competitive Are the Proposed Means?

Many of our university colleagues are quite impatient with cost/effectiveness concerns. Individualized education is an obvious "good" and should be highly valued by all! Of course, this is not how valuation works when policy decisions have to be made. When alternative means are competing for finite resources, the policy-makers' guess as to which ends are most desired, which means are most likely to achieve those ends, and the relative costs of alternative means, will determine which means are selected. The function of evaluative research is to provide information which might improve those guesses.

As far as costs are concerned, LRDC, its collaborator, Research for Better Schools (a regional laboratory in Philadelphia), and its publishers, have made considerable progress in this regard. For example, early versions of our IPI Mathematics program cost 40 dollars per child for materials alone. Today, the costs of materials are quite competitive with conventional texts, especially when the costs of teacher prepared materials which are reproduced to supplement those texts are also considered. Generating such information is part of the evaluative research function.

The main increases in costs for LRDC programs over conventional approaches are the extra adults (para-professionals) who are currently required for operating the programs. Thus, if these new programs are to successfully compete, it is necessary to figure out ways to reduce these costs or show the importance of the increased benefits. Right now elementary schools have to increase costs about 10 percent just to adopt our mathematics program. The consumers must feel that their benefits are increasing correspondingly, or they will not buy.

Let us return now to the question of value with which this chapter began. A complete program of evaluative research aimed at providing information useful to others who would judge the value of innovative education programs must cover the range of issues that have been illustrated here. The demonstration that a new method can in fact achieve the instructional objectives of the developer is only a part of the valuing problem. What we expect our own line of inquiry will eventually reveal is that effective programs of individualized education are an important national need which, when met, will solve other costly problems in our society; that this need is very important relative to others; and that the costs for such programs are reasonable and competitive relative to available alternatives.

Another point which this discussion has illustrated is that evaluation is not a one-shot affair, but rather a program of research. It also illustrates our conviction that evaluative research can and must be done as part of a total research and development effort. The credibility of the results produced by people who are possibly biased toward the innovation must be generated in the same way that credibility is achieved by basic researchers who are biased toward a particular theoretical position, namely, through public display of procedures and results in a manner that allows competent peers to judge the quality of the research and the validity of the results.

Footnotes

1.   The percentage of children present can be considered both a context variable and a process variable. It is a context variable in the sense that a classroom which is somewhat smaller than expected pro-

vides a different environment than one in which all of the children are present. It is a process variable in that low attendance can be considered symptomatic of a poor attitude toward school.

References

Glaser, R. Individuals and learning: The new aptitudes. *Educational Researcher,* 1972, *1,* 5-13.

Jastak, J. F., Bijou, S. W., and Jastak, S. R. *Wide Range Achievement Test.* Wilmington, Delaware: Guidance Association, 1965.

Leinhardt, G. *The boojum of evaluation: Implementation, some measures.* Unpublished Doctoral Dissertation, University of Pittsburgh, 1972.

Thorndike, R. L., Hagen, E., and Lorge, I. *Cognitive Abilities Test.* Boston: Houghton-Mifflin, 1968.

System-Wide Analysis of Social Interaction and Affective Problems in Schools

14

James R. Barclay

Part I

Multiple Needs Assessment in the Elementary Schools

The problem of effecting change in the schools is monumental. This is so because human learning is cumulative and interactive. It is influenced by other students, teachers, curriculum, and parental and environmental factors. Teachers, counselors, school psychologists, curriculum specialists and administrators are all in need of information about individual differences in order to make decisions about the allocation of limited resources. This information must not only consist of achievement scores, but social and affective data. If the school is to prevent rather than respond to problems, it must consider evaluation as a prime means of decision-making. Evaluation must serve a reflective and corrective function in policy decisions.

Specifically, school personnel need information on how to allocate rather limited resources so that the school effort can be maximized. This means that, along the developmental continuum, learning must be viewed as an interaction composed of socio-economic, self-concept, group interaction and self-management variables which are in some way predictive of task-oriented achievement. Moreover, the research supporting policy-making must be capable of replication under many differing circumstances, outside the laboratory, and not only be concerned with changes in achievement test data.

Logically, it follows that there is a need for determining, at an early age, who is presenting learning problems in the school, and then determining strategies of behavior change or intervention. In short, there is a need to (a) identify methods of screening large groups of children by a comprehensive, economical, effective, and non-offensive psychometric method, (b) identify methods of using multiple-input predictors that approximate real life inputs, (c) develop a parsimonious procedure for interpreting these results, (d) relate such results to a logic of intervention, (e) make a set of policy judgments about the allocation of resources, needed training programs and cost-effectiveness, and (f) evaluate both the consequences of research and the process.

This chapter describes a multi-method, multi-trait system for evaluating social and affective variables in the elementary classroom by a computer technology. The system known as the Barclay Classroom Climate Inventory (hereafter abbreviated to BCCI) is appropriate to grades two through six, and is capable of describing individuals and cumulating individual characteristics into descriptions of classroom units. This paper will (1) describe the system, (2) discuss individual inter-district and intra-district analysis methods, and (3) draw some implications for a preventive-intervention model. It is believed that this system provides relevant diagnostic information about affective and social variables that are related to and in fact mediate progress towards task-oriented achievement.

Instrumentation

Over a period of seventeen years I have worked on a multi-method, multi-trait instrument to assess differences in the classroom. It is an inventory that employs three methods of assessment: self-report, peer nominations, and teacher judgments.[1] Under the self-report section it includes a portion relating to self-competency skills (I can run fast, I like to listen to others, etc.), a section relating to reinforcers (candy, money, doing something fun with parents, etc.), and a section relating to vocational awareness (interest in various occupations or skills relating to such occupations). The peer section is composed of 26 group nominations that relate to who can do a specific activity the best within the choice range of that classroom (who can run fast, who likes to listen to others and the like). Only one person can be nominated for each skill. The skills are similar to those contained in the self-competency scales with the exception that there are items relating to reticence and disruptiveness. The final method is the teacher input. This consists of 62 adjectives which are distributed into areas relating to stable and unstable extroversion and stable and unstable introversion. Teachers check only those adjectives that appear typically characteristic of the child.

In addition to the methods, there are a number of common traits distributed throughout the instrument. Interviews with children indicated that skills, competencies, and patterns of liking or not-liking appear functionally similar to Holland's psycho-vocational dimensions (Holland, 1966). Holland enunciated a theory of vocational choice that is based on a pattern of nurturance, initially within the family, and later in conjunction with the environmental press. He identified families of occupations that related to artistic, intellectual, social, conventional, realistic-outdoor, and enterprising characteristics.

After a process of initial experimentation, self and group scales were included in the BCCI that reflect (1) the artistic-intellectual dimension, (2) the social-conventional dimension, (3) the realistic-outdoor-masculinity dimension, and (4) the enterprising area. In addition, items composing a reticence and disruptiveness set of scales were included. The vocational-awareness scales also reflect these same areas. Teacher judgments expressed by adjectives tend to distribute themselves into gradations of extroversion and introversion, stable and unstable behavior. They follow a distribution which is typical as reported by Eysenck and Rachman in their studies (1965). Finally, there are a number of reinforcer-type activities that have been grouped into seven scales, and a measure of satisfaction with the classroom climate. The reinforcer scales are (1) interests in self-stimulating activities, (2) interests in esthetic activities, (3) interests in task-oriented activities, (4) interests in family activities, (5) interests in conventional activities, (6) interests in male peer activities, and (7) interests in female peer activities. In all, there are 32 short scales that are independent of each other plus some summary and total scale scores.

Through the use of principal axis factor analysis and multi-method, multi-trait factor analysis as described by Jackson (1969) it has been possible to group together various scales by factors. There is repeated evidence that self-report, group nominations and teacher judgments converge on basic factors such as affiliation, aggression, seclusiveness and the like (Barclay and Elton, 1973, Tapp and Barclay, 1973).

On the basis of a number of experimental and observational studies, including all the traditional reliability and validity studies together with behavioral observations (Barclay, 1972), it has been possible to develop both an individual computer written report and several scattergram grids and tables for use by school personnel. The programming problems are formidable and work on this aspect of the inventory has proceeded for seven years with continual modifications. Basically, there are two kinds of interpretations required for the programming. The first relates to the individual report. Here judgments about individual scales are made in terms of the standard deviation of the scale with a judgment of *high* reflected at or about the one standard deviation above the mean, and a judgment of *low* reflected at or about one standard deviation below the mean. The second kind of judgment is found in the summary paragraph about the child and consists of a series of conditional "if" statements in the computer that searches for the convergence of discriminant judgment of various scales that are known to fit together through correlational and factor analysis studies.

On the basis of these inferences, an individual report is written by the computer describing the child at three levels. The first level is a summary of the factor scores. The second level provides information about the child as related to his special characteristics. In this portion of the report his self-report information is presented with specific reference to high and low interests. Peer judgments and teacher expectations are then reported as related to the child's special characteristics. The third level is an analysis of the child's summary characteristics and special interests as applied to the context of the learning environment. Here a summary paragraph is included plus possible suspected problem areas. The rationale of the report is that assessment should contain three components: (1) an overview of the individual on major dimensions, (2) a commentary on his unique and special characteristics, and (3) an application of these findings to the special learning setting.

Another output of the computer program is the formation of two scattergram grids. These grids simply compare the total self-competency ratings of the individual with his peer support, and teacher expectations versus peer support. The first grid indicates how the child's self-competency ratings compare with the estimate of his skills from the peer group. This provides an estimate of how realistic the child's own judgments are in comparison with the peer group's. The second grid provides a quick visual outline of the support system that exists in that classroom for the child. By looking at the combination of positive teacher ratings and peer nominations it is possible to determine at a glance who has a lot of support in the classroom and who does not.

A third output of the computer program is a table that summarizes *suspected* problems for all of the individuals in the class and provides percentages of such *suspected* problem areas for both boys and girls. This printout is important in determining whether the frequency of observed problems is greater or lesser in one specific problem area. It also provides a basis for comparing classroom units on frequency of *suspected* problems. The eight suspected problem areas are derived from the factor scores and the summary total scores on self-competency, vocational awareness and attitude toward school. They are: (1) self-competency skills, (2) group skills, (3) self-control skills, (4) verbal skills, (5) physical skills, (6) vocational development, (7) cognitive-motivation, and (8) attitude toward school.[2] *If* conditions are met, an X is placed after the number of the appropriate child and in the proper column. Then the number of Xs are summed by problem area and the percentage of problems in that category is obtained separately for boys and for girls.

Another output of the program is a child's report. This is a report designed to provide information to the child or to his parent about his social interaction in the classroom. This report is phrased in language appropriate to a child's understanding and only summarizes the six factor scores.

On the following pages, illustrations of these printouts are found. **Figure 1** is an example of the individual report. The student report (**Figure 2**) is present also to provide an example of this output. **Figure 3** is the grid created from self and peer comparisons. **Figure 4** is the grid created from teacher and peer comparisons and **Figure 5** presents the summary data on *suspected* problems.

Thus the BCCI provides information about the individual student on several levels. It presents an individual report reflecting differences in the individual scales and summarizing temperament and self versus peer group determinants, then consolidates these scales into a series of personological and environmental judgments, and finally draws some conclusions about suspected problems. What is obtained is the consequence of many multiple observations by the child himself, all of his class peer group, and the teacher.

The BCCI has been administered to approximately 12,000 children in eight states. These children were from central city, suburban, and rural communities. Basic standardization studies were completed with approximately 3400 children.

Method

This study is based on the use of the eight problem categories together with a summary analysis of teacher ratings. Over 4000 elementary school children distributed from the second through the sixth grades were represented in 143 classrooms. The unit of measurement, then, was the summary set of percentages of problems for each classroom unit, separately arrived at for males and for females. The population was drawn from three quite different communities. District A represented a university town in the deep South. District B represented a suburban area of a Northern large city, and District C represented the inner city schools of a large central Southern school district.

Three problems were posed relating to this study: (1) What are the characteristics of classroom groups described cross-sectionally by

Figure 1   Printout of Individual Report

BOY   STUDENT NO 13   TEACHER 3   DATE 0   BCCI CODE B-5

1. OVERALL SUMMARY BASED ON FACTOR SCORES

ACHIEVEMENT–MOTIVATION   VERY INADEQUATE THRUST FOR ACHIEVEMENT AND QUITE DEFICIENT IN PERSISTENCE.
CONTROL–STABILITY   DEMONSTRATES ADEQUATE LEVEL OF PREDICTABLE AND STABLE BEHAVIOR.
INTROVERSION–SECLUSION   ADEQUATE LEVEL OF VERBAL BEHAVIOR.
ENERGY–ACTIVITY   NORMALLY ADEQUATE LEVEL OF ENERGY AND PERSISTENCE IN COMPETITIVE ACTIVITIES.
SOCIABILITY–AFFILIATION   OCCASIONAL REMOTENESS AND INABILITY TO RELATE TO OTHER PEOPLE AND INTERACT WITH THEM.
ENTERPRISING–DOMINANCE   OCCASIONAL NEED FOR LEADERSHIP ROLES.

2. SPECIAL CHARACTERISTICS

A. ESTIMATE OF SELF–REPORT

SELF–COMPETENCY   OVERALL ADEQUATE ESTIMATE OF SELF SKILLS.   HIGH OUTDOOR–MECHANICAL SKILLS.

VOCATIONAL AWARENESS   OVERALL MANIFESTS VERY RESTRICTED RANGE OF VOCATIONAL INTERESTS.
LOW INTELLECTUAL–SCIENTIFIC INTERESTS. LOW OUTDOOR–MECHANICAL INTERESTS. LOW SOCIAL INTERESTS.
LOW CLERICAL INTERESTS. LOW BUSINESS INTERESTS.
PREFERENCE FOR STABLE AND SECURE OCCUPATIONAL INTERESTS.

REINFORCERS   HIGH INTEREST IN MONEY, FOOD, CANDY, POP AS BASIC REINFORCERS.

ATTITUDE TOWARDS SCHOOL   MANIFESTS A USUALLY FAVORABLE ATTITUDE TOWARDS SCHOOL.

B. PEER NOMINATIONS   PERCEIVED OVERALL BY PEERS AS POSSESSING FEW PERSONAL OR SOCIAL SKILLS.
LOW ARTISTIC AND INTELLECTUAL SKILLS. LOW SOCIAL–AFFILIATIVE SKILLS.

C. TEACHER EXPECTATIONS   MANIFESTS OCCASIONAL POOR PERSONAL ADJUSTMENT.
MANIFESTS SOMEWHAT INCONSISTENT PATTERN OF SOCIAL ADJUSTMENT.
MANIFESTS OCCASIONAL POOR EFFORT AND MOTIVATION.

3. SUMMARY: THIS CHILD TENDS TOWARDS A SELF–IMAGE OF NOT POSSESSING MANY PERSONAL OR SOCIAL SKILLS. DOES NOT RECEIVE MANY PEER NOMINATIONS. MAY BE AN ISOLATE OR REJECTED CHILD.

4. SUSPECTED PROBLEMS: GROUP INTERACTION DEFICITS.   LIMITED VOCATIONAL INTERESTS.
LOW COGNITIVE ACHIEVEMENT MOTIVATION.

SELF–RATED SCALES		GROUP NOMINATION SCALES				VOCATIONAL PREFERENCE SCALES				TEACHER ADJECTIVE SCALES				BEHAVIORAL SCALES				FACTOR SCORES	
SAI	3	GAI	1	GR	1	INT	1	ENTR	0	TR7	5	MEL	3	SSR	10	CNV	21	I	40	IV	51
SRM	5	GRM	4	GD	3	REAL	0	CONT	8	TR8	16	CHL	6	ESR	13	PRM	33	II	51	V	42
SSC	0	GSC	0			SOC	0	ST	2			PHL	2	ITR	13	PRF	16	III	49	VI	49
SE	3	GE	2	GTOT	7	CONV	0	VTOT	18			SAN	2	FRR	15	CCI	7				
STOT	15																		

Figure 2 Printout of Student Report

A MESSAGE FROM YOUR COMPUTER FRIEND TO STUDENT NUMBER 13

HI ———————. GEE, I WISH I COULD SAY HI JOHN OR HI SUSAN. BUT I ONLY KNOW PEOPLE BY THEIR CLASSROOM NUMBER. SO YOU FILL IN YOUR NAME FOR ME. THANKS.

I AM A COMPUTER AND I HAVE SOME NEWS FOR YOU. A LITTLE WHILE AGO YOU ANSWERED SOME QUESTIONS ABOUT WHAT YOU LIKE AND WHAT YOU CAN DO. THIS WAS ON THE BARCLAY CLASSROOM CLIMATE INVENTORY. I LOOKED AT YOUR ANSWERS AND THOSE OF YOUR FRIENDS AND YOUR TEACHER. WHEN I GOT ALL THROUGH LOOKING I DECIDED TO WRITE THIS REPORT JUST FOR YOU.

NOW I DO NOT KNOW YOU LIKE YOUR PARENTS, FRIENDS AND TEACHER DO, SO WHAT I WRITE MAY NOT ALWAYS BE CORRECT. IF YOU HAVE QUESTIONS ABOUT WHAT I HAVE WRITTEN PLEASE TALK TO YOUR TEACHER, PRINCIPAL OR COUNSELOR.

YOU ARE NOT DOING SO WELL IN YOUR EFFORTS IN SCHOOL WORK.

YOU ARE DOING OKAY IN THE WAY YOU ACT IN CLASS AND IN YOUR SELF CONTROL IN SCHOOL.

HEY, YOU SEEM TO BE ABLE TO TALK WITH OTHERS PRETTY WELL.

YOU WORK WELL AT THINGS THAT INTEREST YOU. GREAT.

EVEN THOUGH YOU HAVE SOME CLOSE FRIENDS, YOU DONT ALWAYS GET ALONG SO WELL WITH SOME OF YOUR CLASSMATES.

YOU SHOW LEADERSHIP SKILLS.

IF SOME OF THE THINGS I WROTE ABOVE ARE PROBLEMS THAT YOU HAVE THOUGHT ABOUT, MAYBE TALKING TO SOME- BODY WOULD HELP YOU TO DECIDE WHAT TO DO. YOUR TEACHER OR COUNSELOR ARE AVAILABLE TO YOU, IF YOU WANT INFORMATION OR IDEAS.

BYE, BYE FOR NOW FROM YOUR COMPUTER FRIEND.

```
XXXXXXX
 X    X
 X    X
 X    X
XXXXXXXXXXXXX
  X    X     X
  X XX  XX  X  X
   X  XX XX X  X
    X   XX   X  X
     X  XXX  X  X
      X   X  X
       X XX X
        XXXXX
```

Figure 3   Self and Peer Comparisons

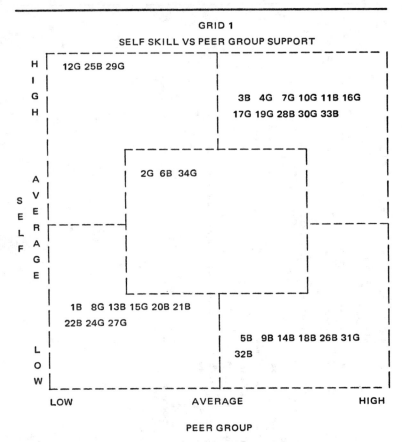

GRID 1

SELF SKILL VS PEER GROUP SUPPORT

THIS GRID COMPARES TOTAL SELF SKILL ESTIMATE WITH TOTAL PEER
NOMINATIONS. STUDENTS ARE IDENTIFIED BY NUMBER AND SEX. THE
UPPER LEFT CORNER REPRESENTS STUDENTS IN THE A CODE. LOWER
LEFT B; MIDDLE C; UPPER RIGHT D AND LOWER RIGHT E.

grade and sex determinants? (2) What can be learned through a comparison of districts by problems? (3) What can be learned through
intra-district comparisons? A number of statistical procedures were
used to ascertain answers to these questions. First of all, a multivariate
analysis of the data using race, grade and sex as factors was obtained.
This multivariate analysis was based on a computer program designed
by Dr. Jeremy Finn of the University of New York at Buffalo. Differ-

Figure 4   Teacher and Peer Comparisons

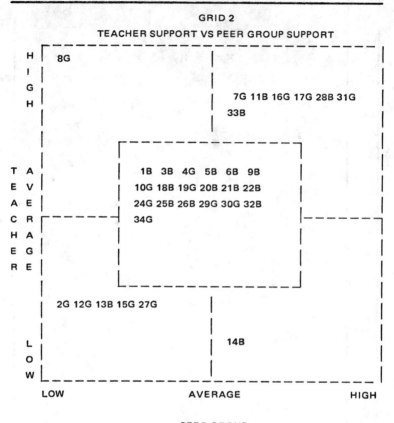

GRID 2

TEACHER SUPPORT VS PEER GROUP SUPPORT

PEER GROUP

THIS GRID COMPARES TOTAL TEACHER POSITIVE ADJECTIVES
(TR7) VERSUS TOTAL PEER GROUP RATINGS (GTOT). UPPER LEFT
CORNER REPRESENTS HIGH TEACHER SUPPORT VS. LOW PEER
SUPPORT; LOWER LEFT CORNER, LOW TEACHER AND LOW PEER
SUPPORT; MIDDLE AREA, AVERAGE SUPPORT FROM ONE OR BOTH
GROUPS; UPPER RIGHT, HIGH TEACHER AND HIGH PEER SUPPORT;
AND LOWER RIGHT, LOW TEACHER VERSUS HIGH PEER SUPPORT.

ences associated with race, grade and sex were looked at on all of the
problems variables. This provided both the statistical comparisons
desired and data for plotting differences.

Second, a principal factor analysis was completed on the eight
problems variables and the three summary teacher ratios (these ratios

Figure 5 Summary Data on Suspected Problems

SUSPECTED PROBLEMS SUMMARY TABLE

CHILD	SEX	SELF-SKILL EVALUATION	GROUP	CONTROL	VERBAL	PHYSICAL	VOCATIONAL DEVELOPMENT	COGNITIVE	SCHOOL ATTITUDE
1	B	X						X	X
2	G			X					X
3	B								
4	G				X		X		
5	B						X	X	
6	B							X	
7	G								
8	G					X			
9	B	X					X	X	X
10	G								
11	B								
12	G					X			
13	B		X				X	X	
14	B	X						X	X
15	G		X			X			
16	G								
17	G								
18	B								
19	G								
20	B	X						X	X
21	B						X	X	X
22	B							X	

Figure 5, continued

CHILD	SEX	SELF—SKILL EVALUATION	GROUP	CONTROL	VERBAL	PHYSICAL	VOCATIONAL DEVELOPMENT	COGNITIVE	SCHOOL ATTITUDE
24	G		X		X				X
25	B							X	X
26	B	X						X	
27	G	X	X				X		
28	B					X			
29	G					X			
30	G								
31	G								
32	B	X							
33	B								
34	G								

PERCENTAGE OF CLASS WITH SUSPECTED PROBLEM

		SELF—SKILL EVALUATION	GROUP	CONTROL	VERBAL	PHYSICAL	VOCATIONAL DEVELOPMENT	COGNITIVE	SCHOOL ATTITUDE
GIRLS		13	19	6	13	31	0	0	19
BOYS		29	6	0	0	0	35	65	29

SEE MANUAL FOR USE OF THIS TABLE IN INDIVIDUAL STRATEGY PLANNING OR CURRICULUM INTERVENTION.

reflect the sum of positive and sum of negative adjectives chosen by each teacher for each child).[3] Third, using a discriminant analysis program by district it was possible to look at differences between school districts. Fourth, using the data obtained discriminant analysis was used to determine differences within a school district as an example of how this procedure can be used for policy planning.

In summary, then, the procedures mentioned above were used to (1) identify cross-sectional differences on grade, sex, and race variables, (2) ascertain differences in problem factors between three school districts, and (3) illustrate differences within one school district.

Results

The results of this study will be reported in three sections. The first section will be concerned with cross-sectional differences by age, sex, and race for the problems percentages. The second section will deal with differences between school districts, and the third section will be concerned with differences within one school district.

1. Cross-Sectional Differences

The multivariate analysis of the problems and teacher judgments provide some interesting information about the relationship between percentages of problems. The intercorrelations for the males (Table 1) may be summarized as follows:

1.   Self-concept problems appear to be related significantly to cognitive-motivation problems and dislike of school.

2.   Group interaction problems tend to be related positively to verbal skill deficits and cognitive-motivation problems.

3.   Verbal skill deficits are related to group interaction, self-management, cognitive-motivation and poor attitude towards school problems. They are also related significantly to positive ratings by teachers in the personal adjustment, social adjustment, and effort and motivation areas. This suggests that verbal skill deficits in males are related to positive teacher evaluations.

4.   Self-control problems are positively related to verbal skill deficits and negative teacher evaluations.

Table 1 Means, Standard Deviations and Intercorrelations for Suspected Problems (Males)

Problem Area	Mean	S.D.	2	3	4	5	6	7	8	9	10	11
1. Self Concept	27.16	16.41	.12	.07	−.07	.10	.16	.18	.22	−.13	−.10	−.11
2. Group Interaction	19.05	11.79		.02	.17	.20	.05	.18	−.07	.01	.06	.01
3. Self Management	14.52	14.14			.27	−.13	−.21	.09	.01	−.21	−.20	−.24
4. Verbal Skills	13.86	11.66				.19	.02	.20	.29	.31	.33	.39
5. Physical Skills	1.34	3.01					.15	.05	.25	−.01	−.08	−.03
6. Vocational Skills	15.90	14.78						.16	.26	−.07	−.13	−.07
7. Cognitive Skills	10.80	10.30							.16	−.28	−.23	−.25
8. Attitude Toward School	21.41	13.99								−.19	−.26	−.31
9. Teacher P.A.	.16	.26									.94	.89
10. Teacher S.A.	.19	.27										.85
11. Teacher E.F.	−.03	.22										

N = 143 Elementary Classroom Means   P<.01 = .208,   05 = .159

Note: decimals omitted and significant correlations underlined.

5.   Physical skill problems appear to be related to group interaction problems and poor attitude towards school.

6.   Vocational deficits tend to be related to self-concept deficits, cognitive-motivation problems and poor attitude towards school.

7.   Cognitive-motivation problems tend to be related to self-concept problems, poor group interaction skills, poor verbal skills, poor knowledge of the world of work and low teacher judgments.

8.   Poor attitude towards school is reflected in a lowered self-concept, poor verbal skills, poor physical skills, lack of knowledge about vocational alternatives and low teacher expectations.

Turning now to **Table 2** relating to the girls, the intercorrelations may be summarized as follows:

1.   Self-concept problems are positively related to verbal, physical, cognitive-motivation and poor attitude towards school deficits. They are also related to lowered mean evaluations by teachers.

2.   Group interaction problems are related positively to verbal, physical, vocational, cognitive and attitudinal deficits.

3.   Self-management deficits are related to verbal and cognitive deficits, as well as to negative evaluations on personal adjustment by teachers.

4.   Verbal deficits tend to be related to almost all other problems.

5.   Physical skill and attitudinal deficits are related significantly to almost all other problems.

6.   Vocational problems are related to group interaction deficits.

A further clarification of the relationship between the problem areas and teacher judgments can be observed in the results of a principal axis factor analysis completed separately for males and females. These data are reported in **Tables 3** and **4**. As can be seen from Table 3, 30 percent of the total variance is accounted for by the summary teacher judgments. Self-management and verbal skill deficits define the second factor. This might suggest that verbal mediation skills and the lack

Table 2 Means, Standard Deviations and Intercorrelations for Suspected Problems (Females)

Problem Area	Mean	S.D.	2	3	4	5	6	7	8	9	10	11
1. Self Concept	24.48	15.41	.13	-.15	.24	.45	.13	.28	.43	-.19	-.21	-.26
2. Group Interaction	15.20	11.18		.13	.33	.32	.19	.33	.27	.13	.09	.14
3. Self Management	8.88	10.46			.30	-.08	.01	.42	.13	-.22	-.04	-.10
4. Verbal Skills	19.44	12.00				.16	.04	.26	.23	-.21	-.17	-.22
5. Physical Skills	12.27	10.87					.14	.22	.22	-.25	-.20	-.28
6. Vocational Skills	10.45	12.19						.14	.09	-.09	-.06	-.12
7. Cognitive Skills	10.42	10.78							.36	-.26	-.15	-.20
8. Attitude Toward School	21.79	15.24								-.28	-.24	-.30
9. Teacher P.A.	.35	.27									.90	.89
10. Teacher S.A.	.40	.25										.84
11. Teacher E.F.	.21	.20										

N = 143 Elementary Classroom Means   P < .01 = .208,   .05 = .159

Note: decimals omitted and significant correlations underlined.

Table 3

Table 3   Principal Factor Analysis (Varimax Rotation)
           Proportion of Suspected Problems (Males)

Factor I		Factor II		Factor III	
Teacher Rating P.A.	.97	Self-Management	.81	Group Inter-	.87
Teacher Rating S.A.	.95	Deficits		action	
Teacher Rating E.F.	.91	Verbal Skill	.64	Attitude toward	
		Deficits		school	.44
30.45% of Variance		15.07% of Variance		11.36% of Variance	
		45.53 Cum. %		56.89 Cum. %	

Factor IV		Factor V		Factor VI	
Physical Skill	.84	Self Concept	.97	Vocational	.78
Deficits		Deficits		Skill Deficits	
Attitude Toward				Cognitive Skill	.66
School	.53			Deficits	
Verbal Skill					
Deficits	.42				
9.33% of Variance		8.32% of Variance		7.45% of Variance	
62.22 Cum. %		74.54 Cum. %		81.98 Cum. %	

Sum of Squares	I	II	III	IV	V	VI
of Factors	2.86	1.35	1.13	1.35	1.06	1.23

Note: Data based on 143 elementary classrooms representing approximately
4000 cases.

thereof play an important role in the manifestation of uncontrolled and impulsive behavior. Factor 3 is a combination of poor group interaction and poor attitude towards school. This is a logical if not causal relationship. Physical skill deficits, poor attitude towards school and verbal deficits define the fourth factor with self-concept problems standing alone as the fifth factor. Finally, the sixth factor appears to be a combination of vocational and cognitive-motivation deficits.

For girls, the summary teacher judgments contribute something over 32 percent of the total variance for the first factor. Factor 2 is a combination of self-concept deficits and poor attitude towards school. Factor 3 is a combination of self-management deficits and cognitive-motivation deficits. Factor 4 stands alone as vocational deficits. Factor 5 is a combination of group interaction and physical skill deficits and factor 6 is verbal skill deficits alone.

What these data infer in regard to the explanation of the variance associated with mean classroom problems in the 143 classrooms constituting the data base for this study appears to be clear:

**Table 4   Principal Factor Analysis (Varimax Rotation)
Proportion of Suspected Problems (Females)**

Factor I		Factor II		Factor III	
Teacher Rating P.A.	.95	Self-Concept	.85	Self Manage-	.84
Teacher Rating S.A.	.94	Deficits		ment Deficits	
Teacher Rating E.F.	.92	Attitude Toward	.73	Cognitive	.73
		School		Deficits	
32.68% of Variance		15.84% of Variance		12.99% of Variance	
		48.52 Cum. %		61.51 Cum. %	

Factor IV		Factor V		Factor VI	
Vocational Deficits	.98	Group Interaction	.78	Verbal Deficits	.92
		Deficits			
		Physical Skill	.75		
		Deficits			
8.89% of Variance		7.71% of Variance		6.56% of Variance	
70.39 Cum. %		78.11 Cum. %		84.67 Cum. %	

Sum of Squares	I	II	III	IV	V	VI
of Factors	2.77	1.62	1.51	1.07	1.36	1.02

Note: Data based on 143 elementary classrooms representing approximately 4000 cases.

1. For both boys and girls in these classrooms, the largest deficit variance is related to teacher expectations.

2. For both boys and girls, verbal skill deficits and self-management deficits are tied together, and generally associated with the frequency of cognitive-motivation deficits.

3. Poor attitude or dissatisfaction with school is associated with a number of other problem areas and may be a byproduct of poor social interaction and lack of teacher support.

The next statistical operation was the multivariate analysis of the suspected problems using the original problems data and the obtained teacher ratios. The program first contrasted blacks and whites using the determinant of the predominant racial group in the classroom. Because the unit of data analysis was the classroom mean, classes having 60 percent or more black students were classified as Black, with the same logic for White classrooms. No significant multivariate F ratio was obtained for this contrast. Second, grade levels were contrasted. Here it was found that grades 2, 3, 5, and 6 showed significant multivariate F ratios when contrasted with the grand mean. Third, the two sexes were contrasted with very significant differences. Finally, race-sex interactions were contrasted. A significant multivariate F ratio was obtained for the second and sixth grades.

The results of the multivariate analysis are more adequately viewed by inspecting graphs of the means of problem variables by race and by sex. These data, however, are cross-sectional.

Figure 6 (p. 357) plots the mean percentage of self-competency problems for the four groups by grade level. It is apparent in this plot that second-graders, with the exception of Black males tend to see themselves as more competent than at any other grade level. In general the level of self-competency deficits holds at about 25 percent during the third and fourth grades with a sharp rise in deficits for all groups noted by the sixth grade.

Figure 7 (p. 358) depicts the percentage of group interaction problems by grade, sex and race. Here it is evident that children in the second grade have a mean proportion of problems in group interaction that is higher. White males end up with the highest percentage of group interaction problems and White females tend to show a marked decline of these problems through the third, fourth, and fifth grades with a slight increase noted in the sixth grade.

Figure 8 (p. 359) compared the percentage of self-control or self-management problems by grade, sex and race. Here there appear to be some common racial trends. Black males and females both tend to show a peak in behavioral management problems in the fifth grade with a marked decline noted towards the sixth grade. Black males show the highest percentage of self-control problems over all groups and start out with the most problems in this area. Both White groups show a gradual decline to the fifth grade. White females show fewest problems in this area and reach a very real low in the fifth grade.

Figure 9 (p. 360) compares the percentage of verbal skill deficits by grade, sex and race. Here again there seems to be some kind of a trend characteristic of Whites and another one for Blacks. Whites tend to show an increase in verbal skill deficits peaking in the fourth grade. This trend declines markedly in the fifth grade and increases

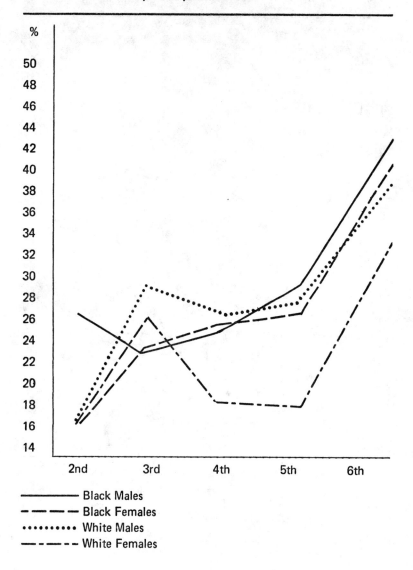

Figure 6 Comparison of Proportion of Self-Competency Problems by Grade, Sex and Race

——————— Black Males
— — — — Black Females
•••••••••• White Males
— - — - — White Females

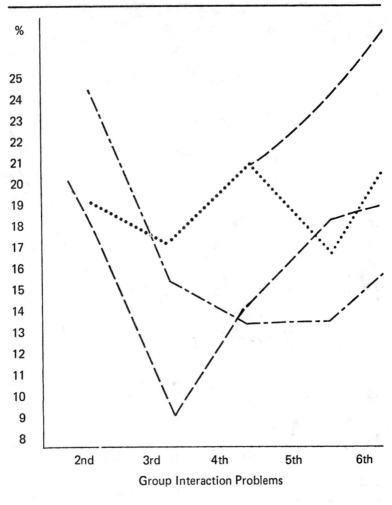

Figure 7   Comparison of Proportion of Group-Interaction Problems by Grade, Sex and Race

Group Interaction Problems

———————— Black Males
— — — — Black Females
•••••••••••• White Males
— · — · — · White Females

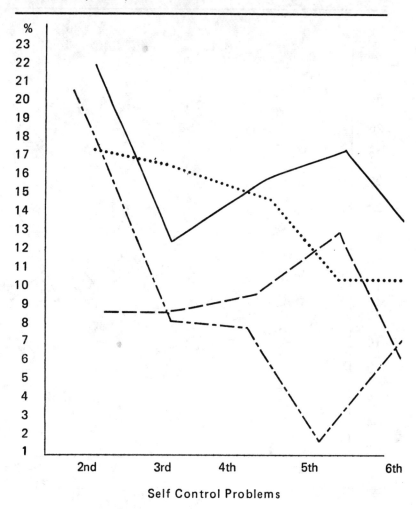

Figure 8   Comparison of Proportion of Self-Control Problems
by Grade, Sex and Race

Self Control Problems

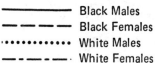

——————— Black Males
— — — — Black Females
•••••••••• White Males
— · — · — · White Females

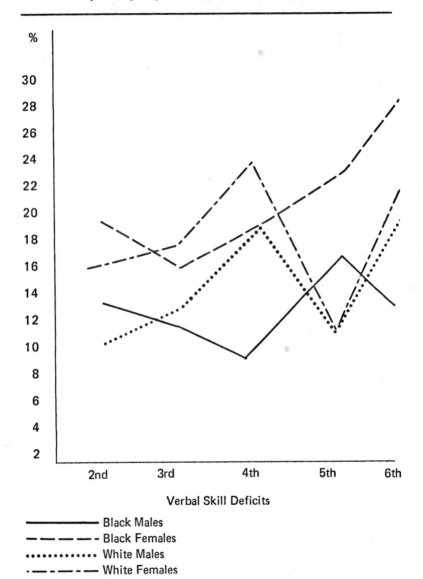

Figure 9 Comparison of Proportion of Verbal Skill Deficits by Grade, Sex, and Race

Verbal Skill Deficits

——————— Black Males
— — — — - Black Females
•••••••••••• White Males
·—·—·—·— White Females

sharply in the sixth grade. Blacks tend to start with higher verbal deficits than Whites. Black females tend to have the overall highest level of verbal deficits rising steadily from the third to the sixth grade where it reaches a mean proportion of almost 30 percent of the girls in Black classes.

Figure 10 (p. 362) represents percentage of physical skill deficits. This percentage represents peer and self-estimations of physical skills, outdoor manual and competitive activities. Very few boys show problems in this area. Girls by contrast tend to show a higher percentage of problems in this area.

Figure 11 (p. 363) compares the percentage of vocational development deficits by grade, sex and race. Results here may be the consequence of more discrimination by sixth graders regarding interest in vocations. This would lead to a decline in choices or a specific focus on one vocational area.

Figure 12 (p. 364) compares the percentage of cognitive motivation deficits by grade, sex and race. This problem area reflects interest in intellectual-scientific and task-oriented activities. With the exception of the White females the trend is clearly towards more cognitive-motivation deficits from the second through the sixth grades. Here again, Black females show the highest percentage of problems in this area.

Figure 13 (p. 365) compares the percentage of poor attitudes toward school by grade, sex and race. The general trend in these data is toward progressively more dissatisfaction with school over the grades. Of specific interest is the fact that Black children in the second grade already have rather well-defined poor attitudes towards school as compared with the generally favorable attitude manifested by Whites. Regardless, it appears from this figure that initial differences are smoothed out in the third grade and there is generally an increasing percentage of dissatisfaction with school.

Figures 14, 15, and 16 show the characteristic trends in mean teacher ratios by grade, sex and race. Here it should be noted that a high mean ratio represents a good set of evaluations with more positive adjectives chosen than negative ones. These figures illustrate the mean proportion of positive adjectives chosen over negative ones. In these graphs it is apparent that the mean teacher expectations as obtained by classroom ratios tend to decline from the second through the fifth grade. Then there is an upswing in the sixth grade. Boys are rated lower than girls and there are some differences observed by racial groups.

Despite the fact that it would be most appropriate to obtain longitudinal data on the same individuals over this period of time, it

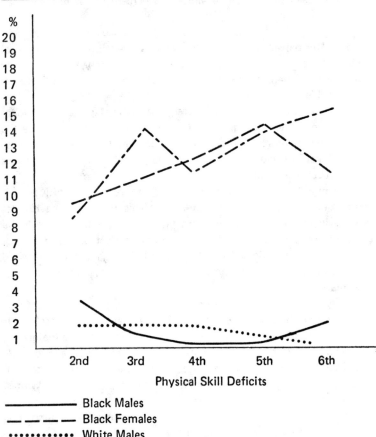

Figure 10   Comparison of Proportion of Physical Skill Deficit by Grade, Sex, and Race

Physical Skill Deficits

——————— Black Males
— — — — Black Females
•••••••••• White Males
·—·—·—·— White Females

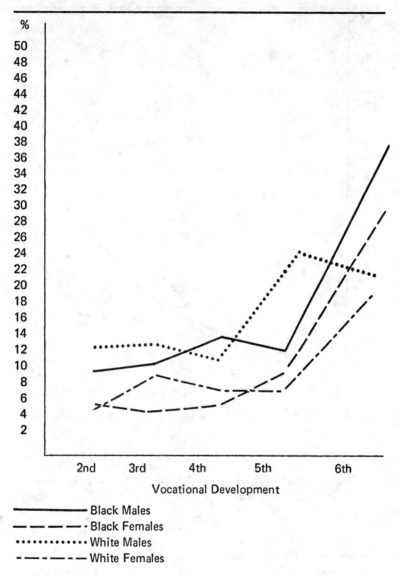

Figure 11   Comparison of Proportion of Vocational Development
               Deficits by Grade, Sex, and Race

Vocational Development

——————————— Black Males
— — — — — · Black Females
··············· White Males
—·—·—·—·— White Females

Figure 12   Comparison of Proportion of Cognitive Deficits by Grade, Sex, and Race

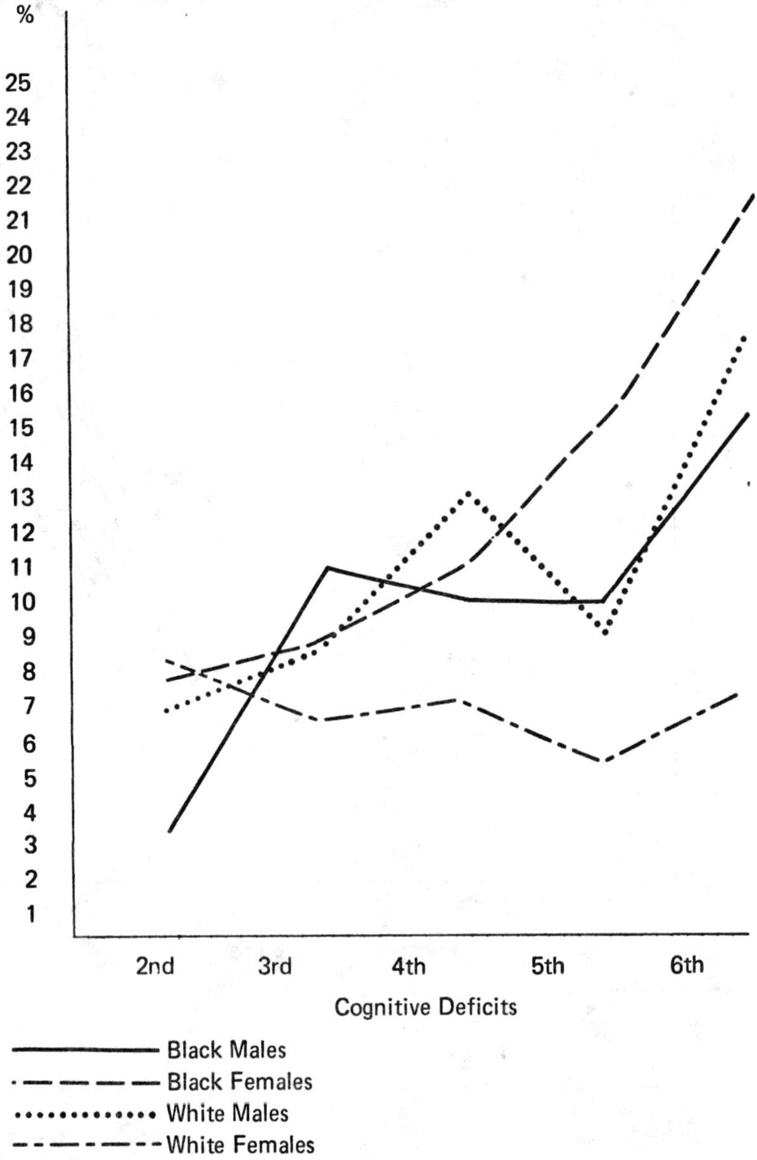

Cognitive Deficits

——————— Black Males
· — — — — Black Females
············ White Males
— — — — — White Females

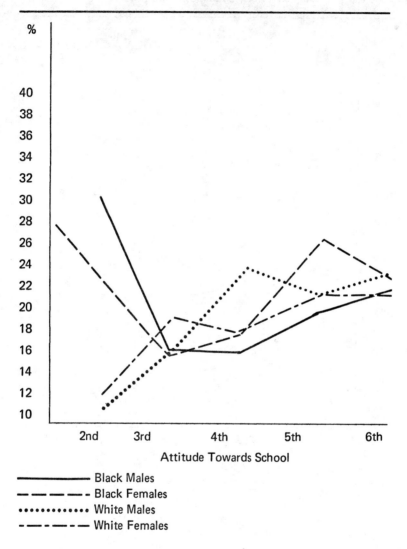

Figure 13   Comparison of Proportion of Poor Attitude Towards
               School by Grade, Sex, and Race

Attitude Towards School

———————— Black Males
— — — — — Black Females
•••••••••••• White Males
—·——·——·— White Females

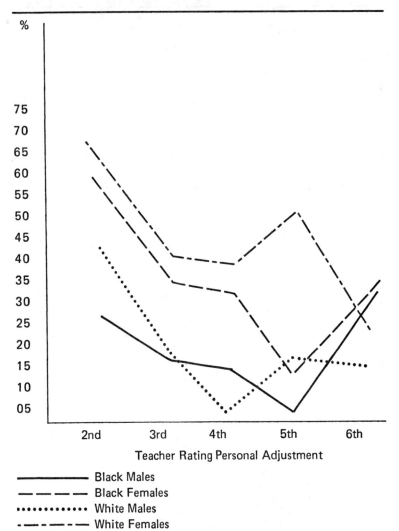

Figure 14 Comparison of Mean Teacher Ratios for Personal Adjustment by Grade, Sex, and Race

Teacher Rating Personal Adjustment

―――――― Black Males
― ― ― ― Black Females
•••••••••••• White Males
•―•―•―•― White Females

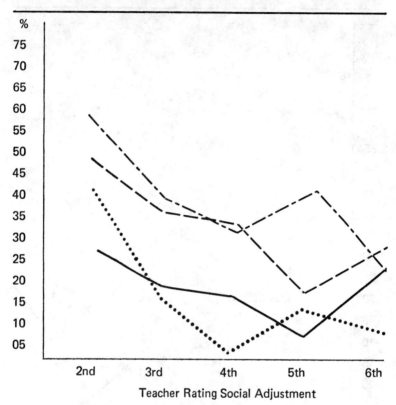

Figure 15   Comparison of Mean Teacher Ratios for Social Adjustment by Grade, Sex, and Race

Teacher Rating Social Adjustment

——————— Black Males
— — — — — Black Females
•••••••••••• White Males
— • — • — • — White Females

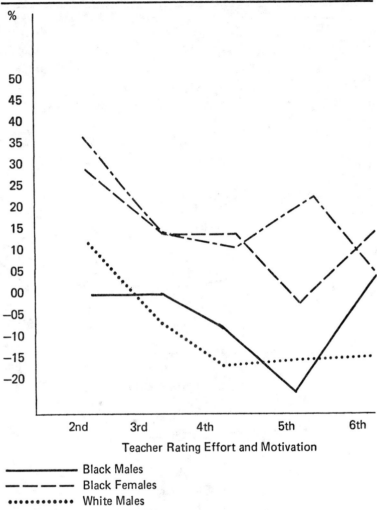

Figure 16   Comparison of Mean Teacher Ratios for Effort and Motivation by Grade, Sex, and Race

Teacher Rating Effort and Motivation

———————— Black Males
— — — — Black Females
•••••••••• White Males
— · — · — · White Females

would appear that there are some significant implications here for affective social variables in schooling. They may be summarized as follows:

1. The process of schooling tends to reduce the self-competency of children over the grades.

2. The process of schooling tends to be relatively ineffective in reducing group interaction problems.

3. The process of schooling tends to reduce the frequency of self-control or self-management problems. Children generally become more restrained.

4. Schooling results in increased verbal and cognitive-motivation deficits in children.

5. Schooling results in increased poor attitudes towards the experience.

6. Boys are treated differently from girls.

7. At the same time children are becoming less self-confident, less verbal, less cognitively motivated and more disillusioned with school; teacher judgments and expectations for them are becoming more negative.

2. Differences Between Districts

A second problem of this study was to determine what might be learned about differences between school districts. There were three districts included in this study. District A was a Southern university city. District B consisted of schools within the suburban area of a Northern City. District C represented the inner-city schools of a large Middle-Southern City.

Differences between school systems have always been a concern to administrators and school boards. The differences are often obtained only on socio-economic or achievement test data. Typically, administrators look at mean student achievement test scores and draw conclusions about the quality of the educational effort from these data. Thus a principal might note that his school is at the 60th percentile on a given achievement test *based on his students' scores.* He might not consider this very good. But if the mean of his school's achievement were arranged in a distribution with other schools, it might be that his comparative rank would be at the 80th percentile since the variability of students' scores is much greater than the variability of mean classroom units. Lindquist (1966) has argued for the determination of special distributions to reflect differences between classroom units and/or schools.

Using the factor score values obtained from the factor analysis of the problems data and teacher ratios (see Tables 3 and 4), a series of discriminant analyses were completed in accordance with a procedure described by Bock and Haggard (D. K. Whitla, ed., 1968). Discriminant analyses were run comparing the three districts by racial groupings, and also by grade levels. To detail all of these findings here would be inappropriate and detract from the major argument of the chapter. However, one example will be given relating to differences obtained between districts on overall racial group means.

One of the by-products of the discriminant analysis program used was a multiple step-wise discriminant analysis. In this procedure the major difference between the districts is identified first, and then covarying the first difference, other differences are indicated. Black and white male classroom units showed significant differences: (1) teacher expectations (Factor 1), (2) physical skill + attitude deficits (Factor 4), (3) vocational + cognitive deficits (Factor 6), and (4) group interaction deficits (Factor 3). For the Black and White female classroom units, only teacher expectations discriminated between districts (Factor 1).

The illustration of the profile of classroom means may facilitate observation of the differences obtained between the districts. **Figures 17-22** provide a visual portrayal of the comparative frequency of problems and teacher ratings between districts. These profile tables include not only the *z* score and *t* score equivalent, but an approximate percentile value for interpreting *z* scores.

With the aid of the multiple step-wise analysis one may observe that District A (Southern university city) shows high teacher ratings for both males and females. The mean level of group interaction and attitude towards class deficits appears to be high for White males. Both White and Black males in this district tend to show a higher mean proportion of cognitive and vocational problems. White females in this

Figure 17 Mean Factor Scores for District A Males

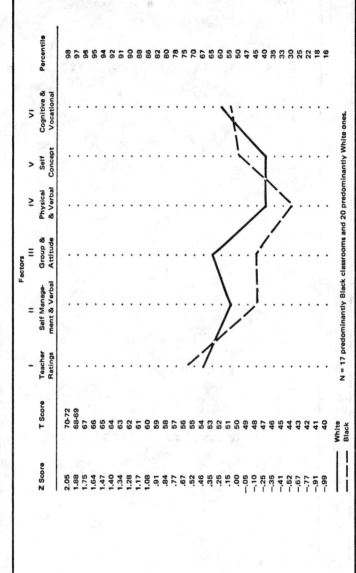

N = 17 predominantly Black classrooms and 20 predominantly White ones.

371

Figure 18　Mean Factor Scores for District A Females

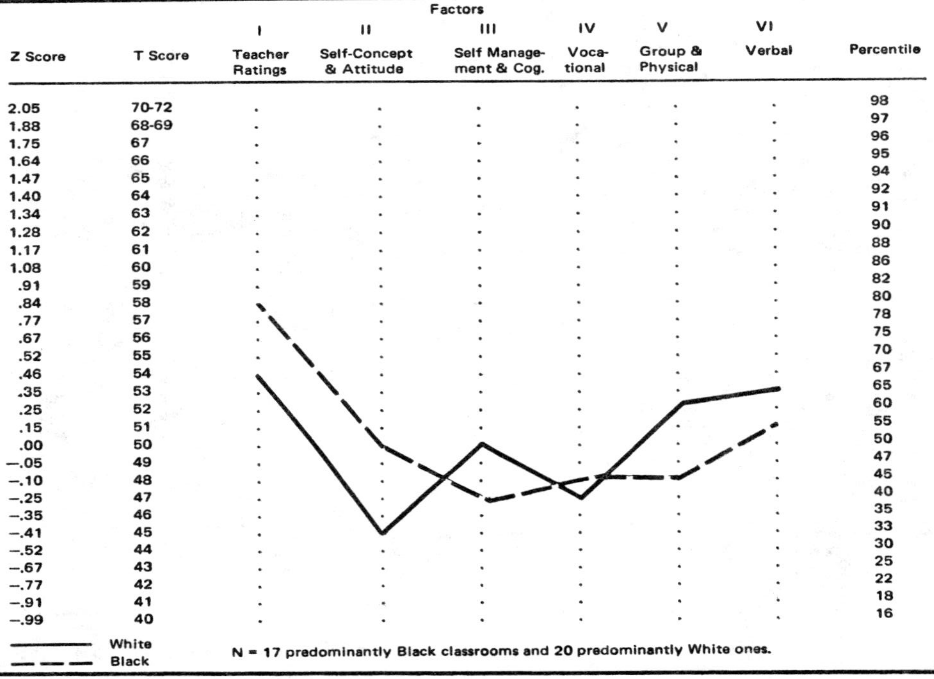

Z Score	T Score	I Teacher Ratings	II Self-Concept & Attitude	III Self Management & Cog.	IV Vocational	V Group & Physical	VI Verbal	Percentile
2.05	70-72							98
1.88	68-69							97
1.75	67							96
1.64	66							95
1.47	65							94
1.40	64							92
1.34	63							91
1.28	62							90
1.17	61							88
1.08	60							86
.91	59							82
.84	58							80
.77	57							78
.67	56							75
.52	55							70
.46	54							67
.35	53							65
.25	52							60
.15	51							55
.00	50							50
−.05	49							47
−.10	48							45
−.25	47							40
−.35	46							35
−.41	45							33
−.52	44							30
−.67	43							25
−.77	42							22
−.91	41							18
−.99	40							16

Factors

——— White
– – – Black

N = 17 predominantly Black classrooms and 20 predominantly White ones.

Figure 19   Mean Factor Scores for District B Males

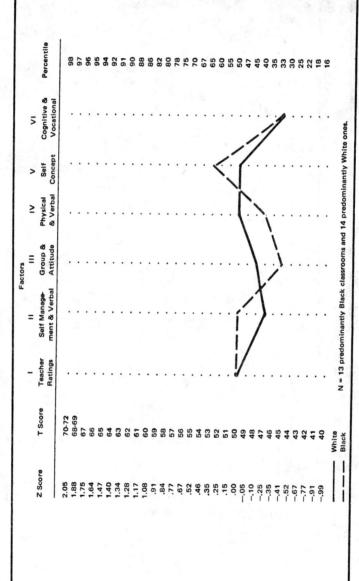

N = 13 predominantly Black classrooms and 14 predominantly White ones.

White ——————
Black – – – – –

Figure 20 Mean Factor Scores for District B Females

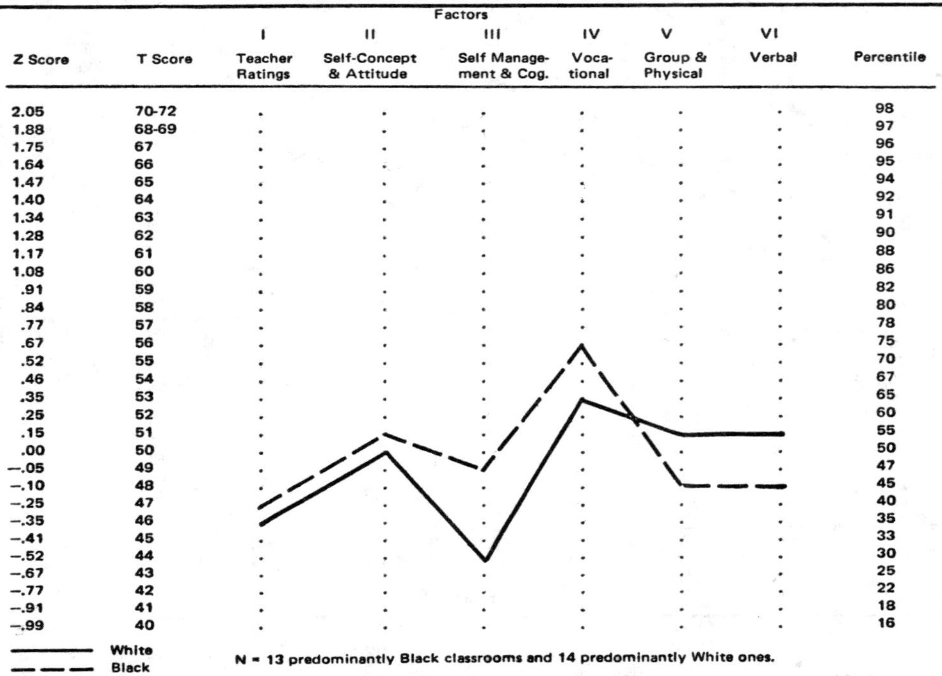

N = 13 predominantly Black classrooms and 14 predominantly White ones.

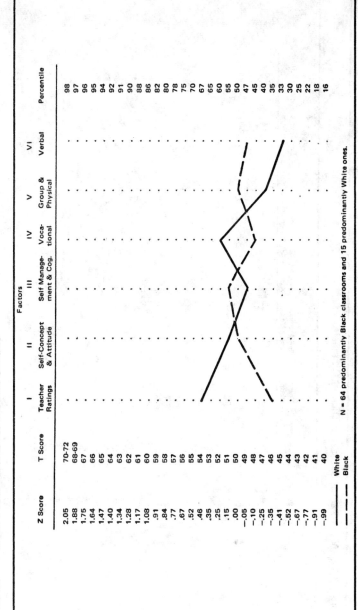

Figure 21   Mean Factor Scores for District C Males

N = 64 predominantly Black classrooms and 15 predominantly White ones.

White
Black

Figure 22   Mean Factor Scores for District C Females

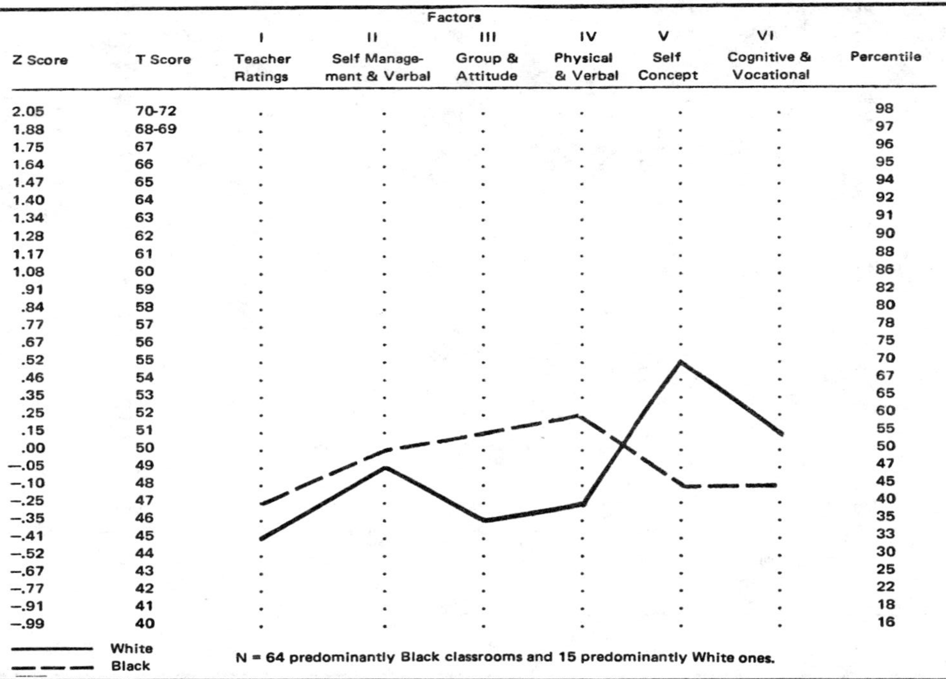

Factors

Z Score	T Score	I Teacher Ratings	II Self Management & Verbal	III Group & Attitude	IV Physical & Verbal	V Self Concept	VI Cognitive & Vocational	Percentile
2.05	70-72							98
1.88	68-69							97
1.75	67							96
1.64	66							95
1.47	65							94
1.40	64							92
1.34	63							91
1.28	62							90
1.17	61							88
1.08	60							86
.91	59							82
.84	58							80
.77	57							78
.67	56							75
.52	55							70
.46	54							67
.35	53							65
.25	52							60
.15	51							55
.00	50							50
-.05	49							47
-.10	48							45
-.25	47							40
-.35	46							35
-.41	45							33
-.52	44							30
-.67	43							25
-.77	42							22
-.91	41							18
-.99	40							16

———— White
– – – – Black

N = 64 predominantly Black classrooms and 15 predominantly White ones.

district tend to have higher mean levels of group interaction, and verbal deficits. District B (Northern suburb) shows average teacher ratings for males and slightly elevated self-concept deficits for Black males. Female mean factor scores for teacher ratings appear low, and vocational development means are high. In District C (Southern Midwestern inner city) the mean teacher ratings are low for males and for Black females. Only White females obtain a high mean teacher rating. In addition, White males appear to have a very high comparative mean on self-competency ratings.

This brief analysis demonstrates how differences between school systems on social and affective variables can be observed. It is also possible to compare grade levels or special groups in this same fashion. The methods exemplified here provide a limited example of how this technique can be used to describe differences between districts. With larger samples, and perhaps by regional samplings, it would be possible to take a look at the affective and social-interaction needs of large areas. With the inevitable restriction that comes with expanded efforts to effect change in the schools, and the short supply of resource personnel, such a technique can provide a means for identifying the overall needs of districts. Still further, specific problem areas can be pinpointed. Other variables such as percentage of racial composition, socio-economic status and achievement data can also be entered into the descriptive analysis of districts.

3. Differences within Districts

The third problem of this study is to describe how intra-district differences can be analyzed. The importance of this problem is obvious since it provides the district with the specific information needed to design interventions. For, though District A in the previous comparisons fared relatively well by comparison with the other two districts, it is still important to consider how grades and schools within this district differ from each other.

In District A, four schools containing 37 elementary classrooms were tested on the BCCI. Again using factor scores of problems and teacher ratings a multiple discriminant analysis was completed. The findings for this analysis will be summarized here.

A look at the discriminant analysis data provided for this District allows the following possible descriptions of the four schools.

School No. 1
This school is characterized by a low mean on teacher judgments. Males

tend to show a high proportion of physical skill deficits. Females show a high proportion of attitude towards school, cognitive-motivation and self-management deficits.

School No. 2
In this school the mean proportion of disruptive and self-management behaviors is high for males. They also show a high proportion of cognitive-motivation deficits. Females show a high proportion of poor attitude towards school and also a high proportion of self-management deficits.

School No. 3
Males in this school tend to have a high proportion of self-concept problems. Females show a high proportion of verbal problems. This school tends to have a low teacher evaluation of males and a high evaluation of females. There are very low levels of disruptiveness or cognitive problems evidence. Males also have a high proportion of poor attitude towards school.

School No. 4
Both males and females receive very high mean teacher ratings. Males tend to show a high mean proportion of self-management problems. Females show the lowest mean percentage of problems for females in the district.

Empirical observations of these schools by the writer and discussions with staff working with these schools in a Teacher Corps program confirmed the accuracy of the data analysis. Schools No. 1 and No. 3 are traditional in the sense that control of behavior and cognitive task-order skills are stressed. The schools themselves are old and arranged in a conventional model. Schools No. 2 and No. 4 are modern in their school plant and curriculum approach.

Differences within the schools themselves can also be looked at using either the generated factor scores for the problems that are unique to the district or the frequency of problems data obtained directly off the printout. The advantage of the first approach in analysis is considerable if the school district is large enough to warrant a separate factor analysis, the generation of factor scores, and a discriminant analysis. For small samples or schools the procedure is not warranted and reference can be made to the normative group of classroom means percentiles.

These data then provide some comparative analysis of differences between districts. The same procedures can be utilized in the district itself comparing either grade levels between schools or total schools. In addition, it is possible to determine the characteristics of special groups of children, for example, children who are in foster homes, children who have been bussed, children who are gifted or who have learning difficulties. Though contrasts between districts may be of prime importance to regional units within a state or to a state, the focus for the local school district is on differences which exist therein. Thus, for example, of the four schools located in the Southern City District, one tends to have many unfavorable teacher judgments and a high incidence of poor attitude and self-concept deficits. Another tends to be very well-controlled but to have problems centering in disruptive behavior. A third shows considerable control of students. A fourth shows that boys and girls are treated differentially. These examples show how the inventory can be used by a school district to ascertain the proportion of specific problems relating not only to individual classrooms, but to grade comparisons between schools, and many other comparisons.

Part II
A Model for Policy-Making

The research that has been detailed here has been directed toward meeting the criteria of a multiple-needs assessment system. There are a number of postulates that specify the strategy of approach. Some of these are as follows:

1. The chief purpose of the school is to promote adaptation to the environment. This includes not only basic skills in the academic area, but also, and perhaps equally as important, social and personal skills.

2. Social skills, self-management skills, verbal skills, and physical skills have a continuing high priority in the elementary school system because without them the academic skills that serve as primary traditional targets of the school cannot be realized effectively.

3. Peer pressures and teacher expectations are major determinants of self-concept in children. The elementary classroom must be

viewed as a constricted life-space in which vital support systems for psychological life and development are dependent on peer and teacher support.

4. Basic change agents of education must be found in the primary psychological support system within the classroom. This includes a support system for meeting teachers' needs and expectations as well as the utilization of the peer group.

5. Characteristic modes of adaptation or accommodation to the classroom interaction environment form the basis of both broad and specific temperament traits and states in individuals. This is not to denigrate the possible contribution of hereditary components, but to suggest that the self-regulating mechanisms of individuals and characteristic modes of approach to problem-solving are strongly mediated by a succession of reinforcement and modeling contingencies as well as a subjective construct system that monitors attempted behavior by the quantity and quality of success or failure experiences.

1. Preventive Intervention

The methods that have been detailed here have been directed towards the first step in a prevention-intervention model. That step is to develop an instrumentation capable of identifying individual characteristics in a group setting. These characteristics must include non-cognitive variables. Traditionally, and with recurrent emphasis in the research literature, the only viable criterion of the process of education has been the achievement test score. And yet, Cohen (1970), Gintis (1971), and Holtzman (1971) state that academic grades and achievement test scores do not predict success in future life. Averch and his colleagues (1972) conclude that achievement tests are by and large unsatisfactory since they are being used repeatedly and increasingly as a measure of accountability and performance objectives.

Though many have recognized the need for measuring variables relating to social interaction, self-esteem, self-management and the like, there simply has been no single battery appropriate at an elementary level. Moreover, what has existed has relied exclusively on single-input measurement systems such as self-report. The existence of the present methodology provides information regarding a diagnostic triad of methods. Obviously the data exist as a set of pooled perceptions, but perceptions lead to expectations, and expectations mediate behavior. These pooled perceptions then provide a set of clues that potentially can approximate medical diagnosis methods.

There is much that we now know about educational diagnosis. We *know* that a pupil's achievement is strongly related to his own educational background and social class as well as to the educational backgrounds and aspirations of other students (Coleman, 1966). We *know* that measurements of achievement and grades do not correlate significantly with success in later life. We *know* that large scale compensatory education projects and intervention programs have short-lived consequences. "Virtually without exception, all of the large surveys of the national compensatory education programs have shown no beneficial results on average. However, the evaluation reports on which the surveys are based are often poor and research designs suspect.... There is considerable evidence that many of the short-run gains from educational intervention programs fade away after two or three years if they are not reinforced. Also this 'fade-out' is much greater for the more highly structured programs, which are most unlike public school practice" (Averch *et al.*, 1972, p. 125). We *know* that expectations at all levels of educational intervention are a mediating force on patterns of covert and overt reinforcement (Brophy and Good, 1970; Beez, 1968; Coleman, 1966). We *suspect* strongly that alternate instructional approaches, teachers' expectations and needs, children's personality and temperament characteristics all interact in some complex manner (Cronbach and Snow, 1969). We *know* from much experience that our orientation towards problems in education has been crisis-oriented with a focus on the reconstruction of monumental problems rather than prevention. Finally, from the extensive survey detailed by Averch (using reviews of educational research grouped under five known methods: (1) the input-output approach, (2) the process approach, (3) the organizational approach, (4) the evaluation approach, and (5) the experiential approach), *we can conclude* that no single approach can provide the necessary research guidelines for educational policy-making.

These judgments lead me to conclude that educational change to be effective will have to be focused on the primary unit of interaction, i.e., the classroom. The diagnostic inferences provided by the present system function as clues. These clues may be compared to medical symptoms. For example, in the question of medical diagnosis relating to coronary problems, there are some definite symptoms or signs. A symptom of possible heart involvement might be shortness of breath in walking upstairs, a sense of pressure in the chest, poor circulation, protracted tension, overweight, excessive smoking, lack of exercise and the like. When all of these clues are put together with age factors and family history there is a rather good predictive possibility of a heart attack. The predictive features of these symptoms and clues are lessened by specific interventions designed to reduce weight, control the diet, provide more exercise and the like. The diagnosis or predictive judgment is fitted not only to what the individual himself does, but to what he does within the constraints and in reaction to his hereditary and social environment.

What this means in the *educational* environment is that diagnostic clues arrived at from a multiple needs assessment system may suggest differential treatments. If within a given district students in school A tend to show a very low teacher evaluation and many poor attitudes towards school as well as behavioral problems, then it may be relevant to aid this school through a behavior modification or structured curriculum approach. If students in school B have many deficits in self-esteem and group interaction, it may be relevant to develop a curriculum or counseling procedure that accents the development of self-competency skills and verbal interaction processes.

In the past we have been prone to try a single new curriculum vehicle for an entire district. Or we may be persuaded to institute this or that approach. What seems evident from the literature is that no single set of approaches works best with all children and teachers. Some children may learn reading best through a kinesthetic approach; others, through a visual modality. Still others may do better with an auditory approach. Probably all will gain something from each approach, but individuals can profit and accelerate their own learning potential by maximizing a specific approach related to their needs and special capabilities.

The existence of the system and our efforts to utilize it in the school setting has led to further conclusions. One of these is that school personnel need to be trained to think in preventive terms. Doing this means that teachers, principals, psychological staff and top administrators must think about education in a "goodness of fit" relationship. Prevention means both identification and intervention. This means that a tentative strategy must be elicited by school personnel not only for dealing with suspected individual problems, but for considering needed curricular interventions for groups of students. Teaching school personnel about prevention means that they must not only be concerned about the overt behavior problems (that can be easily identified by teacher nomination alone), but also about the many children who are shy, passive, reticent and minimally accepted. Another conclusion about intervention is the fact that often intervention based on clues can take place before a problem has reached crisis level. Prevention takes much less intensive effort than remediation and reconstruction. Sometimes it simply means alerting school staff to the needs of individuals, suggesting more attention, specific reinforcement, developmental adjustments and alternate groupings. A third conclusion is that strategies of intervention can be broadly grouped into three categories: (1) information feed-back to school staff and children, (2) social interaction exercises and opportunities for social modeling, and (3) environmental manipulation.

It would be naive on my part to suggest that at our present stage of development we have learned precisely how to fit these three families of strategies to the suspected problems of children as identified through the BCCI. But our experience thus far in working with schools suggests that many of the suspected problems of individuals can be approached on the first level, i.e., information feedback. By this level of strategies is meant providing information back to the student about how he is being perceived through counseling, audio or video feedback, test analysis and the like. A by-product of this feedback is understanding about the child's learning style, his interests and motivation. Often this results in changes of rules, a more flexible learning structure, the use of a resource center and the like. Both student and teaching personnel benefit from the exchange—particularly if teachers are attuned to methods of social reinforcement.

The second level is supplementary to the first and involves the development of social interaction and the use of exemplary models. Here study skills groups, groups relating to specific social skills, vocational exploration and the like can be skillfully used to develop both verbal interaction on a reciprocal level and confidence in problem-solving. In addition, using students as tutors for others with similar problems, and assigning roles in psychodramas, community and teacher-aide roles and simulation games provide excellent opportunities for social reinforcement and social modeling.

The third level is reserved for the more severe problems and includes environmental adjustments that include both the school and home environment. This may involve placement in another group, special reinforcement and social learning techniques designed to develop self-control such as carrels, time-out procedures, desensitization techniques and the like.

Crucial to the implementation of strategies of intervention is the development of learning-development teams in the local school. We recommend that these teams be composed of teachers, the principal, and guidance-psychological consultants. We believe that the logical coordinator of such a team is the school psychologist or a well-trained guidance consultant. The data provided by the BCCI provide a starting point for strategy planning. Learning teams can either identify children they are concerned with independent of the BCCI printouts or look at children who are identified as disruptive and reticent. Since the BCCI does not provide achievement-intelligence test data, the learning team needs to take these data into consideration along with its own observations of the characteristics of children. The computer process then provides assessment data for local learning-development teams to begin their own process of problem-solving. Patent remedies for what ails Susan cannot be suggested from assessment data alone. As in real life, what *is* and what *can be done* moderate what *will be.*

2. Policy-Making

One of the chief laments of federal, state and local administrators, according to Averch (1972), is that educational research fails to provide guidelines for policy-making. Educational research has not addressed itself to considerations of the basic cost per pupil, overall district assessment, training needs and the like. There are many reasons for this deficit. For example, researchers are often split on the merits of *pure* versus *applied* research. They sometimes are not aware that the same ideas and constructs have been researched time and again. Laboratory studies of gains in one method of teaching against another are often not verified by replication in actual teaching situations. Methods of evaluating change have often been tied to differences in achievement scores or mean gains using analysis of variance for groups. Where differential approaches are taken within classrooms or school units, the analogy with planting different types of corn in a field simply breaks down and suggests that analysis of variance, particularly on mean-gain achievement scores, may not be relevant. This is particularly true in the strategy efforts we have attempted to develop. Parenthetically, we believe the aptitude-treatment interaction is the most appropriate of techniques for looking at differences in individual change. Often the criterion of change is not flexible or sensitive enough, the treatment weak or the statistical method inappropriate. All of these problems have contributed to the failure of educational research to develop guidelines for policy-making.

We have postulated that multiple needs assessment beginning with individuals and moving to groups such as classes, grades and schools is the logical point to begin policy-making. The second step is logically dictated by the first: Once the characteristics of the district and groups within the district are known, then this information should be disseminated to various concerned and skilled groups for their discussion and problem-solving. From this process local targets, criteria and resources can be determined. With the determination of some specific objectives, criteria and methods of intervention, the district can proceed to design both the techniques of implementation and the evaluation procedures that will enable it to look at both the quality and quantity of change occurring.

There are obviously many intervening variables that occur in school experimental designs. For these reasons it is not always possible to utilize the most powerful research designs. Even where they are used, the process must be consistently monitored and the history of the effort taken into consideration. Evaluation should not only include some of the typical research methods, but efforts should also be made to arrive at generalizations through the tracking of individuals on a longitudinal base. What is most effective for whom under what circumstances cannot be obtained through the massaging of group data, but by the tracking of individual cases, the obtaining of both psychometric and behavioral base-line data, and the comparison of pre- versus post-treatment changes. By accumulating individual-treatment results we may ultimately arrive at an expectancy table capable of suggesting probable success ratios based on the individual-alternate-treatment equation.

Finally, as a by-product of the assessment-treatment-evaluation paradigm, feedback information can be obtained about cost effectiveness per pupil, training programs needed, differential staffing and many other pertinent educational issues. More and more emphasis, I believe, will be placed on intervention. Moreover, if the district is successful it is most likely that the need for special remediation and reconstruction approaches will diminish. To this end, we may see the development of specialized teams of learning development personnel who will address themselves to problems in self-management, cognitive learning techniques, vocational development, group process approaches and the like. This development would make it possible to allow educational and psychological personnel to concentrate in a specific area of intervention. Such specialization would increase the overall effectiveness of the personnel and also provide the resources needed in the district for specialized interventions.

Summary

This chapter has dealt with the problem of multiple-needs assessment both as it relates to individual and group differences and as it relates to possible conclusions for policy making in the local school. It is believed that the paradigm described provides some real advantages to schools not only in the assessment of non-cognitive and social-interaction characteristics of children, but also in the design of experiments, identification of criteria and alternate strategies of intervention, and allocation of district resources based on the evaluation procedures.

Footnotes

1.   In 1956-59, I served as a school diagnostician in a suburban Detroit school district. It was here that the beginnings of this inventory occurred. There were many problem children that defied attempts at diagnosis and remediation. Consequently, I began a series of studies to utilize peer and teacher judgments to ascertain the characteristics of individual children in the classroom.

In one study the interest patterns of 1,777 elementary and junior high school students were related to a sociometric device and teacher rating (Barclay, 1966a). The subjects were asked their preferences in a variety of class interests, including T.V. watching, music listening, vocational plans and the like. Results of the study showed that teachers' ratings and peer ratings differentiate between interest patterns and these patterns are associated with a broad extroversion-introversion continuum. A follow-up study (Barclay, 1966b) indicated that both the sociometric predictor and teacher ratings identified subsequent dropouts. It was found that 54 percent of the female and 64 percent of the male dropouts had sociometric and teacher ratings below the median on the data from four years earlier.

Using the data from the above first study the mean sociometric ratings and teacher ratings from 70 classrooms were analyzed in relationship to the age and sex of the teacher. Specifically it was hypothesized that social desirability measures such as sociometric ratings and teacher judgments represented a measurement of the environmental "press". Older male teachers tended to be most severe in their ratings of children and older female teachers tended to be most lenient. For boys in particular the best ratings seemed to be associated with young female teachers (Barclay, 1966c).

Still another study (Barclay and Barclay, 1965) related measures of visual perception to sociometric and teacher judgments. In this study six classes of third-graders in the Pocatello, Idaho, Public Schools were tested on a number of devices to determine level of perceptual organization. Of 24 hypotheses made regarding relationships between variables 19 were confirmed. It was concluded that perceptual organization and measured control of responses are factors relating to social desirability in children. On the basis of the foregoing studies, a theoretical article was written (Barclay, 1966d) suggesting that social desirability and social skills are related to motivation for achievement and survival in the classroom.

With the development of the new inventory (the current BCCI) more studies were completed. One of these (Barclay, 1967) utilized the instrument as a criterion of change relating pre-post scores to three treatments tried out with some fifth graders. One treatment was to provide some modeling and social exercises in a classroom to increase the social desirability of isolates. Another consisted of training a teacher how to select out appropriate behaviors in isolates and reinforce them. The third treatment was a placebo one inasmuch as it consisted of changing the regular teacher to a teacher intern for five weeks. The results of the treatments indicated that the greatest changes in poorly accepted children were shown in the experimental group as a result of modeling and social group procedures. However, considerable changes also took place in the classroom where the teacher intern had replaced the regular teacher.

Another study was completed by Brown (1967) and later reanalyzed by Stilwell and Barclay (Stilwell, Brown and Barclay, 1973). This pilot study tried out three different classroom or guidance techniques to help to raise the social desirability of rejected or isolated children in the fifth grade. The children were identified by the global sociometric device used in the earliest studies, and low scoring children were assigned to three treatment groups. The first treatment was group counseling based on a transactional analysis approach. The second approach involved reorganizing children in small social studies groups in which boys and girls of high sociometric status worked with boys and girls of low sociometric status on projects. They were also permitted to sit near each other for this activity. The third approach was one that involved discussing vocational information with groups of low status children. There were six weekly sessions and all students were pre- and post-tested on the BCCI. The original data showed some ambiguous results. However, in reanalyzing the data using the aptitude-treatment-interaction significant results were obtained for the vocational placebo group. The results of this study suggested that vocational information discussions seemed most effective in raising both high and low sociometric scorers' interests in status and mechanical occupations. Peer leadership judgments of unpopular girls rose. Many children became more assertive.

2.   The suspected problem categories were the result of considerable research, and are based on inferences from that research. The steps included typical reliability and validity studies including: internal consistency and test-retest reliability studies; tetrachoric correlations between items in scales; scale correlations with other tests such as the Kuder, the California Test of Personality and the Children's version of the 16 P.F. Test; factor analysis procedures using both the principal axis and multi-method, multi-trait approach.

The convergent and discriminant validity of the BCCI was studied by Barclay and Elton (1973) using the test scores of 2000 elementary school children. A number of factors possess convergent validity in the sense that self, peer and teacher judgments of specific competencies load on a given factor (for example, self-social report, group social nominations, and teacher judgment of stable extroverted behavior are the only variables loading high and significantly on the factor termed affiliation). Tapp (1972) developed another multi-method system and administered it to a sample who had also taken the BCCI. He compared the two systems and found that they generally agree.

However, the most important study for the determination of the suspected problem categories was a behavioral observation study completed in 1972 (Barclay, Stilwell, Santoro and Clark, 1972). This study, done in Corpus Christi, Texas, involved the observation of classroom behaviors of 700 children over a ten-day period. These children had previously completed the BCCI. A number of substitute teachers were trained in three observational techniques and spent ten days in observing student behavior. Approximately 300 of these students had multiple observations and were used in this study. The results of the observations, plus achievement and intelligence test data and BCCI results, were used. Step-wise regressions were obtained using achievement data as dependent variables. Discriminant analyses were used on the basis of temperaments determined via the BCCI with observations the dependent variables. Finally, a multivariate analysis of behaviors was completed using BCCI categories as classifying criteria. Representative of the findings obtained are the following:

1. girls who are judged to be shy and reticent on the BCCI do not often raise their hands in response to teacher questions,

2. boys who are called on often view themselves as above average on enterprising and leadership skills,

3. both boys and girls who are classified as unstable extroverts on the BCCI tend to raise their hands more often, talk out loud, and are more prone to stand up at their seats;

4. girls who do well in arithmetic are viewed by their peers and teachers as possessing outdoor-masculine and intellectual skills, tend to have a higher I.Q., are interested in occupations that call for competition and risk-taking, are less interested in peer female reinforcers, more interested in male reinforcers and tend to receive less favorable ratings by teachers;

5. boys who do well in arithmetic appear to be viewed by teachers as stable introverts, are seen by the peer group as quiet but effective leaders, generally have a higher I.Q., appear to be less interested in artistic and creative occupations, do not appear to attend as well as others to ongoing classroom activities nor do they raise their hands and volunteer as often.

Thus this study tended to confirm the fact that the BCCI variables do possess behavioral correlates as obtained from actual observations.

On the basis of this research, a series of conditional "if" statements were entered into the computer. These conditional statements exist as criteria for decision-making. For example, if a child receives a high number of reticence nominations from his peer group, sees himself as comparatively ineffective in social behavior, and receives a high rating on the unstable-introversion scale as checked by teachers, an asterisk is placed under the category of verbal skills next to his number. The same set of procedures are followed for each of the suspected problem categories.

In the research and User's Manual, the point is emphasized continually that these indicators are suspected problems and need to be confirmed by further observation in the classroom.

3.   The teacher rating scales are formed by grouping various adjectives together. Both positive attributes and negative ones are described by the adjectives. The teacher ratio is obtained by summing the total number of positive adjectives chosen for all children and the total number of negative adjectives chosen and using the following formula.

$$\text{Ratio} = \frac{(\ \Sigma \ \text{Positive})\ -\ (\ \Sigma \ \text{Negative})}{N\ (N\text{-}1)}$$

References

Averch, H. A., Carroll, H. A., Donaldson, T. S., Kiesling, H. J., and Pincus, J. *How effective is schooling?, A critical review and synthesis of research findings.* Prepared for President's Commission on School Finance, Rand Corporation, March, 1972.

Barclay, J. R. Interest patterns associated with measures of social desirability: some implications for dropouts and the culturally disadvantages. *Personnel and Guidance Journal,* 1966a, *45,* No. 1, 56-60.

Barclay, J. R. Sociometric choices and teacher ratings as predictors of school dropouts. *Journal of School Psychology,* 1966b, *4,* No. 2, 40-44.

Barclay, J. R. Variability in sociometric choices and teacher ratings as related to teacher age and sex. *Journal of School Psychology,* 1966c, No. 1, 52-58.

Barclay, J. R. Sociometry: Rationale and technique for effecting behavior change in the elementary school. *Personnel and Guidance Journal,* 1966d, *44,* No. 10, 1067-1076.

Barclay, J. R. Effecting behavior change in the elementary classroom: an exploratory study. *Journal of Counseling Psychology,* 1967, *14,* No. 3, 240-247.

Barclay, J. R. (with the assistance of L. K. Barclay and W. E. Stilwell). *The Barclay Classroom Climate Inventory, a research manual and studies.* Educational Skills Development Inc., Lexington, Kentucky, 1972.

Barclay, J. R. and Elton, C. F. The validity of self-report in elementary children. Manuscript submitted for publication, University of Kentucky, 1973.

Barclay, J. R., Stilwell, W. E., Barclay, L. K. The influence of paternal occupation on social interaction measures in elementary school children. *Journal of Vocational Behavior,* 1972, *2,* No. 4, October, 443-446.

Barclay, J. R., Stilwell, W. E., Santoro, D. A., and Clark, C. Behavioral and achievement correlates of social interaction variables in the elementary classroom. Manuscript submitted for publication, University of Kentucky, 1972.

Barclay, L. K. and Barclay, J. R. Measured indices of perceptual distortion and impulsivity as related to sociometric scores and teacher ratings. *Psychology in the Schools,* 1965, *2,* No. 4, 372-375.

Beez, W. V. Influence of biased psychological reports on teacher behavior and pupil performance. APA Annual Meeting, 1968, San Francisco, California. Also reported in *Proceedings of the 76th Convention of the American Psychological Association,* American Psychological Association, Washington, D. C., 1969.

Brophy, J. E. and Good, T. L. Teachers' communication of differential expectations for children's classroom performance: some behavioral data. Paper presented at AERA National Meeting, Minneapolis, Minnesota, 1970.

Brown, P. W. An evaluation of three counseling approaches. Unpublished Master's Thesis, California State College at Hayward, Hayward, California, 1967.

Cohen, D. K. Politics and research: Evaluation of social action programs in education. *Review of Educational Research,* 1970, *40,* 213-238.

Coleman, J. S. *et al. Equality of educational opportunity.* U. S. Department of Health, Education and Welfare, U. S. Office of Education, OE-38001, Washington D. C., 1966.

Cronbach, L. J. and Snow, R. E. *Final report: Individual differences in learning ability as a function of instructional variables.* Stanford University, Stanford, California, 1969.

Eysenck, M. J. and Rachman, S. *The causes and cures of neurosis.* San Diego: Robert Knapp, 1965.

Gintis, H. Education, technology and the characteristics of worker productivity. *The American Economic Review,* 1971, *61,* 266-279.

Holland, J. L. *Psychology of vocational choice.* Boston: Ginn and Co., 1966.

Holtzman, W. H. The changing world of mental measurement and its social significance. *American Psychologist,* 1971, *26,* 546-553.

Jackson, D. Multimethod factor analysis in the evaluation of convergent and discriminant validity. *Psychological Bulletin,* 1969, *72,* 30-49.

Lindquist, E. F. Norms of achievement by school. In A. Anastasi (Ed.), *Testing problems in perspective.* American Council on Education, Washington, D. C., 1966. Pp. 269-271.

Stilwell, W. E., Brown, P. W., and Barclay, J. R. Effects of three classroom management methods on classroom interaction of fifth graders. *Psychology in the Schools.* 1973, *10,* 365-372.

Tapp, G. S. *Convergent and discriminant validity of the BCCI.* Unpublished Doctoral Dissertation, University of Kentucky, 1972.

Tapp, G. S. and Barclay, J. R. Convergent and discriminant validity of the Barclay Classroom Climate Inventory. Manuscript submitted for publication, 1973.

Whitla, D. K. (Ed.) *Handbook of measurement and assessment in behavioral sciences.* Reading, Massachusetts: Addison-Wesley Publishing Co., 1968.

Evaluating Program Evaluation: A Suggested Approach

15

Charles Windle and Peter Bates[1]

Introduction

The title of this chapter suggests an infinite regression, like the images in two mirrors facing each other, or a magazine cover which has within it a picture of the magazine whose cover has within it, etc. However, it seems poetically just to apply our faith in program evaluation to program evaluation itself. In so doing, we should learn either how to be more effective, or how to be more humble. In this chapter we plan to:

a. present a framework of the values or interests which surround program evaluation research as a basis for evaluating this activity,

b. review several experiences in applying program evaluation research to mental health programs, and

c. suggest some criteria for evaluating the success of program evaluation research in helping programs.

The Framework of Values of Program Evaluation Research

A Value Identification Approach

We want to begin by discussing the many values which surround program evaluation research. This approach of identifying values is similar to that of explicitly specifying program goals to serve as criteria, which many advocates of program evaluation insist upon. It includes whatever program goals can be specified as major values for the program administrator, but it also recognizes that these goals at any point in time fall within a broader system. Societal and technological conditions change over time. Goals specified at the beginning of a program may not be appropriate for determining the worth of the program several years later. Further, some of the values surrounding a program such as its viability and the welfare of the staff are not usually considered as goals, but play a large part in shaping a program. There are also always a number of unplanned impacts and interactions among programs. A full evaluation should determine whether these results are generally helpful or harmful.

The concept of values makes it easier to contrast differences in vested interests of different program elements. And this distinction is important in evaluating the consequences of evaluation.

The Schematic Representation of Values
Surrounding Program Evaluation

The distinctions among the various values involved in program evaluation research may be made clearer by a schematic representation. This representation should start with the service program system (**Figure 1**) which evaluation is supposed to support. In public programs taxpayers provide the funds and citizens provide the votes to officials who establish and support programs which provide services to consumers. Consumers, in turn, feed back their satisfaction and needs to the program, officials and the general populace.

Program evaluation is a portion of the program which formalizes feedback from consumers. In addition, program evaluation includes other kinds of research which lead to reports which go to the service program staff and administrators (**Figure 2**). Much of the input to the program from program evaluation is informal. This applies both to research findings and to incidental information and attitudes. Information generated for one purpose may also serve other purposes. For example, in a study of the feasibility of measuring continuity of care in a mental health center (Bass and Windle, 1972) we needed a roster of all clients served during a sample period and the therapist with primary responsibility for them. When such a list was developed from the records, it was found that there were a number of cases in which the assigned therapist was no longer with the institution. Other cases carried on the books had not been seen for a long time and no further contact was expected. The development of this list provided an opportunity for management to review staff assignments and plans for particular clients. Many of the results of program evaluation research, perhaps the most effective, are transmitted informally to the staff while the research is still going on. This phenomenon is the bane of researchers who wish to do "good" research, reaching conclusive findings. Control groups frequently are found to be receiving the experimental treatments around the mid-point of a study when preliminary results and staff enthusiasm suggest that there really is a benefit to the experimental

Figure 1   Service Program System

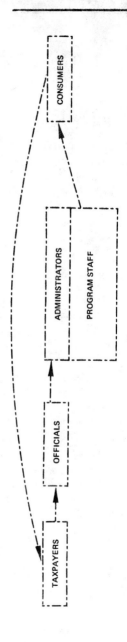

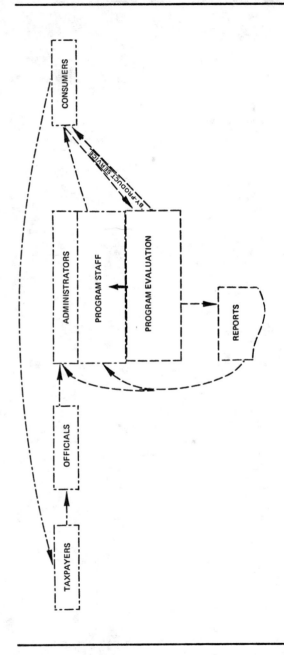

Figure 2 Primary Program Evaluation System

programs. That this is seen as a problem reflects the opposing interests of service staff and researchers. From the viewpoint of the program staff the ultimate purpose of the evaluation, to improve the services, has been accomplished—yet the researcher persists toward the intermediate goal of developing evidence to support a decision that has already been made. In addition to these benefits to program efficacy, evaluation research activities often have direct service effects. The thought that research is good and that change is synonymous with improvement, leads to a general belief among staff and clients that programs connected with research are more effective. The services become, therefore, more effective in fact, increasing benefit for consumers.

In this connection, a recent review of literature (Wilkins, 1973) on expectancy of therapeutic gain failed to discover clear evidence of effects from such a trait or state in the client. However, there was a methodological difference between studies finding or not finding significant differences resulting from expectancy manipulations. Only in the latter were therapists and experimenters assessing outcome blind to the expectancy instructions subjects received. Therefore it appeared that part of the gains observed in studies of expectancy are after all determined by the therapists. If so, this is an additional reason for applied researchers to convince therapists of the potential value of experimental treatments they want to study.

Sometimes there is a benefit simply from the activities associated with research which become a part of service. A particularly dramatic example occurred a quarter of a century ago in the Columbia Graystone Project study of the effects of topectomy on chronic psychotics. A large research team went into the back wards extensively testing a group of chronically hospitalized patients to permit a pre-post comparison. Some of the patients were given topectomy operations to remove selected portions of their brains. Other patients were simply controls. It appeared that the "total push" stimulation of the testing and attention from the research had many effects on the entire group making its history different from what would have occurred had no special program come in to disturb life on the back wards. The topectomy operations showed no benefits beyond the total push stimulation received by the tested "controls." In this case the research program was more therapeutic than the service program.

Most activities associated with program evaluation research may benefit consumers. However, such activities may also have negative effects. For example, follow-up inquiries of released clients to see how they are doing after treatment could be a source of embarrassment to them and reinforce the stigma often associated with mental illness.

Parenthetically we might note that, at least in the experience of the Hennepin County Mental Health Center, most clients who participated in a post-service interview reacted to it favorably (Salasin and Baxter, 1972).

In the dissemination of evaluation research results (**Figure 3**) there is probably an interaction between channels used and type of program implications. The formal system consists of reports which go to a wide range of audiences. These reports are often designed primarily for the scientific community from which mobile, upward moving researchers expect most of their rewards. Service program action implications are likely to be implicit rather than explicit, abstract (i.e., generalized to all services of the type studied rather than described as applying to the particular program studied), and advanced with much caution and scientific qualification. They are, however, because of researchers' greater dependence on the scientific community than on a particular program, likely to be relatively objective—and thus to carry implications for program curtailment as well as for support or change. The information most conducive to change, however, is likely to go informally from the evaluation efforts into the program. This informal process may consist of discussions and may be in the absence of formal reports, or may supplement them.

In addition to this dissemination from the program evaluation unit there is usually a special selective dissemination by the program which can best be thought of as Public Relations to get support from officials and the community. This activity goes on even in the absence of Program Evaluation, but is greatly assisted by the data from program evaluation. Much of this dissemination process, and the selective assemblage of information to advertise or advocate the program may be assigned to the evaluation staff, compromising their functioning.

There is one other subsystem (**Figure 4**) which we should note with special attention in these days when fairly radical (or is the word conservative?) changes in funding mechanisms for human services are being initiated. Third-party reimbursement procedures such as those for Medicare and Medicaid require that facilities use mechanisms to contain costs and assure appropriateness of services. The utilization review procedures required by the Social Security Administration for facilities to qualify for Medicare and Medicaid reimbursement are a form of program evaluation which may, if done conscientiously, improve care for clients and improve program efficiency. This type of program evaluation may become even more important if Professional Standards Review Organizations provided for in the Social Security Amendments of 1972 become effective instruments of program monitoring.

Figure 3   Program Evaluation Report Dissemination System

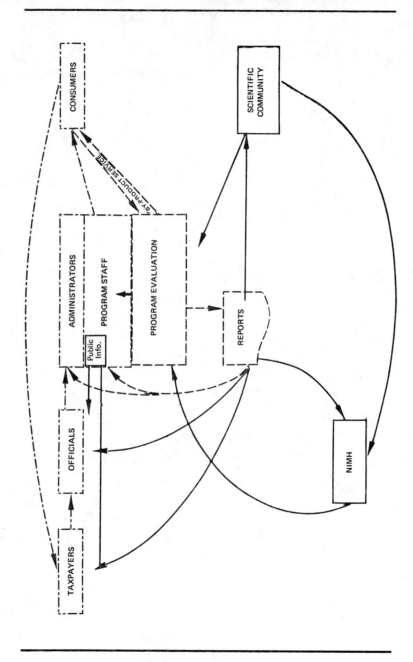

Figure 4   Third-Party Funding System

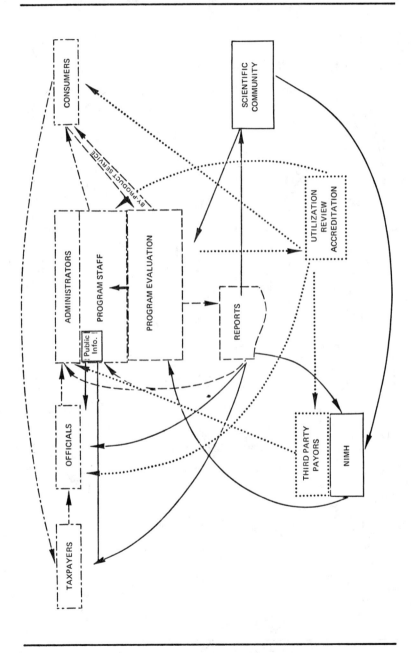

The last feature we would like to include in this now complicated representation is the place of efforts to evaluate the program evaluation activities (**Figure 5**). For easier understanding let us make a distinction in terms. We have been referring to activities designed to evaluate processes occurring within a service program as *program evaluation.* The activities to evaluate the impact of any such program evaluation we shall term *evaluation assessment.* We see evaluation assessment related to program evaluation in the same way that program evaluation is related to the service program. This parallel includes the use of both informal and formal report input to the program evaluators so that they may benefit from what is learned. The channels for distribution of results are also likely to be influenced by the type of action implications, in this case implications primarily for the program evaluation activities. Information which suggests that the program evaluation is helpful and therefore should be supported or expanded by the program administrators is likely to receive special distribution by what might be considered the equivalent of a public information or advertising effort by the program evaluation staff. There are also likely to be third-party supporters of the program evaluation activity, as is the case at the Northwest Denver Community Mental Health Center which has a research grant to develop and demonstrate program evaluation methods for monitoring a large community mental health center.

Experiences with Program Evaluation Research

We want now to describe six experiences with program evaluation and related applied research as a background for suggesting criteria which can be used for evaluating program evaluation research.

These observations were taken from experiences in evaluating mental health service programs, mainly from a perspective within or associated with NIMH. This perspective is, of course, limited. Therefore, it may be helpful to indicate how others have viewed NIMH's evaluation activities in comparison with other program evaluation efforts. The Russell Sage Foundation has done a survey of evaluation studies of social action programs. Preliminary findings, according to the researchers (Bernstein, 1972), indicate NIMH far superior to other agencies in the "research quality" of their grant and contract studies.

Havelock (1972) is studying research utilization on four federal agencies, including the NIMH Mental Health Services Development Branch, the part of NIMH responsible for applied research on mental

Figure 5   Evaluation Assessment System

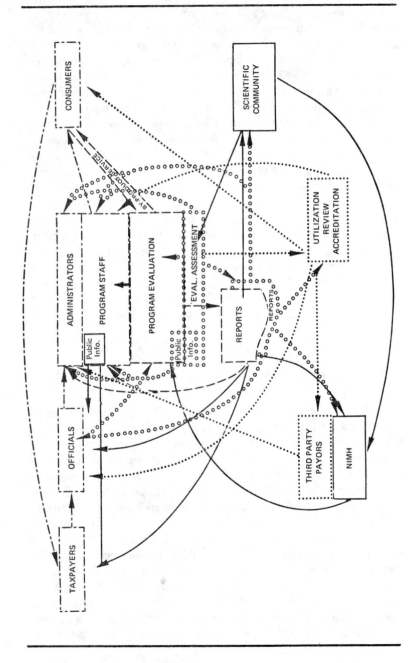

health services. Havelock reported that NIMH falls at one extreme of "relying heavily on individual initiative and creativity in the academic community, minimizing centralized planning and policy-making and allowing the existing 'natural' networks of communication within the mental health professions to carry the major dissemination load."

On the other hand, the former Secretary of HEW, Elliot Richardson, cited the evaluation of community mental health programs as exemplary, "among the most significant efforts at evaluation now underway at HEW" (Salasin, 1972).

These three judgements constitute rather a mixed review. They suggest that NIMH does relatively well in the technical portions of research, but rather little in utilization.

Factors in the Success of Applied Research Grants

The Applied Research Branch of NIMH gave a contract to the Human Interaction Research Institute to determine what factors differentiated five relatively "successful" and five relatively "unsuccessful" research grants. Glaser and Taylor (1969) found the successful projects differed in having high communication to others and high involvement within and outside the immediate environment from the beginning of the project. The principal investigator worked on the project full time. The extensive communication and involvement of others led to commitment and support by the host agency which helped the projects deal with later problems. By contrast, less successful projects were insular, and were resented by administrators and practitioners. In consequence any problem encountered had more severe repercussions.

Literature on Research Utilization

A later contract to the same organization has resulted in a set of publications on research utilization. These include an annotated bibliography of studies in this area, a distillation of principles on research utilization and a manual on how to use research for creative change in mental health services (NIMH, 1972, a,b,c). The authors observed that there is a long time lag between research findings and corresponding changes in practice. New research often doesn't reach practitioners, in large part because scientists and practitioners think differently. Practitioners tend to rely more on precedent, common sense or intuition than on research findings. These authors listed nine characteristics of an innovation which affect the probability of its adoption (Figure 6).

Figure 6 Innovation Characteristics Favoring Adoption

Relevance
Compatibility
Relative Advantage
Observability
Feasibility
Reversibility
Divisibility
Trialability
Credibility

Factors in Success of Evaluation Contracts

The third specific experience we want to examine was first-hand and concerned NIMH's categorical program evaluation activities. Starting in Fiscal 1969, 1 percent of the funds from the Community Mental Health Centers Program was set aside for evaluation of that program. These efforts were organized around determining the extent to which and conditions under which the process goals of the Centers Program were being attained. By process goals we meant the major processes for providing services specified in the Program's concepts, for it was these concepts of how services should be given, rather than any change in ultimate goals, which constituted the novelty of the Centers Program. Therefore, we initiated studies of accessibility, equity, decreased use of state hospitals, community participation, responsiveness to needs, and organization for continuity and efficiency. These studies included both substantive evaluations and methodology development to permit substantive study. We aimed substantive studies toward national program level topics, but aimed methodology development at procedures individual centers, States, or NIMH could use. The rationale for this approach has been described in more detail elsewhere (Feldman and Windle, 1973).

After this evaluation effort had been underway three years, 15 contract studies were examined which had been completed or were so far advanced that products were available. To establish their relative success the senior author had nine NIMH staff and one contractor, all of whom had been involved in administering or studying these efforts, rate the value of the product of each study relative to its cost. Five of the raters were involved in program analysis and evaluation or research, and five were primarily administrators. Not all raters knew all studies, but each study was known widely enough to be rated by at least six raters. Since raters differed in their average level of rating, each raters' ratings were divided as near the median as possible and then the frequency with which each study fell above or below the median of each rater was determined. Across the 10 raters this yielded a bimodal distribution of percent of ratings of the studies as a relative success (**Figure 7**). There was no distinction between technical program evaluation staff and program administration staff in terms of their ratings. The agreement was not higher within these types of raters than between the two types. Having separated the evaluation studies into criterion groups, the

---

Figure 7   **Distribution of Evaluation Studies by Percent of Ratings as Relatively Successful**

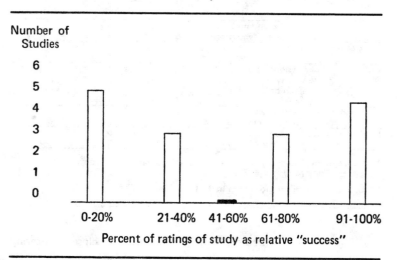

Number of Studies

Percent of ratings of study as relative "success"

---

senior author did two types of comparisons: quantitative and judgemental. The quantitative comparison consisted of the frequency with which particular characteristics differentiated the two criterion groups. Of those examined, the condition which best differentiated was how closely NIMH staff monitored the research (see **Table 1**). Closeness was established by the senior author's judgement of whether NIMH staff spent a relatively large or relatively small proportion of their time in

Table 1 Relationship of Characteristics of Evaluation Contracts and Judged Success in Providing Useful Products

Contract Characteristics	Number Successful	Number Unsuccessful	Significance* to 10% level
Location: near	4	1	
distant	3	7	
Procurement: sole source	6	4	
competitive	1	4	
Monitoring: "close"	4	0	
: not "close"	3	8	P=.06
Project Officer: consistent	6	4	
: changed	1	4	
Project Officer: methods specialist	3	3	
: content specialist	4	5	
Project Officer: Ph.D.	3	6	
: M.D.	3	1	
: other	1	1	
Contract staff: consistent	4	6	
: disrupted	3	2	
Contract: > $50,000	4	6	
: < $50,000	3	2	
Contractor: had mental health expertise	3	3	
: lacked mental health expertise	4	5	
Study: methodological	3	3	
: substantive	4	5	
Report makes: recommendations	2	3	
: no recommendations	5	5	
Contract effective: last week in June	6	4	
: other dates	1	4	
Contractor: professional organization	3	1	
: university	1	2	
: research organization	2	2	
: other	1	3	
Topic relatively: important to NIMH**	4	2	
: unimportant to NIMH	3	6	
Study mainly: program evaluation**	2	5	
: not program evaluation	5	3	

* D. J. Finney, The Fisher-Yates test of significance in 2 x 2 contingency tables. *Biometrika,* 1948, *35.*

** Based on ratings by more than half of four raters.

working with the contractor. In fact, all the cases of close monitoring involved collaboration in collecting data or preparing reports. Over half of the relatively successful studies had NIMH staff collaborating in the study, whereas none of the relatively unsuccessful did. Several related characteristics showed some difference in distributions but were less significant statistically. There was somewhat greater likelihood of a successful product if the contractor was located nearby, if there had been sole source rather than competitive procurement, and if there was a consistency in project officers throughout the study. These findings are consistent with those of Glaser and Taylor concerning success in applied research. However, since we did not make hypotheses in advance, a two-tailed test of significance was used in our statistical test. This study involved few cases and these were interrelated. Thus this study should be conceived of as mainly the start of a data pool to which others can add in order to reach general conclusions.

As a part of the same rating system, raters were asked to judge the quality of contractors' work. We had thought these two questions would differentiate between technical quality and utility of products. However only one study was rated differently in relation to the group mean. This made little difference in the results, but did lead to the loss of even the one finding which had exceeded the .10 level of significance with the two-tailed test. This similarity in ratings of technical quality and utility was also found by Glaser and Taylor for research grants (1969).

The second approach to contrasting the successful and unsuccessful evaluation studies was for the investigator to use his own judgement to identify the factors which had led to the usefulness or limitations of each study. Of the eight less successful studies, two seemed to suffer mainly from lack of harmony between their largely negative results and NIMH's expectations or needs. The studies seem to have been done adequately within their constraints and on the problems to which they were directed, but in one the procedures being tested for feasibility turned out to be non-feasible, and in the other the correlations computed turned out to be negative or insignificant. This proportion of non-fruitful studies seems consistent with what a fairly adventuresome research effort into unknown areas could be expected to result in. The other six relatively less successful studies suffered from technical inadequacies of four types. Several contractors lacked knowledge of the complexity of the Center's program. Thus, if investigators were not already familiar with this program, either they had to spend a fair amount of time learning about it or they were likely to make errors of over-simplification or distortion. By contrast, one of our successful studies included a one-month period for orientation for the investigators about the service program. The second problem of the less successful studies was that the task as defined was too difficult to accomplish within the scope of study. Sometimes this was because the task was beyond current technology, such as developing procedures for determining the success of indirect services or developing procedures for utilization review. In other cases the contract was under-funded for the amount of work required. The third problem was that several contractors were not oriented toward NIMH's goals. Sometimes researchers had too academic and collegial an orientation to organize themselves for a unified applied task. Sometimes contractors had a narrow social action commitment which precluded an objective examination of some issues. In a couple of cases the contractors' orientation toward the type of research approach proved a barrier, either because they were too hard data oriented or because they were alienated from hard data. The last problem appeared to be insufficiently close monitoring by NIMH staff to redirect errant contractors. In our program, most project officer assignments were imposed as additional duties.

Determination of why studies were successful is more difficult because success may involve simply carrying through the original plan of study. However the most important special characteristic of the seven successful studies appears to be the unusual amount of NIMH staff involvement. As previously mentioned, this was often so close that the monitor collaborated in conducting the research.

We should note that this study was done soon after many contracts were completed—before there had been much opportunity for utilization. Therefore the ratings of expected value of the products were in part predictions.

Disjunction Between Program Decisions and Formal Evaluation Efforts

Another experience with program evaluation research is the senior author's (hereafter called CW) personal and second-hand observations during the three-year period since NIMH's first 1 percent evaluation study was completed. This appraisal requires awareness of personal biases. CW has been a consistent and sometimes shrill advocate of the use of "TRUTH," as produced by research, unalloyed by other considerations. He has tried to sell this product. This selling is based on both convictions and self-interests. We will try to desist from selling now in giving you an assessment of the results of our research.

You should also recognize that history is unfolding so rapidly for the Centers Program that a status report now is of doubtful long-term validity. In fact, the week before this talk in the U. S. Senate Subcommittee on Health, Senator Kennedy was questioning HEW Secretary Weinberger about apparent inconsistencies between evaluation study results and the Administration's proposed termination of Federal funding for community mental health centers.

However, several tentative and personal observations can be suggested:

1. There have been a wide variety of minor impacts from our studies. They include, for example:
   (a) providing methods individual centers can use for evaluation or cost-finding,
   (b) showing program critics that NIMH is concerned with problems such as sources of funds,
   (c) providing information NIMH staff can use for technical assistance during monitoring site visits,
   (d) and reminding centers of the importance of program goals.
2. There is a major disjunction between formal program evaluation and program decisions. This has been true at 3 echelons of potential implementation for a variety of reasons.

First, let us describe a little more our evaluation study results. By the end of 1972, 17 evaluation studies had been completed. Eleven studies were primarily substantive, studying the extent to which or conditions under which the Centers Program was achieving its process goals. An overall summary of the major findings is that on most process goals the Centers Program has been making progress, for none has it achieved these goals, and for some process goals we have found facilitating conditions. These are unsurprising results, and they leave unresolved whether the extent of progress is great enough to warrant the expenditure in support of the Centers Program. Especially, they do not speak to the issue of the relative advantage of this benefit compared to other possible expenditures in other domestic programs or in military defense. This manner of presenting our results in terms of both progress and whether there has been achievement of goals stems from the two different types of study designs we have used. Some use a before/after or a with centers/without centers comparison. These typically find that there has been progress and this progress is usually attributed to the Centers Program. The other type of design, however, is one where a condition such as accessibility or citizen participation is examined in a number of community mental health centers. It is always found that there are many ways in which these processes are not being carried out completely. This contrast in viewpoints, in judging whether a glass is half-full or half-empty, is nicely illustrated by a set of articles in the Fall 1972 issue of MH. Chu and Trotter, the co-authors of the Nader Report, cited evidence of lack of citizen participation in centers. On the other hand, the Director of NIMH said that this is only one of many program goals and that progress was being achieved in it through the Centers Program.

Lowest echelon of possible implementation. Use of results by individual centers has been limited by the lack of a determined effort to diffuse and encourage local adoption of results. We have set up a procedure to make contractors' final reports available to the public without adulteration by agency hands. For three to six dollars the Department of Commerce will send the full report plus a summary and a critique prepared by NIMH.

Further, several methodology reports have been sent to all federally funded centers. However, NIMH staff felt that substantive evaluation reports require editing and added information to be of educational value. The extra staff time for this purpose has not been available. Such staff time may be one of the often unanticipated overhead burdens required by evaluation efforts.

NIMH Program Staff. At the level of NIMH program staff there has been some use of results. But in relation to the costs of the studies the use by staff seems disappointing. In part this is because studies failed to make a compelling case for clear and feasible changes. They evaluated existing activities much more than they analyzed potential changes, thus doing only part of even the rational part of the decision-making task. However, much of this task of analysis is what program staff must do to use research results. Fairly low priority was given to ear-marking resources for utilization. This, in turn, was due partly to changing responsibilities within NIMH and HEW for Centers Program management and evaluation study management.

Supra Program echelons. The third echelon is the policy initiatives of the Nixon Administration and the actions by Congress. In the interaction between the Administration and Congress the evaluation study results appear to be involved. What contribution they will make is less clear. There seems to be some disjunction between these results and current Administration thinking.

While NIMH staff were worrying about whether the Centers Program was looking successful enough in its evaluation studies and considering how improvements might be made, they were disconcerted to learn that the Administration was proposing to terminate Federal support for centers on the grounds that, "the workability of the community mental health center concept has been thoroughly demonstrated." To the knowledge of the NIMH program staff evidence for this "workability" under conditions of no seed-money stimulation has not come from the categorical 1 percent evaluation studies. In fact, one of these studies several years ago indicated that centers were going to face serious problems in finding financing after federal staffing grants were terminated. Although this problem was alleviated for the time being by the Community Mental Health Center Act Amendments of 1970, there has been no later formal study that suggested a substantial change in the financial problems centers would have as federal funding ceases. Thus our formal evaluation studies taken by themselves seem inconsistent with the actions proposed by the Administration. Such an inconsistency does not, of course, indicate that the Administration's judgements are necessarily wrong. It rather indicates that a different perspective for evaluation is being used for the most important decisions of the program than was used for planning the evaluation studies.

Let us make clear that we are not passing a judgement on the Administration's evaluation of the Centers Program nor on its orientation toward our evaluation studies. Instead we are trying to derive the implications for the function of program evaluation from its role in current decisions.

We see three implications. The first concerns relevance.

It appears that we needed more study of the types of options now being proposed by the Administration. Whether an agency could reasonably be expected to guess what type of options to study, and whether it would be feasible to design the conditions to study them in a convincing fashion are questionable. However, it suggests that topics for study chosen by a program staff tend to be of limited perspective. Especially in times when radical program redesign is likely, program evaluation should be directed mainly at large scale problems, and thus mainly planned by superordinate echelons.

The second implication has to do with the role of program evaluation in demonstrations. The Administration is now saying that the Centers Program is a demonstration program, wherein the experience of the 515 initially funded centers will not only stimulate them to continue, but convince the rest of the country to do likewise without Federal seed-money. There has been a fairly low level of evaluation accompanying the Centers Program—and little of it has been directed at assessing the relative value to a community of initiating a center, especially under conditions of no seed-money.

The third implication is, we think, the most serious—it concerns objectivity or credibility. Let us quote Secretary of HEW Casper Weinberger from a recent press interview (Broder, 1973).

> Q: Is it one of the objectives of the President's reorganization plan for government to break up what you call the natural alliances between people administering programs and the beneficiaries of the program?

> A: One of the goals of the administration reorganization is to enable the chief executive to have more control over the administration and the direction of these programs. I think the present structure makes it difficult for him to get that, because these alliances do develop and therefore the reports that come in from the people running the programs are basically designed to support their continuation and their increase in size.

> Q: How do you get an honest program evaluation, so you know which programs should be cut and which should be spared?

> A: I don't think you have any problem getting it. It is a matter of techniques and skills and getting the people who are equipped to do it.

And in reacting to our evaluation studies he said,

> Our figures are more impressive...than a lot of ordered studies. (He said he) doesn't lean too heavily on studies obviously designed to bring out the results wanted by the people who ordered them initially. (Weinberger, 1973)

This appraisal is quite disturbing for program evaluation. We personally do not believe there was bias in the study Weinberger was discussing. Both the first principal investigator and the NIMH project officer (the senior author) have some reputation in the program staff as being overly critical of the Service Programs, not overly supportive. But if these studies are really seen as biased, there's need for additional procedures to assure objectivity. Secretary Weinberger has suggested using his own staff. This seems to be an advocacy model of evaluation—a tool for the political process. At the moment, Program Evaluation technocrats do not appear to threaten to displace the political process.

Feedback from Evaluation Research Feedback

We would like at this time to provide a concrete example of one approach to the evaluation of program evaluation research. Although this is but one example, we report it to illustrate the philosophy of the benefit from reciprocal feedback. This case also may be used to focus discussion on some of the problems and considerations which must be dealt with in order to apply evaluative techniques to program evaluation research.

The program evaluation activity reported here is currently in operation, under the direction of James Ciarlo, in the Northwest Denver Community Mental Health Center. The evaluation section spent about two years in designing reporting forms, computerizing data collection and retrieval processes, designing and initial testing of a therapeutic outcome assessment instrument, and training of Center personnel in the procedures of data reporting. Then in the last eight months it began its main evaluation task.

In general, the Denver Center evaluation project can be described as oriented toward the assessment of treatment outcomes generated by the various services within the Center (e.g., inpatient, day care, crisis intervention, vocational rehabilitation, etc.). In addition, process measures are monitored by evaluation personnel and accessibility indicators are studied. Goal determinations are not made by program evaluation personnel. Rather, information collected and processed by evaluation personnel is reported to Center personnel for their assessment and evaluation regarding goal attainment and goal modifications.

The Northwest Denver Center initiated its research under the assumption that one of the outcomes of the research should be the ability to demonstrate the extent to which such evaluation affects the system under study. Feedback of evaluation results to system personnel must be assessed in terms of both its utility to decision makers and its helpfulness to caregivers. While every aspect of program evaluation will not be equally important to all individuals in the system, Program Evaluation Research should attempt to discern what information, at what points in the system, can be used for program change and improvement.

Basically, two groups may be identified toward whom research feedback might be directed. One group, direct caregiver clinicians, is usually composed of individuals ranging in education, experience, and research sophistication from volunteers and paraprofessionals to psychiatrists and psychologists. This group, charged with the everyday "production" of mental health care activities, may be limited in their interest, concern, and understanding of many research activities. A second identifiable group constitutes management, or administrative personnel. Within most mental health facilities this group normally is composed of individuals with less variability of experience and training, usually on the order of social workers to psychiatrists and psychologists. Here too, however, may be found a substantial range of interest, concern, and understanding of research activities.

Study of the effect of program evaluation research on these groups presents problems both of strategy and of content. The caregiver group, while greater in number and therefore potentially more desirable from a data gathering standpoint, may lack the overview necessary to perceive the importance and relevance of program evaluation results. Their primary concern, the individual clients whom they see, is often not the immediate focus of research and evaluation of *programs* carried on in the system. Also, the time delay necessitated by collection and processing of data may often make program evaluation research feedback outdated for individual caregiver use except in some general summary manner. Assessment of research feedback must therefore first be directed to the relevance of the feedback to those receiving it.

The effect of research feedback to administrative personnel also presents difficult assessment problems. The size of the administrative staff in any one mental health system is usually quite small, from a research and data gathering standpoint. Therefore, statistical tests of feedback responses are made difficult. In addition, this group, charged with the main decision-making responsibility, consists of individuals whose formal training is mainly in service delivery of mental health care. They are not, by training, managers and administrators and may experience difficulty in orienting themselves toward an organization-wide assessment of the operation of their center. Such an orientation by management is necessary for wise decisions concerning cost effectiveness, distribution of resources, etc.

The difficulties which may be experienced by either of these groups in the utilization and improvement of research feedback include a basic, initial aspect of research which cannot be overlooked if research feedback is to be relevant to system personnel. Sympathy for, and cooperation with, research personnel is vital to the gathering of evaluation data and to its successful integration into the decision-making processes of the system. Such assistance from system personnel, in view of the problems mentioned above, cannot be taken for granted. Additionally, the mere existence of a separate or semi-separate group of individuals designated as "evaluators" can be expected to increase, rather than diminish, the resistance of system personnel to provide evaluation information because of the implications for individual evaluation and the possibility of "cutting one's own throat."

What then are the prospects for evaluating the effects of feedback of research information? Our initial assessments of results of feedback provide a general baseline of immediate and expected utility. We will continue to make assessment over time to determine when and why changes may occur. Assessment at multiple points in the system, at multiple times and with different types of indicators such as attitudinal reactions, rated utility and process and outcome measures, will permit us to determine the extent of convergence of evidence.

To date, four studies have been conducted in the Northwest Denver Center which try to assess the effects of the program evaluation unit on the Center.

The first of these concerned the concept of continuity of care. The program evaluation unit conducts quarterly studies of the effectiveness of client transfers from one serving element in the Center to another. Program evaluation results fed back to Center personnel concerned the success rates of such transfers as a function of the use of formally prescribed procedures (these consist of entering the transfer on the client's file and sending a transfer form directly to the receiving element). Evaluation assessment consisted of questioning Center personnel to determine three things: (1) where in the system the staff perceived responsibility for the transfer to rest, (2) the effect which knowledge of the success rate had in effecting changes in this area, and (3) the perceived accuracy of the success rate information.

The data from the evaluation assessment revealed that caregivers (who do the actual transferring of clients) perceived themselves as having a greater effect on the outcome of client transfers than did administrators. In addition, administrators perceived the feedback as more accurately reflecting the magnitude of transfer rates than did caregivers. Neither group reported that program evaluation feedback had affected the manner in which transfers of clients were handled. However, data from actual client encounters as well as the use of transfer forms have shown somewhat increased transfer rates and much better adherence to prescribed transfer procedures since the beginning of program evaluation efforts in this area. Further research is planned to attempt a reconciliation between the rated responses of staff personnel and the more objective transfer information.

The second evaluation assessment study which was done in the Denver Center attempted to find any effects which could be detected from an informational (as opposed to evaluative) report generated by the program evaluation unit. The report dealt with the degree of utilization by alcoholism clients of the services available in the Center. Staff members were asked to indicate the extent to which knowledge of such information helped them in making program decisions and was useful to them in assessing the alcoholism program's effectiveness. Results of this evaluation assessment showed that, although no detectable changes had occurred attributable to the program evaluation, the caregiver group perceived the value of the program evaluation, as well as their ability to affect future service utilization by clients, as higher than did administrators.

A third evaluation assessment study dealt with the subjective impressions of Center personnel to six areas of therapeutic outcome assessment developed by the program evaluation unit. These areas of assessment were designed for use in determining the current level of functioning of clients regardless of their particular problem, diagnosis, or treatment history. The areas measured related to the client's psychological discomfort, interpersonal isolation, non-productivity, abuse of intoxicating substances, dependency on social aid organizations, and satisfaction with the Center in meeting his needs and inspiring his confidence. For the evaluation assessment, respondents were asked to indicate their personal feelings of the utility of each of the six areas for the evaluation of clients. Those questioned were asked only for their opinions of the areas, and were not concerned with any problems of validity or reliability of the assessment device. Data from administrators and caregivers (identified as either professionals or paraprofessionals) showed: (1) acceptance by all system personnel of the importance of the six therapeutic outcome areas developed by the evaluation staff, (2) greater rated importance of the four clinically oriented areas than of the economic (dependence upon numerous caregiving agencies) or satisfaction (with the caregiving system) areas, and (3) a tendency for paraprofessionals (involved nearly entirely in caregiving) to be most concerned with client satisfaction. The concern for client satisfaction declined steadily from paraprofessionals, who showed moderate to extremely high concern for client satisfaction, through professionals, who showed moderate concern, to administrators, who evidenced only slight to moderate concern for patient satisfaction.

The fourth evaluation assessment study, not yet complete, being conducted by the Denver CMHC program evaluation staff concerns the processes used in Center decision-making. Center personnel are being asked what factors are influential in helping them arrive at various kinds of decisions made throughout the Center. The number and kind of factors found will be compared across organizational levels. Similarities and differences in information use and requirements may help to determine the expected value of various forms of feedback to different points within the system.

The preceding data and the theoretical position from which the studies were designed have begun to indicate a difference in the receptivity to, and utilization of program evaluation by personnel in the Northwest Denver Center. Administrators and caregivers have evidenced the greatest differences in terms of attitudes and utilization of feedback. These data are continuing to accumulate and, although limited in statistical significance by the size of the sample available, tend to be quite consistent across studies thus far undertaken.

One subset of individuals whose data are less consistent than those of administrators and caregivers are the unit leaders of the various caregiving teams in the Center. These individuals are at once administrators of their own teams and direct caregivers within them. In general, their responses have tended to fall between those of the administrative and caregiver groups. Such a finding should not be surprising, but further research will be necessary to clarify the role and attitudes of unit leaders before their needs and opinions relevant to program evaluation can be described.

In terms of the utilization of program evaluation and the assessment of the impact of evaluation research findings, the data from this Center provide support for the following hypotheses: (1) different definable groups within the Center will value different types of evaluative feedback, (2) program evaluation designed to assess Center strengths and weaknesses will be seen as more valuable to administrators than to those at the caregiving level, and (3) the relevance of evaluative findings for decision-making in the Center should be a dynamic, increasing function of adaptations by evaluation research staff to findings regarding group differences and organizational feedback requirements.

Support for Automated Psychiatric Record Systems

Another experience which has colored our thinking about program evaluation research is that which NIMH has gained from supporting automated psychiatric data systems. The most ambitious of these have been the Multi-State Information System at Rockland State Hospital and several Psychiatric Case Registers. In brief, the original hopes for these systems, especially as tools for clinicians, have not been fully realized, and they have not demonstrated their value for practice in a way to lead to wide-spread adoption or support by other states or regions (Windle, 1972). A major part of the problem seems to be that these systems have not focused on or developed simple procedures for enabling their use by administrators or practitioners. This problem seems very like that of most applied research.

These six experiences are among those which convince us that program evaluation research should be conceived of as more than simply traditionally designed research on topics which lead to assessing the value of a program. Such a narrow conception has resulted in a history of relatively low application of research to program improvement. This history is leading us to feel it may be more useful to regard program evaluation as an orientation which administrators can take to help them in their decisions, if they are so minded and if we can develop sufficiently simple and compelling techniques to assist them.

Criteria for Program Evaluation Research

Let us now turn to a possible product of these considerations, namely criteria which can be used to judge the value of program evaluation research. We will here focus on benefits from only the substantive results of research, recognizing that there are many other indirect impacts from conducting research which should be considered. The suggestions that follow need more work to become a cost-benefit formula for decision-making of the type presented by Neenan (1974). We would welcome your suggestions toward that goal.

There seem to be four factors in the value of program evaluation research for decision-making.

420

(a) *Scientific quality.* By scientific quality we don't mean the elaborateness of experimental designs, but rather the use of procedures and attention to control for expected major biases in order to learn what is really going on. This has two aspects. The first is the use of insightful program hypotheses. The investigator must choose options to contrast which will reveal possible benefits from the use of knowledge. Most research methodology focuses upon procedures for validation and measurement. Probably the most important aspect of the research should be hunches, ideas, and good guesses about how events are inter-related or how to increase effectiveness.

The second aspect of quality of research is validity. This is usually considered a technical topic. However for program evaluation research there are also often philosophical or ethical questions of even more importance in determining validity. Much of the truth about a program may be embarrassing to program managers. The program evaluator must sometimes choose between allegiance to the program manager and the truth as revealed in his data.

(b) *Utilization.* Unless the findings from research are put into practice, either to make changes in a program or changes in others' understandings of the program (as may occur if a program is found better than other options which are being considered), there may be no practical benefits from the research. This factor of utilization must take into account, however, that findings derived from one program may be applied to benefit others. Such a spreading of benefits is one aim of research, and one reason why it is more reasonable for research to be funded by governmental or professional bodies responsible for a wide range of applications than by specific agencies.

(c) *Cost of implementation.* This is essentially the problem of how difficult it may be to implement change, including its frequently wide-ranging impacts.

(d) *Cost of research.* If research is looked upon as an investment which a program can make to improve its future functioning, the cost of this investment must be taken into account. Since the cost is im-mediate and the benefits in the future, these benefits must be dis-counted at whatever rate seems appropriate, after considering the factors which Neenan has discussed. We must also consider other kinds of costs than those which show up in the budget for program evaluation units. There is often a cost for subjects and staff who must participate. Whether such participation involves more fringe benefits to them in the form of education or services than it does annoyance will depend upon the way in which the evaluation is carried out as well as their prior history of involvement in such activities. We find many community mental health centers suffering, as do the Eskimoes described by Neufeldt (1973), from an excess of attention from researchers. Since centers have been looked upon as a model for futuristic mental health services, they have been a prime target for study. The ethical responsibility of researchers to give the subjects something for their trouble is only gradually coming to researchers' awareness. The lag between how quickly it comes to the subjects' awareness and to the researchers' awareness may be one measure of cost of the research.

We feel these considerations should be assessed for each of two levels of follow-up of program evaluation efforts. It is obviously desirable if one can wait a sufficiently long time to learn what actually ensues. However, the difficulty and the time delay required in measuring changes in program evaluation research suggest that we should also develop criteria at the level of intermediate processes and effects which we believe associated with ultimate benefit. Thus we will describe possible criteria for two levels of outcome: ultimate program benefits and intermediate processes.

Ultimate Criteria

If the ultimate purpose of the program evaluation is to improve benefits to clients in relation to costs to taxpayers, an assessment of whether a particular program evaluation study ultimately facilitated this goal would require: (1) an evaluation of the program in question before the program evaluation effort, (2) an evaluation of the change in the program subsequent to the evaluation, (3) an assessment of the extent to which the program evaluation was responsible for the change, and (4) the benefits of the portion of the change produced by the program evaluation, relative to the cost of the evaluation. This would be much more difficult than the original program evaluation. And because it benefits the service program only indirectly evaluation assessment is probably of much less value than efforts to improve the program.

Ultimate criteria may be useable only under special circumstances:

(1) The first is when enough time has elapsed that a general judgement of the value of a program and changes in it have been made by history. Then the assessment of the role of program evaluation research can be made relatively simply. Unfortunately this is likely to be many years later and the evaluation of the particular program

evaluation effort is likely to be of little value in improving that effort.

(2) The second circumstance is when one is content with determining simply what effect the program evaluation research had. If it is found that the program evaluation research did influence a decision, produce a change, or retard an otherwise impending change, it suggests there may have been an ultimate value from the research. On the other hand, if there is *no* effect, the research can have had no *direct* value. We should bear in mind, however, that there may be a longer range indirect benefit. For example, if the research produces findings consistent with a decision which has already been made it may establish the credibility of research so that a future finding can more readily have impact.

(3) The third circumstance when ultimate criteria may be useable is when the cost of the evaluation effort appears to far exceed the amount of benefit likely from the sort of change in program which the evaluation could effect. This would be the case when a fairly large study is undertaken on a program which is unlikely to change or is likely to be phased out. However, such an evaluation may generalize to other similar programs, and thus be useful in the future. Thus to use the ratio between costs for evaluation and likely opportunity for use of results requires a judgement of what programs will look like in the future and how much concern for this future is the responsibility of those planning the evaluation.

(4) Another special case where ultimate criteria of service program improvement may be feasible concerns the results from continuous monitoring systems which provide feedback to a service program concerning problems observed. When the monitoring is continuous, changes in a program's problems can be detected, and perhaps traced to evaluation feedback. The evaluation system at Northwest Denver Center is designed for this purpose. Such an assessment is also possible from utilization review statistics if these are used with a serious intent to improve the service program.

Process Criteria

A feasible alternative for evaluating program evaluation research is the less satisfying one of focusing on process criteria. Since we are restricting our interest in program evaluation to its use for program improvement, these criteria should be measures of the research processes which are expected to facilitate program improvement. Again, we need to remind ourselves that program improvement must be defined broadly to include increasing effectiveness of a program, continuing an effective program, or eliminating ineffective activities.

We suggest process criteria consisting of two types of variables: those concerning the research process and those concerning utilization of the results.

(1) Variables related to the research process. The first characteristic of research should be validity. Program evaluation research is like a man torn between loyalty to his wife and desire for a mistress. The goal conflict between fidelity to scientific rigor and a lust to aid programs immediately is exacerbated by close contact with the program to be evaluated. If it is assumed that the program to be evaluated is good, necessary, and generally effective, studies may be designed to support these contentions, or information may be disseminated in a distorted form which gives the impression that there is harder or more consistent evidence than actually exists to support them.

The distinguishing feature between program evaluation research and the type of evaluative judgements about programs which everyone makes off-the-cuff is the degree to which certain procedures have been followed to systematize and objectify information collection and analysis. The main characteristics of these methods is not their sophistication or precision as much as it is, first, their *integrity* or control for subjective bias, and second, the care with which program outcomes, cost and purposes or values are interrelated.

The chain of activities in program evaluation research is long—and often the most crucial parts such as drawing the action implications must be quite crudely done. The researcher is likely to feel that in view of the crudeness of the implementation phase it does not make great sense to be highly rigorous at other stages. However, this temptation must be carefully avoided. Because program administrators often express more enthusiasm than accuracy in presenting their programs does not mean that researchers should use similar standards. One of the researcher's main assets is objectivity; if he relinquishes this asset he may find himself, like traditional innocent virgins who have yielded to the entreaties of those with differing interests, devalued even in the view of those whom they have served.

What we're trying to say is that it is important for evaluative research to remain *research,* in the sense that the procedures used to reach the evaluation are free from implicit program values. The safest way to express the program values is in terms of the criterion of the research, that is to use the program goals as the dependent variable to which program options are related as independent variables.

A major validity problem is to assure that measures or estimates are free of bias. In many cases the most economic way to make a complex assessment will be by the judgement of an informed participant. Methods to free such assessments from being self-serving may be necessary. This is one reason why consultants, contractors and research staff divorced from close contact with operating programs are often used for research. It is also a reason why it is often advisable to get evaluative ratings from a set of judges of prespecified characteristics. The degree of confidence one can put in the results often depends upon the procedures which have been used to rule out biased assessments. In the end, however, much of the responsibility for interpreting the results and stating how much confidence can be put in them will fall on the researcher. This gets into the second point we mentioned as a characteristic of research validity, namely the care and comprehensiveness with which the observations are interrelated. Perhaps the most vulnerable point will be the assumptions underlying the analyses. This vulnerability requires that the assumptions be made explicit. Williams (1972) pointed out that evaluative research because of its complexity and likelihood of generating controversy often requires multidisciplinary and high-level administrative skills. This suggests that a process measure of the validity of the study as applying to real world concerns might be the range of topics examined within the research and in negotiations between the researchers and program administrators.

I want to stress only one other point under the heading of validity. Many techniques for controlling bias within studies are well known to researchers. This is not, it seems to us, where most problems are encountered. More difficulty occurs in the conceptualization and interpretation stages—the interface between program and research. Consequently it is in these activities that special efforts must be taken. For example, it may be wise to aim for convergent validation of a result rather than a single crucial test. Data from independent sources which corroborate each other may be more convincing and less liable to error than even very carefully collected data from a single source.

James Wilson of Harvard has been said[2] to have formulated two laws:

> First Law: All policy interventions in social problems produce the intended effect—if the research is carried out by those implementing the policy or their friends.

Second Law: No policy intervention in social problems produces the intended effect—If the research is carried out by independent third parties, especially those skeptical of the policy.[2]

All too often these two laws appear to account for differences in results from evaluative studies. When they do they undermine the credibility and hence the future utility of evaluation research. Perhaps the best process measures of validity are: (a) the reliability of findings when undertaken by investigators of differing sponsorship, and (b) the extent to which a given study has included investigators, advisors or judges of diverse or non-program interest group affiliation.

A second characteristic of the research process should be mentioned to help us keep a systems perspective. If we assume that program evaluative research does improve programs, then the continuation or increase of this research is a process measure of likely program improvement. In fact viability is commonly used as a measure of success, in spite of the circularity of its rationale.

It may be worthwhile to make a distinction between the particular evaluation research activity for a specific program and program evaluation as a general function. If there has been a fruitful evaluation study on a specific program, there may no longer be any evaluation effort connected with the program, since there may be little remaining need for one. Yet there should be more favorable attitudes toward the general function of evaluation. This suggests that the attitudes of program staff and taxpayers about the value of program evaluation as a general activity might be a useful process measure of its past effectiveness.

However, we should note that favorable attitudes can often come from extraneous factors. Buchanan and Wholey (1973) observed that "there is definitely more money budgeted for evaluation" of federal evaluation programs now than three years ago, but that "the impact of evaluation results on program development and improvement over the last two years has been disappointing, when compared with the amount of money and effort that has gone into evaluation." They conclude that "this increasing support must be due to a continuing recognition by the government that evaluation is needed...rather than to the recognition that evaluation as currently practiced is the answer to these needs." This suggests that use of attitudes toward evaluation as a criterion of its effectiveness should be specific enough to differentiate the reasons for advocacy.

426

Variables Related to Research Utilization. Let us now consider process criteria for measuring how well evaluative research facilitates utilization. The nine characteristics (Figure 6) of innovations which the Human Interaction Research Institute (NIMH, 1972) found to favor their adoption offer a promising frame of reference for use as process criteria.

The rationale for using these is that these are moderating conditions which facilitate the ultimate utilization of results in programs. The actual utilization is not under the program evaluator's control, and is influenced heavily by other factors beyond his control.

Thus the best appraisal of how well the program evaluator accomplished what he was responsible for can be done by examining how well the conditions enhancing utilization were attained.

Relevance to Program Decisions. Those who recognize the danger of losing their integrity by becoming too close to programs are likely to err in the direction of irrelevance. They usually do this by identifying with the academic community and aiming their products for this community. This often leads to gathering data with a high degree of precision, and presenting it with a high degree of abstruseness and generality. The questions answered however are often not those of the program administrators. Studies of greatest relevance should be both program specific and comprehensive. They should deal with the program studied in all the detail necessary for informed decisions. This means that they should treat all relevant program options, treat costs as well as effectiveness, and use enough cases to be, and to appear to be, reliable. A major problem in many evaluation studies is that they treat only actions to make the program more effective, but do not consider whether these actions are worth the additional cost, or what other parts of a program should be curtailed to permit the proposed expansions. One of the best indices of a relevant evaluation report is whether or not the costs for implementing proposed recommendations have been calculated and presented. As our experiences with applied research grants and evaluation contracts have shown, linkages between researchers and program staff and administrators are important to encourage utilization, both to win staff commitment and to assure relevance of the study. Wholey (1970) has estimated that adequate monitoring requires one fairly high level staff member for each two to four (or half million dollars) contract studies. The level of a program's liaison to research may be among the most useful process criteria.

An important part of relevance is the timing between the availability of information and when decisions must be made. Since there is often little advance awareness of when a decision must be made, program evaluation research must often sacrifice certain approaches, such as longitudinal study designs and thoroughness, for speed. A rating of concordance between when results are expected and when program decisions have to be made would be one item on a scale of process criteria of goodness of evaluations. On this criterion continuing monitoring activities are likely to score highest. Data are less likely to be decision-specific, but more likely to be available when decisions are made.

Compatibility and feasibility are both related to relevance. They apply specifically to the program options examined and the recommendations made. To be useful, program evaluations should focus upon conditions which the program administrators are able to change, or influence. We should note that this includes evidence about the overall effectiveness or benefits from the program. Even though the program administrator does not control the amount of funds his program has, he can, and usually greatly desires to, influence such decisions. Good program evaluation may increase his influence by giving him better data on which to base his influence attempts. Compatibility also includes the congruence the program staff perceive between their values and those of the researchers. If the program evaluators appear to represent potentially hostile decision-makers such as a budget cutting supervisor or a critical public, or if they conduct a hit-and-run collection of information without feeding back rapidly what is learned to the program staff, these staff will have a negative set toward whatever is concluded. This negative set will also create resistance toward future evaluation efforts, thus limiting the possibilities of future impact.

The relative advantage of various action options studied by program evaluation studies should be made clear. This includes not only their relative effectiveness, but also their relative costs.

Observability refers to communicating the innovations or changes implied by the evaluation in a way which convinces the program manager. This may best be done by getting the program manager involved in the analysis, perhaps by specifying what factors should be considered or checking the reasonableness of interpretations as the researcher drafts the report.

The packaging of a report which includes much data or thoughtful weighing of options and conditions is a major problem when we are concerned with utilization. Efforts must be made to encourage program staff to read enough to be able to make informed judgements. These include both ways of preparing and presenting reports and other forms of communication. Written reports should use brief summaries, graphic presentations, headings which summarize, appendices for detailed data, and lively writing style. Oral presentations, both formal and informal, and usually interactive are of even more value. As a popular bumper-sticker puts it, "Eschew Obfuscation."

Reversability, divisibility and trialability all relate to the likelihood that a recommended action is likely to be tried. This consideration should be taken into account in evaluation studies aimed at program improvement. Program conditions and options which lend themselves to gradual and tentative implementation should be given priority in study design.

Credibility is related to the first point considered, the apparent validity of the research. In this case however the researcher has to be concerned with how persons relatively unsophisticated in research methods would regard the study conditions. It may be useful to take steps which sound good, even when they do not increase research validity in order to be consistent with firmly held, if invalid, program assumptions. For example, sampling across work units or geographic locations may be more appealing to a program manager than stratifying by variables correlated with the factors being studied.

We've now gone over a set of criteria for research which can be applied to evaluating program evaluations. This has been fairly abstract; we have not presumed to try to operationalize these criteria for immediate use. Probably the most feasible way to apply such process criteria would be to have informed judges who are acquainted with a set of evaluations rate each project on each characteristic. Our suspicion is that many of these characteristics would prove highly correlated, and that therefore a smaller number could be used in practice.

Since utilization of program evaluation results depends upon the conditions of the service programs as well as upon the research, we should include among the process criteria some consideration of whether the program conditions are receptive to suggestions for change from research. There should probably be a demerit against program evaluation researchers who undertake an effort unlikely to succeed, unless there are strong countervailing factors. Zusman and Bissonette have made a convincing case, based on the difficulties so frequently encountered in trying to do useful evaluating, against attempts to do evaluative research under any but the most favorable conditions. The entire attempt to make policy decisions more amenable to results of research suffers from each effort which fails.

In this respect the planning and "selling" of evaluation research is similar to that for social service programs. Those who believe in them often find themselves overpromising in order to convince reluctant funding sources. Their claims depict what is, at best, possible, not what is likely as an outcome. When program managers are sold on such expectations, it is very likely that the evaluation will fail to live up to the expectations and must therefore be considered a failure from the program manager's perspective. Prevention of unrealistic expectations of evaluation research may be the most important way of increasing success in the short-run. In the long-run, evaluating our program evaluation efforts, using both ultimate and process criteria, should help us if, as we profess, it helps others.

We have one last thought. Since it doesn't fit well into the structure of this chapter, we will append it as a benediction to the conference. Last month CW heard a Unitarian address which paralleled our concepts of evaluation research. Our theme has been that program evaluation research can be evaluated by using process criteria based on the two primary orientations which evaluation research should have to improve programs: willingness to adapt research to fit program needs and interests, and encouragement of the use of accurate information about programs for making decisions. The Unitarian address reviewed the history of Western liberal religions. Many religions have stressed other-worldly conditions, ignoring "present-worldly" social ills. Liberal religions which identify with social action for social reform often become tied too closely with particular movements which usually are valid only for a limited range of conditions. Thus liberal religions, in trying to be relevant, may confuse means and ends; they may lose their transcendent quality and flexibility. The minister advised that we should, "Be in this world, but not of it."

A similar injunction applies to program evaluators. Be attuned to program concerns, but maintain the transcendent value of truth, as revealed glimmeringly, by research.

Footnotes

1. The views in this chapter are those of the authors and do not necessarily represent those of the National Institute of Mental Health. The work of the late Dr. Bates, who was working with the Denver Mental Health Systems Evaluation Project, is partially supported by NIMH under Research Grant No. MH 20954.

2. Washington Post, February 18, 1973.

References

Abt Associates. A study on the accessibility of community mental health centers. Final report on contract HSM-42-70-92, June 30, 1972.

Bass, R. D. and Windle, C. A preliminary attempt to measure continuity of care in a community mental health center. *Community Mental Health Journal,* 1973, *9,* 53-62.

Bernstein, I. Personal communication, November 1972.

Broder, D. S. Presidential power: An interview with Casper W. Weinberger. Washington Post, February 18, 1973.

Brown, B. S. A look at the overlook. *Mental Hygiene,* Fall, 1972.

Buchanan, G. N. and Wholey, J. S. Federal level evaluation. *Evaluation,* 1972, *1,* 17-22.

Caplan, N. and Nelson, S. D. On being useful: The nature and consequences of psychological research on social problems. *American Psychologist,* 1973, *28,* 199-211.

Chu, F. B. and Trotter, S. The fires of irrelevancy. *Mental Hygiene,* Fall, 1972.

Davis, H. R., Larsen, J. K., and Stout, R. *Planning for change.* American Institutes for Research, Palo Alto, California, 1973.

Feldman, S. and Windle, C. The NIMH approach to evaluating the Community Mental Health Centers Program. *Health Services Reports,* 1973, *88,* 174-180.

Finney, D. J. The Fisher-Yates test of significance in 2 x 2 contingency tables. *Biometrika,* 1948, *35.*

Glaser, E. M. and Taylor, S. H. Factors influencing the success of applied research. *American Psychologist,* 1973, *28,* 140-146.

Glaser, E. M. and Taylor, S. H. Factors influencing the success of applied research. A study of ten NIMH funded projects. Final report on contract to NIMH, Human Interaction Research Institute, Los Angeles, California, January, 1969.

Health Policy Advisory Center. Evaluation of community involvement in Community Mental Health Centers. Final Report on NIMH contract HSM-42-70-106. Accession No. PB-211 267. U. S. Department of Commerce National Technical Information Service, Springfield, Virginia, 1971.

Havelock, R. G. Research utilization in four federal agencies. Paper presented at American Psychological Association Convention, Honolulu, Hawaii, September 1972.

Kelly, B. C. *Central Utah Community Mental Health Center Impact Study.* Report to NIMH on Contract No. NIH-70-505, November 1970.

Martens, H. S. and Warren, C. G. The multi-agency community mental health center: Administrative and organizational relationships. Final report on NIMH contract HSM-42-70-55 by the National Academy of Public Administration, Accession No. PB-210 094. U. S. Department of Commerce National Technical Information Service, Springfield, Virginia, December 1971.

Missett, J. Untitled report on a study to determine the effect of the federally funded portion of a community mental health center on the services provided in its catchment area and the State mental hospital. Connecticut Mental Health Center, New Haven, Connecticut, Report to NIMH on Contract No. HSM 42-70-35, February 1971.

Montague, E. K. and Taylor, E. N. Preliminary handbook on procedures for evaluating mental health indirect service programs in schools. Human Resources Research Organization, Alexandria, Virginia, 1971.

Moors, W. R. Unitarianism: Which way? Address at the Unitarian Church of Rockville, Rockville, Maryland, February 18, 1973.

National Institute of Mental Health. A manual on research utilization. PHS Publication No. (HSM) 71-9059. U. S. Government Printing Office, Washington, D. C., 1972.

National Institute of Mental Health. A distillation of principles on research utilization. Vol. 1, PHS Publication No. (HSM) 71-9060. U. S. Government Printing Office, Washington, D. C., 1972.

National Institute of Mental Health. A distillation of principles on research utilization. Vol. II: Bibliography with annotations. PHS Publication No. (HSM) 71-9061. U. S. Government Printing Office. Washington, D. C., 1972.

National Study Service. The relative impact of various factors, including community mental health centers, in the development of mental health resources. Final report on NIMH contract HSM-42-170-108. Accession No. PB-210 027. U. S. Department of Commerce National Technical Information Service, Springfield, Virginia, 1971.

Neenan, W. B. Benefit-cost analysis and the evaluation of mental retardation programs. In P. O. Davidson, F. W. Clark, and L. A Hamerlynck (Eds.), *Evaluation of behavioral programs in community, residential, and school settings.* Champaign, Illinois: Research Press, 1974.

Neufeldt, A. H. Considerations in the implementation of program evaluations. Presentation at the Fifth Banff Conference on Behavior Modification, March 1973.

Nichols, J. S. Impact of a comprehensive mental health center on the utilization of State hospital facilities. Range Mental Health Center, Virginia, Minnesota. Report to NIMH on Contract No. NIH-70-72, October 1971.

Orden, S. R. and Stocking, C. B. Relationships between community mental health centers and other caregiving organizations. Final report on NIMH contract HSM-42-71-7 by National Opinion Research Center, Accession No. PB-210 026. U. S. Department of Commerce National Technical Information Service, Springfield, Virginia, December 1971.

Riedel, D. C. *et al.* Developing a system for utilization review and evaluation in community mental health centers. *Hospital Community Psychiatry*, 1971, *22*, 229-232.

Salasin, S. Conversational contact...with Elliot L. Richardson. *Evaluation*, 1972, Fall, 9-16.

Salasin, S. E. and Baxter, J. W. Client response to community mental health services. Presentation at American Psychological Association Convention, Honolulu, Hawaii, September 1972.

Stuart, R. B. Strategies and techniques for the evaluation of community health services for delinquents. Presentation at Fifth Banff Conference on Behavior Modification, March 1973.

U. S. Bureau of Census. Survey of State and local mental health finances. Report to NIMH, October 1970.

U. S. Department of Health, Education, and Welfare. Press Release, February 1, 1973.

Weinberger, C. S. Testimony before the U. S. Senate Subcommittee on Health, March 22, 1973.

Wholey, J. S. *et al.* Federal evaluation policy. Urban Institute, Washington, D. C., 1970.

Wilkins, W. Expectancy of therapeutic gain: An empirical and conceptual critique. *Journal of Consulting and Clinical Psychology*, 1973, *40*, 69-77.

Williams, W. The capacity of social service organizations to perform large-scale evaluative research. In P. H. Rossi and W. Williams (Eds.), *Evaluating social programs: Theory, practice, and politics.* New York: Seminar Press, 1972, 287-314.

Windle, C. NIMH perspectives and frustrations. Presentation at American Psychological Association Convention, Honolulu, Hawaii, September, 1972.

Windle, C., Bass, R., and Taube C. PR aside—NIMH's evaluation study results. Presentation at American Psychiatric Association Convention, Honolulu, Hawaii, May 1972.

Zusman, J. and Bissonette, R. The case against evaluation (with some suggestions for improvement). *International Journal of Mental Health* (In press).

AUTHOR INDEX

Abramson, M., 227, 250
Adamek, J., 264, 295
Adams, H. E., 30
Adams, S. 142, 170
Aldrich, C. K., 230, 237, 245
Aleksandrowicz, D., 230, 245
Alexander, F., 239, 245
Allen, K. E., 26
Anastasi, A., 393
Anderson, M. L., 39, 52
Andrews, F. M., 18, 30
Angrist, S. S., 91, 98
Antonovosky, A., 99
Archibald, R. D., 63
Argyris, C., 63
Aronson, S., 295
Arrill, M. B., 94, 99
Arrow, K. J., 192
Auerbach, A. H., 159, 172
Ault, M. H., 205, 220
Averch, H. A., 380, 381, 384, 391
Avnet, H. H., 148, 168, 170
Ayllon, T., 67, 80, 132, 136, 226, 245
Azrin, N., 132, 136, 226, 245

Bacal, H. A., 47, 53
Bachrach, H. M., 159, 172
Badal, K., 300
Baer, D. M., 20, 26, 137
Bailey, J. S., 162, 170
Bailey, W. C., 287, 297
Balfour, F. H. G., 47, 53
Ball, S., 11, 26
Baker, F., 96, 100, 101
Bandura, A., 20, 22, 26
Barclay, J. R., 339, 341, 386-388, 391-393
Barclay, L. K., 387, 391
Barker, L. S., 204, 220
Barker, R. G., 204, 220
Barten, H. H., 139
Bass, R. D., 86, 98, 396, 431, 435
Bates, P., 395, 431
Battle, C. C., 35, 36, 49, 52
Baum, M., 296

Baxter, J. W., 400, 434
Beattie, W. M., 241, 245
Becker, G., 195
Becker, W. C., 20, 29
Beez, W. V., 381, 392
Beigel, A., 137
Beisser, A. R., 103, 137
Bellak, L., 139
Benefiel, D., 204, 220
Bereiter, C., 49, 52
Berenson, J., 249
Bergin, A. E., 49, 52, 53, 54, 92, 98, 101, 102, 147, 149, 150, 154, 170, 171, 237, 245
Berkman, P. L., 235, 249
Bernstein, I., 403, 431
Berrien, V., 66, 73, 81
Bijou, S. W., 4, 5, 6, 7, 26, 205, 220, 330, 338
Birnbrauer, J. S., 20, 26
Bissonette, R., 429, 435
Blatt, B., 202, 220
Blenkner, M., 223, 227, 228, 238, 243, 245, 249
Bloom, M., 245, 249
Bloom, W., 197
Bogatz, G. A., 11, 26
Bonner, C. D., 241, 248
Boren, J. J., 91, 101
Borgatta, E. F., 270, 298, 299
Boulanger, D. G., 63
Boulding, K., 195
Bower, S. M., 5, 30
Bracht, G. H., 72, 80
Brady, J. P., 173
Brandon, S., 88, 99
Briggs, J., 151, 171
Brim, O., 296
Broder, D. S., 414, 431
Brody, E. M., 229, 236-237, 245, 248
Brophy, J. E., 381, 392
Brown, B. S., 431
Brown, G. W., 227, 251
Brown, P. W., 387, 392, 393
Browning, P. C., 63

437

Buchanan, G. N., 426, 431
Buchanan, J. M. 193
Bucher, B., 20, 26
Buckley, N. K., 20, 31
Bullock, J., 241, 245
Burghardt, S., 255, 296
Burkhead, J., 194
Burns, J. W., 3, 28
Burton, A., 220
Bushell, D. B., 204, 221
Butter, I., 198

Campbell, D. T., 4, 13, 26, 72, 75,
 81, 149, 174, 259, 296
Canton, R., 121, 137
Caplan, N., 431
Caro, F. G., 258, 287, 296
Carroll, H. A., 391
Carter, R. D., 160, 165, 169, 170
Carter, R. M., 298
Cassell, W. A., 97, 98
Cataldo, M. F., 201, 204, 220
Cattell, R. B., 49, 52
Cautela, J. R., 225, 237, 246
Chandler, M., 159, 170
Chase, Jr., S. B., 195
Chien, C., 96, 99
Christie, N., 296
Christophersen, E. R., 204, 222
Chu, F. B., 103, 137, 412, 431
Cicourel, A., 255, 296
Clark, C., 388, 392
Clark, F. W., 433
Clements, C. B., 225, 249
Clemmer, D., 253, 296
Cobb, J. A., 3, 14, 15, 16, 18, 20,
 26, 27, 28, 30
Cohen, D. K., 224, 225, 246, 380,
 392
Cohen, J., 6, 27, 159, 170, 198
Cole, C. B., 196, 236, 245
Cole, J. O., 96, 99
Coleman, J. S., 381, 392
Cook, D. L., 63
Cooley, W. W., 323
Coons, D., 246
Conley, R. W., 94, 99, 184, 186,
 188, 193, 199
Connett, A. V., 297
Conwell, M., 94, 99
Cosin, L. Z., 224, 225, 246
Costello, C. G., 48, 52
Cotton, J. W., 28
Couzens, M., 258, 300
Cowen, E. L., 101
Cressey, D. R., 296

Cronback, L. J., 1, 27, 381, 392
Crow, W. J., 297

Dager, E. Z., 264, 295
Daniels, R. S., 234, 246
Davidson, P. O., xv, 433
Davis, H. R., 431
Davis, J., 132, 138
Davison, G. C., 226, 246
Davitz, J. R., 197
Davitz, L. J., 197
DeAlessi, L., 193-194
Deline, S. E., 198
Dembo, T., 205, 220
Deniston, O. L., 297
DeRisi, W., 103, 106, 117, 137, 138,
 278, 298
Dodson, R., 196
Doke, L. A., 134, 137, 204, 220, 222
Donabedian, A., 89, 99
Donahue, W., 224, 246
Donaldson, T. A., 391
Downs, T., 249
Drabman, R., 20, 29
Dreikurs, R., 142, 172
Duhl, L. J., 250
Dumpson, J. R., 302
Dupuit, J., 192

Eckman, T. A., 103
Edwards, A. L., 155, 170
Elashoff, J. D., 9, 27
Ellis, R. H., 91, 99
Ellsworth, R. B., 91, 99
Elton, C. F., 341, 391
Endicott, W., 132, 137
Emerson, R., 297
Empey, L., 256, 275, 283, 297
Epstein, L. J., 233, 237, 240, 246
Erickson, M. T., 256, 297
Erickson, R. C., 225, 246
Erickson, R. J., 297
Ericson, R., 257, 299
Evans, J. W., 1, 31
Eyberg, S., 9, 27
Eysenck, H. J., 45, 52, 341, 392

Fabian, V., 117, 137
Fairweather, G. W., 225, 246
Farndale, J., 53
Farrald, R. A., 312, 313, 321
Fein, R., 43, 44, 52
Feldman, S., 406, 432
Filer, R. N., 225, 246
Fink, M., 248
Finn, J., 346

438

Finney, D. J., 432
Fisher, J., 237, 246
Fiske, D. W., 10, 27, 142, 148, 150,
151, 154, 155, 170
Flomenhaft, K., 100
Fogel, D., 297
Foley, A. R., 129, 137
Ford, D. H., 45, 54
Forstenzer, H. M., 129, 137
Forsyth, R. P., 225, 246
Foster, S. C., 301
Fox, P. D., 43-44, 53, 89, 95, 99
Frank, J. D., 35, 49, 52, 142, 143,
170, 171
Franks, C. M., 172
Fraser, H. N., 98
Freeman, H. E., 53, 91, 99
Fried, M., 86, 99
Furby, L., 1, 27

Gafni, M., 297
Gaitz, C. M., 235, 247
Gallon, S. L., 3, 27
Garabedian, P. G., 301
Gardner, E. A., 101
Garfield, J. C., 151, 171
Garfield, S. L., 5, 27, 52, 53, 54, 98,
101, 102, 154, 171, 245
Gentile, J. R., 5, 27
Gerhard, R. A., 97, 101
Getting, V. A., 297
Gibbons, D. C., 301
Gintis, H., 380, 392
Glaser, D., 297
Glaser, E. M., 405, 409, 432
Glaser, R., 326, 338
Glass, G. V., 72, 80
Glasscotte, R., 129, 137
Gliedman, L. H., 142, 143, 170, 171
Goffman, E., 230, 234, 247
Gohlke, C. A., 296
Goldberg, C. A., 86, 99
Goldfarb, A. I., 227, 240, 242, 247
Goldstein, A. P., 150, 171
Good, T. L., 381, 392
Gore, C. P., 40, 53
Gottesman, L. E., 224, 237, 247
Gottfredson, D., 297
Grace, D., 39, 52
Grad, B., 249
Grad, J., 236, 243, 247
Granger, C. H., 63
Grob, G. N., 234, 247
Gruber, R. P., 20, 27
Gruenberg, E. M., 88, 89, 103, 137
Grunberg, F., 98

Gump, P. V., 149, 172, 204, 205,
220, 221
Guttentag, M., 259, 297

Haberland, H., 237, 247
Hacker, S. L., 235, 238, 247
Hagen, E., 334, 338
Hall, T. L., 75, 81
Hamburg, D. A., 227, 250
Hamerlynck, L. A., 433
Hamilton, M. W., 40-41, 53
Harberger, A. C., 176, 183, 192,
193, 195
Harding, J. S., 249
Harris, C. W., 1, 2, 27
Harris, F. R., 26
Harris, R. E., 220
Hart, B. M., 204, 221, 222
Haughton, E., 80, 310, 321
Havelock, R. G., 403, 432
Haveman, R. H., 192, 195
Hawkins, G., 299
Hawkins, N., 143, 172
Head, R., 63
Heath, E. S., 47, 53
Heck, E., 151, 171
Heller, K., 150, 171
Henderson, J. D., 173
Hiebert, S., 33
Hinrichs, H. H., 194
Hoch, P., 247
Hochman, H. M., 195
Hoehn-Saric, R., 35, 49, 52
Hoenig, J., 40-41, 53
Hogarty, G. E., 91, 100
Holland, J. L., 340, 392
Hollingshead, A. B., 242, 247
Holmes, T. H., 86, 100
Holtzman, W. H., 2, 28, 380, 393
Homburger, F., 241, 248
Hopkins, C. E., 82
Hops, H., 15, 16, 18, 20, 27, 28, 31
Huetteman, M. J., 151, 171
Hunt, H. F., 27, 142, 170
Hunter, W. W., 246
Hurley, R., 199
Hursh, D. E., 204, 221
Hutchison, G. B., 87, 100

Imber, S. D., 35, 49, 52, 142, 143,
170, 171
Ingraham, B. L., 260, 298
Ittelson, W. H., 133, 137, 138, 204,
221
Jackson, D., 341, 393
Jackson, D. G., 197

439

Jacobson, J. M., 204, 221
Jahn, J., 245
James, E. V., 204, 221
James, G., 298
Jasnau, K., 230, 248
Jastak, J. F., 330, 338
Jastak, S. R., 330, 338
Jayaratne, S., 141, 160, 165, 167, 173
Jesness, C. F., 148, 171, 278, 282, 298
Johnson, S., 20, 31
Johnston, M. S., 26
Jones, D. C., 225, 248
Jones, K., 40, 53
Jones, R. R., 1, 3, 5, 14-18, 20, 27, 28, 29
Jones, W. C., 270, 298, 299

Kadushin, C., 34, 53
Kahana, B., 230-231, 248
Kahana, E., 230-231, 248
Kahn, R. L., 66, 81, 223, 229, 234, 235, 236, 242, 246, 248, 250
Kahneman, D., 2, 29
Kandel, D. H., 298
Kanfer, F. H., 22, 29, 38, 53, 91, 100, 160, 171
Kaplan, F., 202, 220
Kassebaum, G., 257, 258, 298, 301
Kasterbaum, R., 249
Katz, D., 66, 81
Kazdin, A. E., 29
Kelly, B. C., 432
Kelman, H. R., 227, 229, 248
Kershaw, D. N., 141, 171
Kiesler, D. J., 10, 29, 33, 53, 147, 150, 171
Kiesling, H. J., 391
Kiker, B. F., 195
Kilpatrick, D., 287, 299
King, L. W., 20, 26, 103, 106, 138
Kitano, H. N. L., 298
Kitsuse, J., 255, 296
Kittrie, N., 298
Kleban, M. M., 229, 237, 245, 248
Kleemeier, R. W., 230, 234, 248
Klein, R. D., 27
Klerman, G. L., 97, 99
Koenig, C., 303, 308, 321
Kornreich, M., 142, 172
Kosa, J., 99
Kosberg, J. I., 241, 249
Kounin, J. S., 149, 172, 220
Kral, V., 230, 249
Kramer,B. M., 250

Krantz, P. J., 204, 221
Krasner, L. A., 39, 54, 260, 298
Krause, M. S., 33, 45, 53, 159, 172
Krutilla, J. V., 192
Kuldau, J. M., 43-44, 53, 95, 99
Kuypers, D. S., 20, 29

Langner, T., 250
Langsley, D. G., 86, 100
Larsen, J. K., 432
Lawton, M. P., 245, 248
Lee, A., 39, 52
Leeds, M., 245
Leighton, A. H., 249
Leighton, D. C., 242, 249
Leinhardt, G., 323, 334, 335, 338
LeLaurin, K., 204, 221
Leopold, R. L., 250
Lerman, P., 259, 287, 298
Levenson, A. I., 137
Levy, R. L., 160, 165, 169, 170
Lewin, K., 205, 220
Libb, J. W., 225, 249
Liberman, R. P., 103, 106, 108, 132, 138
Lichtenstein, E., 38, 50-51, 53
Lieberman, M. A., 224, 230, 232, 249, 250
Lindquist, E. F., 370, 393
Lindsley, G., 225, 249
Lindsley, O. R., 304, 308, 309, 321
Linn, R. L., 9, 31
Lohman, J. D., 298
Lord, F. M., 9, 29
Lorge, I., 197, 334, 338
Lott, Jr., L. A., 148, 158, 165, 173
Lowenthal, M. F., 235, 249
Lubeck, S., 256, 275, 297
Luborsky, L., 27, 142, 159, 170, 172

Mabry, J., 321
Machotka, P., 100
Macmillan, A. M., 249
Macmillan, D., 227, 234-236, 238, 243, 249
Mahoney, M. J., 22, 29
Malan, D. H., 47-48, 49-50, 53
Mandell, N., 298
Marcus, E., 230, 232, 249
Margolis, J., 192, 195
Markus, E., 249
Marks, J., 44, 54
Marsh, J., 296
Martens, H. S., 432
Martin, P. L., 114, 132, 133, 139
Martin, M., 87, 100

Masuda, M., 86, 100
Matarazzo, J. D., 86, 101
Maurice, H., 246
McCaffree, K. M., 95, 100
McClannahan, L. E., 204, 221
McConnell, J. V., 151, 171
McCormick, P. M., 278, 298
McLean, P. D., 83
McNeal, S., 143, 172
Mecklin, D. B., 249
Meehl, P. E., 2, 4, 29
Meltzoff, J., 142, 172
Mendkoff, E., 230, 237, 245
Meyer, H. J., 270, 282, 283, 299
Michael, J. L., 29, 136
Michaux, W. W., 91, 101
Miles, D. G., 97, 101
Miller, J. G., 66, 81
Miller, W. B., 257, 299
Millikan, M. F., 199
Miner, J., 194
Mischel, W., 24, 29, 36, 45-47, 49,
  51, 54
Mishan, E. J., 198
Missett, J., 432
Mitchell, K. M., 94, 102
Moberg, D. O., 257, 299
Montegue, E. K., 433
Moors, W. R., 433
Moos, R., 90, 101, 299
Morris, A., 299
Morris, N., 299
Morrow, W., 132, 138
Mort, M., 246
Mosak, H. H., 142, 170
Moskowitz, E., 227, 249
Moss, G. R., 91, 101
Mott, P., 255, 261, 299
Mullen, E. J., 302
Musgrave, R. A., 195

Nash, E. H., 35, 49, 52, 142, 143,
  170, 171
Neenan, W. B., 175, 195, 420, 433
Nelson, S. D., 431
Neufeldt, A. H., 65, 66, 73, 81, 97,
  101, 422, 433
Neuringer, C., 29
Nichols, J. S., 433
Nielsen, M. A., 245
Niskanen, A., 192, 195
Nutter, R. E., 198

Ochberg, F. M., 227, 250
O'Connell, D. D., 225, 246
O'Leary, K. D., 20, 29

O'Leary, V., 297
Olexa, C., 300
O'Neill, F. J., 230, 250
Orden, S. R., 434
Orne, M. T., 27, 142, 170
Otto, J., 90, 101

Paige, H., 63
Panzetta, A. F., 103, 138
Pappenfort, D., 287, 299
Parker, A. W., 87, 101
Parloff, M. D., 27, 142, 170
Patterson, G. R., 3, 12, 20, 30, 143,
  172
Paul, G. L., 132, 134, 138, 168, 172
Pelz, D. C., 18, 30
Penchansky, R., 225, 250
Pennypacker, H. S., 303, 308, 310,
  321
Perlin, S., 234, 236, 250
Perrow, C., 287, 301
Peterson, R. F., 26, 205, 220
Phelps, R., 143, 172
Phillips, E. L., 162, 170
Phillips, J. P. N., 37, 54
Phillips, J. S., 160, 171
Pierce, C., 204, 222
Pincus, J., 391
Pittman, F. S., 100
Polak, P., 34, 39, 52, 54
Polansky, N., 302
Pollack, E. A., 151, 171
Pollock, M., 248
Popper, R., 3, 29
Porter, A., 11, 30
Post, F., 246
Prager, R. A., 154, 171
Pratt, S., 76, 81
Prest, A., 191
Proshansky, H. M., 133, 137, 138,
  205, 221

Quilitch, H. R., 204, 222

Rachman, S., 341, 392
Radner, M., 29
Rappaport, M., 89, 99
Raush, H. L., 220
Ray, R. S. A., 3, 30
Redd, W. H., 20, 30
Redlich, F. C., 242, 247
Reid, J. B., 3, 5, 29, 30
Reid, W. J., 142, 172
Rein, M., 4, 31
Reinke, W. A., 74, 81
Reiser, M. F., 27, 142, 170

Reynolds, F. W., 227, 250
Reynolds, N. J., 204, 222
Riecken, H. W., 300
Riedel, D. C., 434
Rioch, M. J., 86, 101
Risley, T. R., 20, 21, 26, 134, 137,
    138, 201, 204, 220, 221, 222
Rivlin, L. G., 133, 137, 138, 205,
    221
Robinson, J., 300
Roden, A. H., 27
Rodgers, J. D., 195
Roen, S. R., 86, 87, 101
Rosenstock, I. M., 297
Ross, E. R., 89, 90, 102
Rossi, P. H., 4, 30, 31, 171, 254,
    258, 287, 294, 300, 434
Rubin, R. D., 173

Sainsbury, P., 236, 243, 247
Salasin, S. E., 400, 434
Sanders, D. 129, 137
Santoro, D. A., 388, 392
Saretsky, G., 130, 138
Sarri, R. C., 148, 173, 253, 255,
    285, 296, 300
Saslow, G., 91, 100
Schafer, W. E., 148, 173, 300
Schaefer, H., 114, 132, 133, 139
Schaie, K. W., 36, 54
Schalock, R., 44, 54
Schiefelbusch, R. L., 222
Schmid, C. F., 321
Schoggen, M., 204, 220
Schrag, C., 255, 300
Schulberg, H. C., 96, 100, 101
Schultz, T., 117, 137, 195
Schwartz, D. A., 103, 139
Schwartz, R. D., 149, 174
Schwitzgebel, R., 260, 300
Scitovsky, T., 192
Scott, W. A., 237, 250
Seaver, W. H., 303
Sechrest, L., 149, 150, 171, 174
Seidman, D., 258, 300
Selo, E., 253
Shapiro, M., 35-37, 260, 300
Sherwood, C. C., 295, 301
Sheldon, A., 100
Shine, II, L. C., 5, 30
Shlien, J. M., 142, 172
Shore, H., 245
Shoup, D. C., 182, 194
Shyne, A. W., 142, 172
Sidman, M., 4, 5, 30
Silberman, M., 300

Silverman, H. A., 245
Simmons, D. G., 91, 99
Simon, A., 233, 235, 240, 246
Skeels, H. M., 231, 250
Skindrud, K., 20, 30
Skinner, B. F., 303, 321, 322
Sklar, J., 230, 250
Slawson, M. R., 89, 102
Slosar, J., 253, 301
Small, L., 86, 101
Smith, B. C., 63
Smith, G. L., 260, 298, 300
Smith, L., 66, 73, 81
Snow, R. E., 381, 392
Solomon, L., 250
Sonoda, B., 44, 54
Spitzer, R. L., 92, 101
Staats, E. B., 194
Stachnik, T., 321
Stanley, J. C., 4, 13, 26, 72, 81, 222,
    296
Steiner, P. O., 194
Stillwell, W. D., 297
Stilwell, W. E., 387, 391, 392, 393
Stocking, C. B., 434
Stone, A. R., 35, 49, 52, 143, 170
Stotsky, B. A., 233, 250
Stout, R., 431
Street, D., 287, 301
Strole, L., 242, 250
Strupp, H. H., 91, 101
Stuart, R. B., 141, 142, 143, 148,
    149, 151, 155, 156, 158, 159, 160,
    162, 165, 167, 171, 172, 173, 434
Suchman, E., 255, 301

Tapp, G. S., 341, 388
Taube, C., 435
Taubenhaus, L. J., 225, 250
Taylor, E. N., 433
Taylor, G. M., 194
Taylor, S. H., 405, 408, 409, 432
Taylor, W., 40, 53
Teigen, J., 132, 138
Terry, R. M., 301
Tharp, R. G., 143, 173
Thomas, C., 301
Thomas, E. J., 300
Thorndike, R. L., 334, 338
Tischler, G. L., 87, 102
Tobin, S. S., 250
Tooley, J., 81
Tripodi, T., 155, 156, 159, 160, 162,
    165, 167, 171, 173
Tropman, J., 300
Trotter, S., 103, 137, 411, 431

Truax, C. B., 94, 102
Tuma, A. H., 27, 142, 170
Turner, B. F., 237, 250
Turvey, R., 191

Ullman, L. P., 39, 54, 67, 81, 261, 301
Ulrich, R., 321
Unikel, I. P., 30
Urban, H. B., 45, 54

Valdiviesco, L., 204, 222
Valett, R. E., 313-315, 322
Vaught, R. S., 5, 29
Villoria, R. L., 63
Vinter, R. D., 148, 173, 285, 287, 300, 301
Vorwaller, D. J., 148, 172

Wahl, A., 298
Wahler, R. G., 20, 30, 162, 173
Walker, H. M., 20, 31
Wallace, C., 132, 138
Ward, B., 40, 53
Ward, D., 258, 298, 301
Warren, C. G., 432
Warren, M., 301
Wasser, E., 245
Webb, G. E., 302
Webb, E. J., 149, 174
Wechsler, H., 250
Weckworth, V. E., 69, 82
Wedge, R. F., 278, 298
Weed, L. L., 91, 102
Weinberger, C. S., 414-415, 434
Weiner, N. L., 302
Weinstein, M. S., 76-77, 82
Weisbrod, B. A., 195
Weiss, C. H., 168, 174, 258, 287, 294, 300, 301, 302
Weiss, J. M. A., 36, 54
Weiss, R. L., 4, 31
Weiss, S. L., 151, 171
Welsh, B., 297
Werts, C. E., 9, 31
Westrupp, C., 246
Wetzel, R. J., 143, 173
Wheeler, S., 296
Whitehead, A., 234, 250
Whitla, D. K., 370, 393
Wholey, J. S., 198-199, 426-427, 431, 434
Wildavsky, A., 189, 198
Wilkins, W., 399, 434
Willems, E. P., 220
Williams, A., 190, 198
Williams, M., 246

Williams, R. H., 298
Williams, W., 1, 30, 31, 171, 254, 258, 287, 294, 300, 301, 425, 434
Willie, C. V., 302
Wilner, D., 257, 298
Wilson, N. C. Z., 91, 99
Windle, C., 86, 98, 395, 396, 420, 431, 432, 435
Wing, J. K., 227, 251
Winokur, S., 29
Wisecarver, D., 183, 195
Wolberg, L. R., 170
Wolf, M. M., 20, 26, 137, 162, 170
Wolfgang, M., 302
Wolins, M., 302
Wood, D., 103
Wright, H. F., 204, 220

Young, A., 250

Zarcone, V., 227, 250
Zarit, S. H., 223
Zax, M., 101
Zeckhauser, R., 192, 195
Zola, I. K., 99
Zubin, J., 5, 31, 247
Zurcher, L. A., 297
Zusman, J., 89, 90, 102, 429, 435

SUBJECT INDEX

Achievement test scores, 380
Accuracy of performance, 308-309, 319
Aged, 232-234; community programs, 234-235; evaluation of programs for, 223-243
Age-integrated ward, 231
Age-segregated ward, 231-232
Amelioration vs. prevention, 240
Analysis, functional, 58; path, 336; system, 57-59; task, 58
Analysis of variance models, 12-13
Apathy, 132, 133
A posteriori decisions, 141
Attitude changes, 148

Barclay Classroom Climate Inventory, 340-343
Baseline conditions, 5-7
Behavior therapy, evaluation of, 4
Behavioral change, 304-305; assessment of, 1; causes of, 1
Behavioral measurement, 103-133, 303-307; Behavioral Observation Instrument, 108, 114-128, 135-136; Behavioral Progress Record, 107-114, 130, 135-136
Behavior modification techniques, 109-114, 142-167, 225-226, 279
Benefits, consumption, 179, 187; direct, 178; efficiency, 183; indirect, 178-179; investment, 179, 187-188; marginal, 183, 186
Benefit-cost analysis, 175-191; criteria for choice, 181-182
Bias, 425

Canadian Mental Health Association, 42, 52
Change and control programs, 289-290
Celeration, 304, 308
Classification, 90, 91
Classroom groups, characteristics of, 343
Client transfers, 417-418
Client satisfaction, 90
Cognitive-motivation problems, 352, 361
Community-based psychiatric services, 83-88

Community mental health, center programs, 103-106, 415-419; program models, 85-88
Community-Oriented Programs Environmental Scale (COPES), 90
Comparison group, use of, 8
Comparative assessment, 285-287
Constraint, budgetary, 181-182
Contracts, 76, 158; fixed and open, 158-159
Contingencies, environmental, 23
Control groups, 8; importance of, 4-6; untreated, 142; "wait-list", 142
Correctional programs, evaluation of, 253-295
Cost, accounting, 96; benefits, 51; effectiveness, 303, 311, 316-318, 320, 336, 385; effectiveness analysis, 175; efficiency, 303, 311; opportunity, 179-181
Costs, direct, 43, 44; indirect, 43
Cost-yield ratio, 98
Crime statistics, 258
Criteria, categories of, 255-256, for evaluation, 287; institutional vs. individual, 241; observable, 38-40; of adjustment, 225; of improvement, 225; operational, 285-286; subjective, 37, 42
Critical incidents, 276
Critical Path Method, 59-60
Curricular interventions, 382
Custodialism, 240-241

Decision-making, processes, 419
Dependency needs, 239-240
Dependent variables, 33, 34, 42, 47, 49
Design, comparison group, 142-143; contrast group, 143; implementation, 144-154; quasi-experimental, 259; treatment vs. no-treatment, 143
Designs, control group, 142
Detention programs, 288-289
Developmental schools, new program in, 329-331
Discount rate, 180-181, 421-422
Discriminant function analysis, 350-379; multiple step-wise, 370-377

Dissemination of results, 400

Educational diagnosis, 381
Effectiveness, 259-260; analysis,
11-25
Efficiency, 188-190
Effort variables, 263-265, 268, 272,
276, 279-280, 283
Equity weights, 183
Evaluating program evaluation,
395-430
Evaluation, assessment, 403; contracts, success of, 406; dilemmas
in, 254-261; expressive elements
of, 66, 69, 73-79; individualized,
310; instrumental elements of, 66,
69-73; politics of, 294-295;
rationale of, 223-243; resistance
to, 65, 73-79, 87; signals, 177
Evaluation criteria, 236-243; community mental health programs,
236; covert deterioration, 239;
deterioration, 237; value judgments, 237
Evaluation designs, 3-11
Evaluation strategies, 88-97; choice
of evaluation procedure, 97-98;
cost-effectiveness analysis, 94-96;
evaluation by outcome, 90-94;
program process, 89-90; program
structure, 89; systems analysis,
96-97
Evaluation research, feedback, 415-
419
Excess disability, 229
Exit management and reintegration
programs, 290-291
Expectancy manipulations, 399
Experimental designs for individual
patients, 109-114

Face validity, 90
Factor analysis, 341; principle axis,
341, 354-355; multi-method
multi-trait, 341-342
Fading procedures, 158
Failure rates, 277
Fixed instigations, 165
Follow-up, 92-94, 152; evaluation,
84
Frequency of response, 303-305

Geographically defined service areas,
86
Geriatric population, definition of,
226-227
Global measures, 149
Goal, attainment, 415; determinations, 415; modifications, 415
Goals, economic, 34; humanitarian,
42; non-patient clients, 39, 41;
patients, 34, 38; process, 261;
societal, 41, 45; therapists, 45, 51;

treatment, 33, 36; ultimate, 261
Gordon Personal Profile, 185
Group interaction problems, 350-
352, 356, 378
Guided group interaction, 275-276

Hawthorne effect, 56, 225-243
Holiday relief program, 243
Hospital in-patient care, 86
Hospitalization, long-term, 40
Human investment, 184-185
Humaneness, criteria for, 286

Idiographic, 24
Implementation measures, 331-334
Impression management, 87
Improvement index, 307, 318-319
Individualized education, evaluation
of, 323-337
Innovative education programs,
value of, 337
Input-output, 177; process, 331, 334
Institutions, admission to, 230; for
the retarded, 202-203
Institution relocation, 230
Instruction, individualization of, 314
Interdependency program, 191
Inter-organizational processes, 285,
293
Intervals, of causation, 18-20; of
remeasurement, 18-20
Intervention, setting, 263, 264-265,
267, 271, 275, 278-279; stability
of, 152
Interview, standardized, 35, 45;
structured, 35, 36
Intra-institutional, characteristics,
267; studies, 224-229

Jesness Social Maladjustment Scale,
148-153
John Henry effect, 130
Joint Commission on Accreditation
of Hospitals, 203
Joint Commission on Mental Illness
and Health, 103
Juvenile corrections, a critique, 262
Juvenile justice system, 253

Learning abilities development program, 311
Learning, development teams, 283-
284
Living environments, evaluation of,
201

Manifest description of resident
activity, 201, 205; activity measure,
213-215; interaction measure, 210-
213; stimulation measure, 206-210
Macro-systems, evaluator of, 66
Means and ends, confusion of, 234
Measurement, reactivity in, 149-150

Measures, evaluative, 151; group, 150; individualized, 150; non-obtrusive, 149; obtrusive, 149
Mental disease, 46, 48
Mental retardation, 175, 185-189
Methodological issues, 141
Micro-systems, evaluator of, 66
Mission, analysis, 58; profile, 58
Multi-method multi-trait systems, 340-343
Multiple needs assessment, 339-379, 382, 384

N=one designs, 5-11; efficacy of, 6
Need, assessment, 57; evaluation of, 324-327; perception of, 326; priorities, 327-330
Network techniques, 59-62
Nomothetic, 24
Nonprofessional manpower, 86
Nursing home, parameters, 234; population, 233

Objective burden, 41
Objectivity, 424; need for, 79
Observer reliability, 118, 206-207
Observations of staff behavior, 126-128; 130-131
Operational problems, 141
Oregon Research Institute, 12
Organic pathology, 46, 47-48
Organizational, goals, 291; processes, 285; structures, 292
Outcome, measures, 160, 264; normative measures, 261; variables, selection of, 148
Outcomes distributional, 182-184
Outcome research, 141

Parent-child interactions, 12
Pareto criterion, 182, 183
Parole, 269
Patients, charts, 227; chronic, 227; nursing home, 227-228
Peer, culture, 267-268; nominations, 340; review, 84
Physical skill problems, 352, 367
Planned Activity Check, 134
Planning-programming-budgeting system, 175
Policy-making, a model for, 379, 384-386
Poor attitude, 352, 367
Potential therapy, impact of, 236
Pre-intervention measures, 9
President's Committee on Mental Retardation, 202
Prevention, 87
Preventive intervention, 379-384; strategies, 383
Price signals, 177-178
Prisonization, 253
Private-practice psychiatry, 82-87

Problem-oriented approach, 91
Process, control, 55, 62; criteria, 423-430; evaluation, 84; goals, 406, 411-412; variables, 263, 272-274
Processing programs, 289
Program, benefits, 178-179; costs, 179-180; goals, 261-262; implementation, technological aspects, 72-73, 75; outcomes, 285-287
Program evaluation, and review technique, 59; confidence in, 75-76; consequences of, 76, 79; cost of implementation, 421; cost of research, 421-422; credibility, 73-75; criteria for, 420-422; dimensions of implementing, 68-69; implementation of, 65; implications, 413; negotiations, 78; receptivity to, 419; scientific quality of, 421; utilization, 421; value aspects, 69-71, 73-80
Psychodynamic processes, 46, 49-50
Pupil behavior inventory, 148-152

Quasi-control groups, 144, 155, 156, 159

Race differences, 282, 356-361, 370-377
Recidivism, 256-258
Record systems, automated, 420
Rehabilitation, 42
Reinforcers, 340
Remedial diagnostic form, 312
Research, design flexibility, 167-168; feedback, 417; grants, success of, 405; pure vs. applied, 384
Research utilization, 405; variables related to, 427-430; compatibility, 428; credibility, 429; feasibility, 428-429; observability, 428; relevance, 427; reversability, 429
Reversal designs, 4
Ripple effect, 149

Scattergram grids, 342
School, achievement differences, 324-325; performance, 148
School district, differences between, 369-377; differences within, 377-379
Schooling, social variables in, 369
Selective assignment, 255
Self-concept problems, 350-352, 356, 378
Self-control problems, 350-352, 356, 378
Self-management, 22-23
Self-report, 340
Service, quality profile, 89
Sex differences, 350-361, 370-378
Simulation, 58
Situational specificity, 24
Social, behavior theory, 47, 51;

breakdown syndrome, 103; class, 242; cost, 96; engineering, 86; time preference, 181
Social work, intervention, 269
Source credibility, 77
Staff training, 105-108
Standard behavior chart, 305-310, 313,320.
Status offenses, 256
Stigmatization, 285
Subject population, 262-281
Subjects, random assignment, 165
Subjective burden, 40-41
Sub-optimazation, constraints, 182
Survival skill behaviors, 15-18
Symptom change, 49
Systems, adaptive vs. fixed, 326-327; approach, 56-57

Target complaints, 35
Teacher, input, 148, 151-152, 340; Judgments, 340
Testability criterion of, 232
Tests, personality, 49
Therapeutic outcome, 418
Therapists, opinions, 45; uniformity, 147; variation, 159-160, 164-166
Token economy, 106
Tracking, 255
Trait-state labels, 36
Transactional analysis, 279-280, 387

Treatment, effectiveness and causation, 12; effects, carry-over of, 7-8; efficacy, 92; generalization effects, 20-25; predicting outcome of, 10; short- and long-term, 142-143; technology, 263, 265, 267, 271, 275-276, 279; time constrained, 156
Truancies, 268

Ultimate criteria, 422-423
Utilization review, 409; procedures, 400

Validity, 425; face, 37; patients' reports, 37; process measures of, 426
Value identification, 395-403
Variables, context and process, 329, 335
Verbal skill deficits, 350-352
Vocational, deficits, 352, 361; rehabilitation 186-189

Wide Range Achievement Test, 330

Zero-sum games, 75-76